Antiseizure Medications

Antiseizure Medications

A Clinician's Manual

Third Edition

Ali A. Asadi-Pooya, MD

Professor of Epileptology
Director, Epilepsy Research Center,
Shiraz University of Medical Sciences;

Jefferson Comprehensive Epilepsy Center,
Department of Neurology,
Thomas Jefferson University

Michael R. Sperling, MD

Baldwin Keyes Professor of Neurology
Director, Jefferson Comprehensive Epilepsy Center
Vice Chair for Research, Department of Neurology,
Thomas Jefferson University

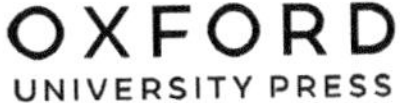

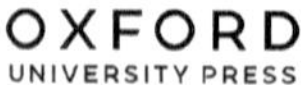

Oxford University Press is a department of the University of Oxford. It furthers the University's objective of excellence in research, scholarship, and education by publishing worldwide. Oxford is a registered trade mark of Oxford University Press in the UK and certain other countries.

Published in the United States of America by Oxford University Press
198 Madison Avenue, New York, NY 10016, United States of America.

Library of Congress Cataloging-in-Publication Data
Names: Asadi-Pooya, Ali A., 1973– editor. | Sperling, Michael R., author.
Title: Antiseizure medications : a clinician's manual /
Ali A. Asadi-Pooya, Michael R. Sperling.
Other titles: Antiepileptic drugs
Description: Third edition. | New York, NY : Oxford University Press, [2023] |
Preceded by Antiepileptic drugs / Ali A. Asadi-Pooya, Michael R. Sperling.
Second edition. 2016. | Includes bibliographical references and index.
Identifiers: LCCN 2022002086 (print) | LCCN 2022002087 (ebook) |
ISBN 9780197541210 (paperback) | ISBN 9780197541234 (epub) |
ISBN 9780197541241
Subjects: MESH: Anticonvulsants—therapeutic use |
Epilepsy—drug therapy | Handbook
Classification: LCC RM322 (print) | LCC RM322 (ebook) |
NLM QV 39 | DDC 615.7/84—dc23/eng/20220209
LC record available at https://lccn.loc.gov/2022002086
LC ebook record available at https://lccn.loc.gov/2022002087

DOI: 10.1093/med/9780197541210.001.0001

This material is not intended to be, and should not be considered, a substitute for medical or other professional advice. Treatment for the conditions described in this material is highly dependent on the individual circumstances. And, while this material is designed to offer accurate information with respect to the subject matter covered and to be current as of the time it was written, research and knowledge about medical and health issues is constantly evolving and dose schedules for medications are being revised continually, with new side effects recognized and accounted for regularly. Readers must therefore always check the product information and clinical procedures with the most up-to-date published product information and data sheets provided by the manufacturers and the most recent codes of conduct and safety regulation. The publisher and the authors make no representations or warranties to readers, express or implied, as to the accuracy or completeness of this material. Without limiting the foregoing, the publisher and the authors make no representations or warranties as to the accuracy or efficacy of the drug dosages mentioned in the material. The authors and the publisher do not accept, and expressly disclaim, any responsibility for any liability, loss, or risk that may be claimed or incurred as a consequence of the use and/or application of any of the contents of this material.

9 8 7 6 5 4 3 2 1

Printed by Marquis, Canada

Contents

Chapter 1

Diagnosis and Evaluation of Patients with Seizures

Approximately 10% of the general population will experience at least one seizure within their lifetimes in most Western countries, and even higher rates are observed in developing countries. However, not all individuals go on to develop epilepsy, which is characterized by recurring epileptic seizures. The prevalence of epilepsy is 7.1 cases per 1,000 people (range 4.0 to 8.9) and its incidence is 47.4 cases per 100,000 people per year worldwide (Hirtz et al., 2007; Kotsopoulos et al., 2002). An *epileptic seizure* is the transient occurrence of signs or symptoms due to abnormal, excessive, hypersynchronous firing of neurons in the brain. The practical clinical definition of epilepsy proposed by the International League Against Epilepsy (ILAE) considers epilepsy to be a disease of the brain defined by any of the following conditions: (1) at least two unprovoked (or reflex) seizures occurring more than 24 hours apart; (2) one unprovoked (or reflex) seizure and a probability of further seizures, similar to the general recurrence risk after two unprovoked seizures (at least 60%), occurring over the next 10 years; and (3) diagnosis of an epilepsy syndrome (Fisher et al., 2014). Epilepsy may be due to genetic causes (possessing an inherited trait to have seizures), brain tumors, infections (meningitis or encephalitis), brain trauma, stroke, developmental anomalies (e.g., cortical dysplasia), brain malformations (tuberous sclerosis, neurofibromatosis), vascular malformations (arteriovenous malformations), and other causes.

To properly diagnose "epilepsy" a physician must do more than simply establish that recurrent seizures have occurred or are highly likely to occur after the first one. It is important that an attempt be made to diagnose a specific *epilepsy syndrome*. This syndrome forms the basis for the healthcare provider to decide on therapy. The syndrome reflects the constellation of historical features, symptoms, signs, and laboratory test results that define a distinct condition. Hence, the syndromic diagnosis involves more than just the seizure type: frontal lobe seizures, for instance, do not constitute a syndrome. In contrast, benign Rolandic epilepsy of childhood does constitute a distinct syndrome, with its characteristic etiology, natural history, seizure type, developmental history, neurological examination, and electroencephalogram (EEG) abnormality (Table 1.1). An *idiopathic (genetic) epilepsy syndrome* is the direct result of a known or inferred genetic defect. Seizures are the core symptom of the disorder. It appears at a specific age (age-dependent) with no underlying structural brain lesions or related neurological abnormalities. Examples of idiopathic (genetic) syndromes include benign Rolandic epilepsy

Table 1.1 Important epilepsy syndromes based on the International League Against Epilepsy (ILAE) classification

General classification	Syndrome	Description
Idiopathic (genetic) generalized epilepsies	Childhood and juvenile absence epilepsies	Childhood absence epilepsy (pyknolepsy) occurs in children of school age (peak manifestation age 6–7 years), with a strong genetic predisposition in otherwise normal children. It is characterized by very frequent (several to many per day) absences. The EEG reveals bilateral usually 3 Hz, synchronous spike waves or polyspikes and waves, on a normal background activity. During adolescence, generalized tonic-clonic seizures often develop. Juvenile absence epilepsy develops insidiously in physically and mentally healthy adolescents. Age at onset is usually between 10 and 17 years (peak between 10 and 12 years). Because the frequency of the absences is low and the symptoms are relatively trivial, the disorder may go unnoticed until generalized tonic-clonic seizures appear.
	Juvenile myoclonic epilepsy	Juvenile myoclonic epilepsy typically appears in the second decade of life. The age at onset often ranges from 8 to 24 years, with peak onset between 14 and 16 years. It is characterized by myoclonic seizures, associated at times with generalized tonic-clonic seizures or absence seizures.
	Epilepsy with myoclonic-astatic seizures (Doose syndrome)	Prior to the onset of myoclonic-astatic seizures, most affected children show normal development. The seizures usually begin between 2 and 5 years of age. The first seizure is most often a generalized tonic-clonic seizure and rarely a myoclonic, astatic, myoclonic-astatic, or absence seizure. Drop attacks may result from pure astatic, myoclonic-astatic, or atypical absence seizures.
Epileptic encephalopathies (in which the epileptiform abnormalities may contribute to progressive brain dysfunction)	West syndrome	West syndrome is an age-dependent epilepsy syndrome that comprises a triad of epileptic spasms in clusters, mental retardation, and diffuse and profound paroxysmal EEG abnormalities in infancy.

Table 1.1 (Continued)

General classification	Syndrome	Description
	Severe myoclonic epilepsy in infancy (Dravet syndrome)	Severe myoclonic epilepsy begins during the first year of life. Development is normal prior to the onset of seizures. Affected infants develop either generalized or unilateral clonic seizures without prodromal signs. Myoclonic jerks, absence seizures, and focal seizures usually appear later. The occurrence of status epilepticus is frequent. Psychomotor retardation and other neurological deficits occur in affected children.
	Lennox-Gastaut syndrome	The Lennox-Gastaut syndrome is, with rare exception, a condition of children. It is characterized by the clinical triad of multiple types of seizures, including especially atypical absences and tonic and atonic seizures, diffuse slow spikes-and-waves and/or generalized paroxysmal fast activity on an abnormal background activity in EEG, and intellectual disability (intellectual disability is not a mandatory element).
	Landau-Kleffner syndrome	Age at onset for Landau-Kleffner syndrome ranges from 3 to 8 years, and boys are more frequently affected than girls. Acquired aphasia (verbal auditory agnosia) is the most prominent feature because seizures are present in only 70–80% of these patients.
Progressive myoclonic epilepsies		These include ceroid lipofuscinosis, sialidosis, Lafora disease, Unverricht-Lundborg disease, neuroaxonal dystrophy, MERRF, and dentatorubropallidoluysian atrophy.
Idiopathic (genetic) focal epilepsies	BECTS (Rolandic epilepsy)	Benign epilepsy of childhood with centrotemporal spikes (BECTS) has five criteria for the diagnosis: (1) onset between the ages of 2 and 13 years; (2) absence of neurological or intellectual deficit before the onset; (3) focal seizures with motor signs, frequently associated with somatosensory symptoms or precipitated by sleep; (4) a spike focus located in the centrotemporal (rolandic) area with normal background activity on the interictal EEG; and (5) spontaneous remission during adolescence.

(continued)

Table 1.1 (Continued)

General classification	Syndrome	Description
	Benign occipital epilepsies	Panayiotopoulos syndrome is best described as early-onset benign childhood seizure susceptibility syndrome with mainly autonomic seizures (e.g., ictus emeticus) and autonomic status epilepticus.
		The cardinal features of late-onset childhood occipital epilepsy (Gastaut type) are visual seizures predominantly manifested with elementary visual hallucinations, blindness, or both. They are usually frequent and diurnal, and they usually last from seconds to 1–3 minutes.
Symptomatic (or probably symptomatic) focal epilepsies	Limbic epilepsies	These include mesial temporal lobe epilepsy with hippocampal sclerosis and mesial temporal lobe epilepsy defined by specific etiologies.
	Neocortical epilepsies	These include Rasmussen syndrome, hemiconvulsion-hemiplegia syndrome, and migrating focal seizures of early infancy.

Note: Febrile seizures (febrile convulsions) are the most common convulsive events in human experience. Febrile seizures can be categorized as either "simple" (generalized tonic-clonic seizure, duration <15 minutes and without recurrence within 24 hours) or "complex" (focal seizure, lasting >15 minutes or occurring in a cluster of 2 or more convulsions within 24 hours). Febrile seizures are generally benign and only 2–3% of children will later develop epilepsy, primarily those who have complex febrile seizures.

From Shorvon SD. The etiologic classification of epilepsy. Epilepsia. 2011 Jun;52(6):1052-7 with minor modifications.

of childhood, childhood absence epilepsy, and juvenile myoclonic epilepsy. A *symptomatic (structural-metabolic-genetic) epilepsy syndrome* is the result of an identifiable structural or metabolic lesion of the brain, such as cerebral infarction, brain tumor, cortical dysplasia, or ceroid lipofuscinosis. A *probable symptomatic (unknown) epilepsy syndrome* is synonymous with cryptogenic epilepsy, and this term defines syndromes that are believed to be symptomatic but for which, no etiology has been identified (Berg et al., 2010; Blume et al., 2001; Engel, 2006).

The ILAE classifies seizures as either focal or generalized. *Focal epileptic seizures* are conceptualized as originating within (focal) networks (often) limited to one hemisphere. These may be discretely localized or more widely distributed. *Generalized epileptic seizures* are conceptualized as originating at some point within, and rapidly engaging, bilaterally distributed networks (Berg et al., 2010).

Definitions for the major seizure are summarized in the following lists (Blume et al., 2001; Fisher et al., 2017):

Motor Seizures

- *Tonic*: A sustained increase in muscle contraction lasting a few seconds to a few minutes.
- *Clonic*: Myoclonus that is regularly repetitive, involves the same muscle groups, usually at a starting frequency of 2–3 jerks per second, and is prolonged.
- *Tonic-clonic*: A sequence consisting of a tonic phase followed by a clonic phase. Variants such as clonic-tonic-clonic may be seen.
- *Myoclonic*: Sudden, brief (<100 milliseconds) involuntary single or multiple contraction(s) of muscles(s) or muscle groups of variable topography (axial, proximal limb, distal limb).
- *Focal impaired awareness motor seizure*: Formerly *complex partial seizure with automatism (automatic behavior)*.
- *Hyperkinetic*: Irregular sequential ballistic movements, such as pedaling.
- *Atonic*: Sudden loss or diminution of muscle tone without apparent preceding myoclonic or tonic event lasting 1–2 seconds or longer, involving head, trunk, jaw, or limb musculature.
- *Epileptic spasm* (formerly *infantile spasm*): A sudden flexion, extension, or mixed extension-flexion of predominantly proximal and truncal muscles that is usually more sustained than a myoclonic movement but not so sustained as a tonic seizure (i.e., 1 second). Limited forms may occur (e.g., grimacing, head nodding). Epileptic spasms frequently occur in clusters.

Nonmotor Seizures

- *Absence seizure*: Eyes open and loss of awareness/responsiveness from 4 to 20 seconds.
- *Aura*: A subjective phenomenon that precedes an observable seizure and for which memory is retained afterward. This may consist of a sensory, psychic, autonomic, or other nonspecific subjective symptoms. Because of retrograde amnesia, some patients may not recall the experience of an aura.
- *Sensory seizure*: A perceptual experience not produced by stimuli from the external world.
- *Cognitive seizures*: Events in which disturbance of cognition is the prominent or most apparent feature, with alterations in perception, attention, emotion, memory, or execution function.

The ILAE 2017 operational classification of seizure types is shown in Figure 1.1 (Fisher et al., 2017).

Continuous Seizure Types

- Generalized status epilepticus
- Generalized tonic-clonic status epilepticus
- Clonic status epilepticus
- Tonic status epilepticus
- Absence status epilepticus

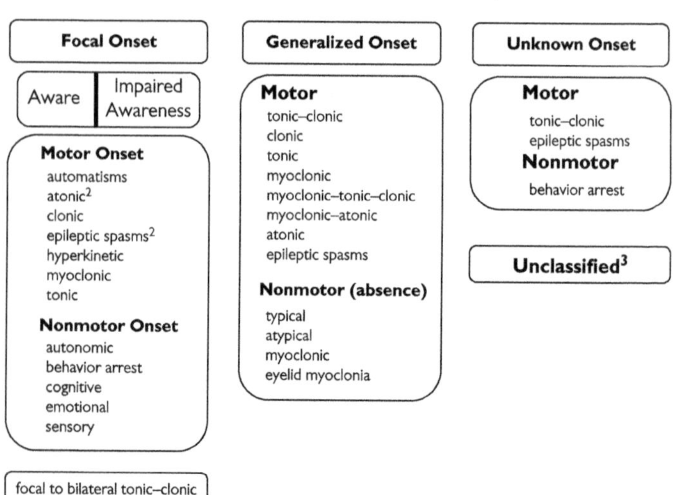

Figure 1.1 The expanded International League Against Epilepsy (ILAE) 2017 operational classification of seizure types. The following clarifications should guide the choice of seizure type. For focal seizures, specification of level of awareness is optional. Retained awareness means the person is aware of self and environment during the seizure, even if immobile. A *focal aware seizure* corresponds to the prior term "simple partial seizure." A *focal impaired awareness seizure* corresponds to the prior term "complex partial seizure," and impaired awareness during any part of the seizure renders it a focal impaired awareness seizure. Focal aware or impaired awareness seizures optionally may further be characterized by one of the motor-onset or nonmotor-onset symptoms, reflecting the first prominent sign or symptom in the seizure. Seizures should be classified by the earliest prominent feature, except that a focal behavior arrest seizure is one for which cessation of activity is the dominant feature throughout the seizure. In addition, a focal seizure name can omit mention of awareness when awareness is not applicable or unknown, and thereby classify the seizure directly by motor-onset or nonmotor-onset characteristics. Atonic seizures and epileptic spasms would usually not have specified awareness. Cognitive seizures imply impaired language or other cognitive domains or positive features such as déjà vu, hallucinations, illusions, or perceptual distortions. Emotional seizures involve anxiety, fear, joy, other emotions, or appearance of affect without subjective emotions. An absence is atypical because of slow onset or termination or significant changes in tone supported by atypical, slow, generalized spike-and-wave on the EEG. A seizure may be unclassified due to inadequate information or inability to place the type in other categories. 1. Definitions, other seizure types, and descriptors are listed in the accompanying paper and glossary of terms. 2. Degree of awareness usually is not specified. 3. Due to inadequate information or inability to place in other categories.

Reprinted with permission: Fisher RS, et al. Instruction manual for the ILAE 2017 operational classification of seizure types. *Epilepsia*. 2017;58(4):531–542.

- Myoclonic status epilepticus
- Focal status epilepticus
- Epilepsia partialis continua
- Aura continua

- Limbic status epilepticus (psychomotor status)
- Hemiconvulsive status with hemiparesis

Evaluation of a Patient Suspected to Have an Epileptic Seizure

Diagnosis of Epilepsy

Epilepsy is a clinical diagnosis. Unless one happens to observe a seizure while recording the EEG, which is a rare event in general clinical practice, the diagnosis relies on the judgment of a physician or other healthcare provider. This judgment ultimately rests on the history provided by the patient and others. Therefore, careful attention must be paid when obtaining the relevant historical details, and one must systematically establish whether a seizure has really occurred and what type of seizure it was. Hence, when evaluating a patient with a possible seizure, one must first determine whether epileptic seizures have truly occurred or whether a disorder exists that mimics epilepsy. The differential diagnosis includes convulsive or nonconvulsive syncope, transient ischemic attacks, complicated migraines, hypoglycemia, panic attacks, sleep disorders, functional seizures (psychogenic nonepileptic seizures), and movement disorders. In children, one must also consider night terrors, breath-holding spells, colic, and tics. An incorrect diagnosis may have many negative consequences. Symptoms that precede the seizure or occur when it begins, as well as behaviors exhibited during the seizure, offer clues about the type of the seizure and therefore the diagnosis (Asadi-Pooya et al., 2012; Asadi-Pooya et al., 2013).

Neurologists and other physicians occasionally must distinguish seizures from *syncope*. Syncope is the impairment of cardiovascular autonomic control, which results in gradual failure of cerebral perfusion. Syncope is often associated with pallor, cold and clammy skin, and perhaps electrocardiographic or blood pressure abnormalities. However, syncope may be associated with one or more jerks at the onset of loss of consciousness or even convulsive activity, leading to ambiguity in diagnosis (Asadi-Pooya et al., 2011). With generalized tonic-clonic seizures, patients typically have increased tone (tonic phase) followed by clonic repetitive jerks associated with labored respiration, flushed color, and incontinence or tongue biting. To differentiate epileptic seizures from other possible diagnoses, details about timing may also be helpful. Most focal-onset seizures last from 30 seconds to 3 minutes, while movement disorders and panic attacks may last longer. Breath-holding spells and panic attacks typically have an inciting event. Sleep state may help distinguish between different diagnoses, because some conditions occur only while a person is asleep and others do not. One must also consider whether there are risk factors that would heighten suspicion for epileptic seizures, such as developmental delay, antecedent brain injury, preexisting neurological impairments, family history of epilepsy, and so forth. Therefore, history is the key step in diagnosing epileptic seizures.

History

The key element in making the correct diagnosis of an epilepsy syndrome is obtaining a detailed clinical history. This includes:

- *Seizure description*: It is critical that a history be obtained from the patient as well as a witness. You should begin by asking the patient and observer to describe in detail the events that occurred before, during, and after the seizure. While individuals may have more than one type of seizure, seizures are typically stereotyped. Other useful clues include sleep–wake cycle, concurrent symptoms (e.g., fever, headache, vomiting), precipitating factors, other comorbidities, and family history of epilepsy.
- *Risk factors for seizures*: It is important to know the risk factors for seizures. However, while there are many risk factors for epilepsy (e.g., perinatal insults, developmental delay, head trauma, infections, genetic tendency, acquired brain lesions), many patients have no obvious risk factors.
- *A complete history*: Past history and medical, psychiatric, family, and social history can be useful.

Physical Examination

Most individuals with epilepsy have a relatively normal general and neurological examination unless they have an underlying significant focal structural abnormality. Usually, if deficits are present, they are subtle and often appear solely as a variety of cognitive and language deficits. It is important to evaluate for skin lesions and other congenital abnormalities, such as adenoma sebaceum associated with tuberous sclerosis. It is also helpful to examine for body hemiatrophy. On occasion, hyperventilation in the office will trigger an absence seizure in individuals with generalized epilepsy.

Electroencephalography

The EEG is a test that evaluates the electrical activity of the brain. The EEG provides information concerning the presence or absence of abnormal electrical activity, as well as information that aids in classification of the disorder and location of the seizure focus. The EEG should be recorded during wakefulness and sleep to optimize chances of detecting an abnormality. Activation procedures such as photic stimulation and hyperventilation may help elicit epileptiform activity as well.

A normal EEG does not rule out the clinical diagnosis of epileptic seizures, and, for approximately 50% of patients with epilepsy, a single routine EEG will be normal. If the suspicion of epilepsy is high, additional EEG recording after sleep deprivation or an ambulatory 24-hour EEG may improve the yield to approximately 90%.

Laboratory Tests and Neuroimaging

These studies are performed to determine the cause of a newly diagnosed seizure. They may include electrolyte and liver function tests, toxicology screen, and chemistry panel if a patient is seen acutely after a seizure. Lumbar puncture is performed only if an infection or malignancy is suspected.

Magnetic resonance imaging (MRI) is the most important test for many patients. It is appropriate to obtain an MRI scan to assess for a structural lesion if epilepsy is not believed to be due to a genetic cause (e.g., childhood absence epilepsy, juvenile myoclonic epilepsy, benign Rolandic epilepsy). An MRI is preferable to a computed tomography (CT) scan because it has greater sensitivity. It detects macroscopic structural lesions, such as tumors, encephalomalacia, cortical dysplasias, and mesial temporal sclerosis (atrophy of the hippocampus). The latter abnormality is the most common finding in individuals with medial temporal lobe epilepsy, a common type of epilepsy characterized by recurrent focal-onset seizures. Coronal sections using fluid-attenuated inversion recovery (FLAIR) sequences and coronal thin-section sequences using T1 sequences optimally display mesial temporal sclerosis. An MRI scan is recommended after a first seizure in anyone who does not have a clear genetic cause for the seizure. In particular, MRI is required if a patient had a focal seizure, a focal neurological deficit, persistently altered mental status, a history of trauma, persistent headache, a history of cancer or anticoagulation therapy, suspected infection, HIV infection, or cognitive or motor impairments. Emergency neuroimaging should be performed on all patients with a postictal focal deficit or change in mental status that does not quickly resolve.

When Should Treatment Be Started?

If the diagnosis of epilepsy cannot be established, one should obtain further testing and diagnostic information. One option is to obtain additional EEG recordings, although often one must simply wait and observe a patient over an extended period of time before reaching a diagnosis. Once epilepsy has been diagnosed, an antiseizure medication (ASM) appropriate for that condition may be prescribed. If only one seizure has occurred, then the decision to treat rests on both the probability of recurrence and type of seizure experienced. Patients who are at significant risk for recurrence are usually offered treatment, whereas patients who have a low probability of recurrence may not be started on medication. The seizure type also influences the decision. Tonic-clonic seizures or other seizure types that cause loss of consciousness or falling are intrinsically more dangerous than seizures without those characteristics. For example, a patient who experiences a tonic-clonic seizure is far more likely to fear the consequences of another seizure than a patient whose seizure consisted of tingling or twitching of a hand for several seconds. Therefore, the decision to treat must be made by the physician in consultation with the patient because the patient is the one who will suffer the risks of seizures, the adverse effects of medication, and the psychosocial consequences of additional seizures. Children usually live in a somewhat sheltered environment; a second seizure therefore has different consequences for a child than for most adults who must function independently and have weightier responsibilities. Therefore, physicians often advise waiting until a second seizure has occurred when seeing a child after a first seizure unless the probability of recurrence is high. In contrast, adults more often desire treatment to minimize the risk of recurrence, thereby maximizing their chances of continued full function in society.

A patient who has had a *single* seizure, with a normal developmental history, neurological examination, EEG, and neuroimaging study and no family history of epilepsy, is often simply observed, and medication is not prescribed. The risk of a recurrent seizure after a single seizure in this circumstance is approximately 25–30% (Figure 1.2). After one seizure with an abnormal EEG or evidence of some other neurological abnormality, the risk for recurrence may be 50% or greater. After two seizures, the risk of recurrent seizures increases to 75–85%, and treatment is often advised after a second seizure has occurred and may be started after one seizure if an individual has a heightened risk for recurrence. Predictors of recurrence after the first seizure are summarized in Box 1.1. If more than one seizure has occurred, then the probability of recurrence is quite high, and treatment is usually offered, although this also depends on seizure type, because some seizures might be so mild and inconsequential that they merit simple observation without treatment (e.g., Rolandic seizures).

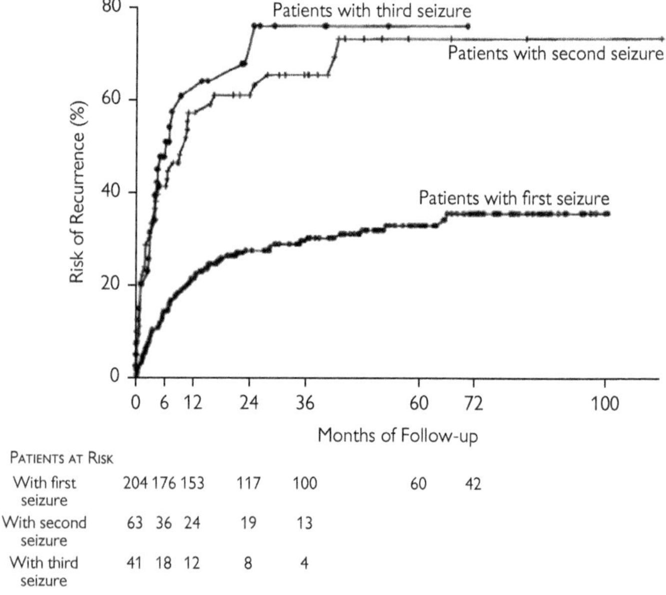

Figure 1.2 Risk of a second, third, and fourth unprovoked seizure after a first, second, and third unprovoked seizure.

Reprinted with permission (Hauser, 1998).

Box 1.1 Predictors of Increased Risk for Recurrence After the First Seizure

- Prior neurological insult (mental retardation, cerebral palsy): The most powerful predictor of recurrence
- Focal-onset seizures
- Abnormal electroencephalogram
- Prior acute seizures including febrile seizures
- Status epilepticus or multiple seizures at the index episode (in adults)
- Postictal Todd's paralysis

From Chadwick (2006), Hauser (2006), and Shorvon and Luciano (2007).

Selection and Adjustment of Medication

The goal of treatment is to prevent future seizures from recurring. Treatment is typically started with one of the first-line ASMs (see Chapters 2 and 5). First-line drugs should be effective and well-tolerated. For focal-onset seizures, these drugs include carbamazepine, lacosamide, lamotrigine, levetiracetam, and oxcarbazepine, among others. For generalized-onset epilepsies, first-line drugs include ethosuximide, lamotrigine, levetiracetam, topiramate, and valproate, among others. If a first-line drug controls seizures and does not cause adverse effects, then therapeutic adjustments are not needed. Should seizures persist, the medication regimen should be adjusted (see Chapter 8). If a patient has significant adverse effects, then the physician should advise switching to an alternative ASM. One should aim for treatment with a single agent (monotherapy) to lessen the chances of adverse effects and drug interactions.

A therapeutic range of serum concentration exists for all drugs. This range, in theory, provides a guideline for determining the appropriate dose. Serum levels below certain concentrations are undoubtedly ineffective. Excessively high serum levels will certainly produce unwanted adverse effects. However, the therapeutic range may differ from one patient to the next, and the lower limits are not well-established for any drug. It is critical that patients be treated based on symptoms—prevention of seizures and lack of adverse effects—and not the plasma drug level (see Chapter 4).

Other Treatment Possibilities

Approximately, 35% of individuals with epilepsy have persistent seizures despite the use of appropriate ASMs. Once adequate trials of two tolerated, appropriately chosen and used ASM schedules (whether as monotherapies or in combination) have failed to achieve sustained seizure freedom, other treatment options should be considered (Kwan et al., 2010). First, diagnostic testing should be performed to verify the diagnosis of epilepsy and to ensure that the patient does not have functional seizures (psychogenic nonepileptic seizures) or some other disorder. If *drug-resistant epilepsy* is confirmed, then several treatment options exist. *Epilepsy surgery* is the only treatment that offers a good chance of stopping seizures completely, and other options are usually palliative. Epilepsy surgery usually involves either excising the cortical area that causes seizures or disconnecting epileptogenic regions of the brain from other areas. Removal of part of the temporal lobe, anterior temporal lobectomy, or anteromedial temporal resection are the operations most commonly performed, but surgery can often be carried out in other lobes of the brain as well. Disconnection procedures, such as a corpus callosotomy, also can be done. This is generally palliative and works best for refractory tonic, atonic, and tonic-clonic seizures. Other treatment options include *vagal nerve stimulation* (VNS), a mainly palliative treatment that electrically stimulates the left vagus nerve in the neck. *Deep brain stimulation* (DBS) for epilepsy is another similar treatment option that electrically stimulates the anterior nucleus of the thalamus. *Responsive neurostimulation* (RNS) is another epilepsy surgical palliative treatment that does not require the removal of brain tissue. The neurostimulator monitors the brain's electrical activity, and, when activity that may lead to a seizure is detected, it delivers a pulse of electrical stimulation through the leads. Figure 1.3 shows a general algorithm for appropriate device selection in patients with drug-resistant epilepsy.

The *ketogenic diet* is a diet that excludes carbohydrates and consists of foods with a fat-to-protein ratio of 3.5:1 or 4:1, so that the body metabolizes ketones instead of glucose. This may lessen seizure frequency in about half of the people who use it and occasionally stops seizures completely; it is mainly used in children but can be prescribed for motivated adults. New treatments are in the pipeline.

Discontinuing ASM Therapy

Once a patient has been free of seizures for an extended period of time, withdrawal of medication may be considered. However, risk of recurrence of seizures should be discussed with the patient (Figure 1.4). The decision to stop medication must be individualized and is based on the epilepsy syndrome and probability of seizure recurrence (Box 1.2), the associated risks (both medical and psychosocial) of seizure recurrence, and the risks of continuing medical therapy. It is typical to require a minimum of 2 years without seizures before considering discontinuation of medical therapy, although some physicians prefer to wait longer. Medication dosages are usually gradually reduced and withdrawn over a period of at least 6 weeks, but longer periods are often advised. Rapid withdrawal of some medications, particularly the barbiturates, is potentially dangerous because this can precipitate seizures (see Chapter 2).

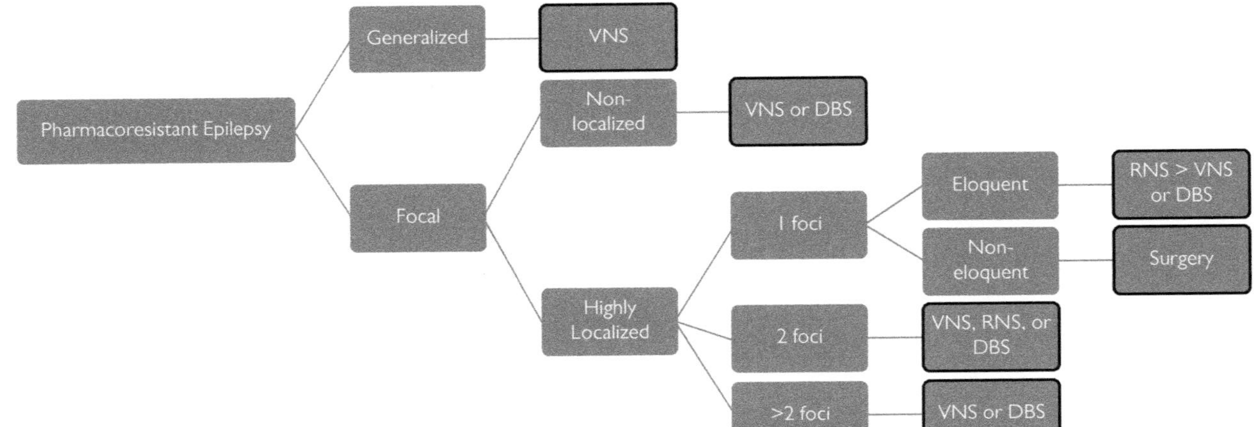

Figure 1.3. Decision algorithm for device selection in patients with drug-resistant epilepsy.

Reprinted with permission: Wong S, Mani R, Danish S. Comparison and selection of current implantable anti-epileptic devices. *Neurotherapeutics*, 2019;16(2):369–380.

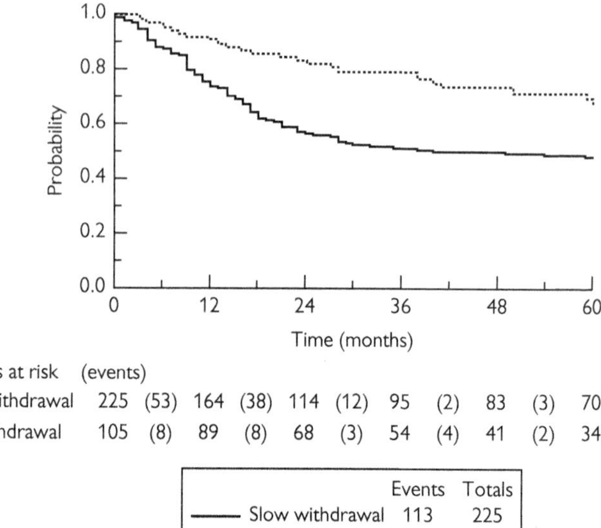

Figure 1.4 Actuarial percentage of seizure-free patients stopping treatment or continuing treatment.

Reprinted with permission (Specchio et al., 2002).

Box 1.2 Predictors of Increased Risk for Relapse After Drug Withdrawal

- Older age at onset: Onset as an adolescent or adult
- Seizures after initiation of treatment
- Long interval between onset and initial control
- Many generalized seizures before control
- Focal-onset seizures
- Myoclonic seizures
- Need for multiple ASMs
- Short duration of remission before medication taper
- Abnormal neurological examination (cerebral palsy, mental retardation)
- Known cause for epilepsy
- Abnormal EEG at diagnosis, particularly a spike-wave pattern
- Presence of abnormal EEG after starting treatment
- Worsening of EEG findings during medication taper

From Chadwick (2006), Hauser (2006), and Shorvon and Luciano (2007).

When to Seek Specialist Consultation

Neurology consultation is useful when the diagnosis is uncertain or if one ASM has failed to completely control seizures. Other indications for consultation include family planning or if the patient has a form of epilepsy that is particularly difficult to treat. An epilepsy specialist should be consulted if two ASMs fail to control seizures or the diagnosis remains in doubt.

References

Asadi-Pooya AA, Emami M. Reasons for uncontrolled seizures in children: The impact of pseudointractability. *Epilepsy Behav*. 2012;25(3):341–344.

Asadi-Pooya AA, Emami M, Ashjazadeh N, et al. Reasons for uncontrolled seizures in adults: The impact of pseudointractability. *Seizure*. 2013;22(4):271–274.

Asadi-Pooya AA, Emami M, Sperling MR. A clinical study of syndromes of idiopathic (genetic) generalized epilepsy. *J Neurol Sci*. 2013;324(1–2):113–117.

Asadi-Pooya AA, Nikseresht AR, Yaghoobi E. Vasovagal syncope treated as epilepsy for 16 years. *Iran J Med Sci*. 2011;36(1):60–62.

Berg AT, Berkovic SF, Brodie MJ, et al. Revised terminology and concepts for organization of seizures and epilepsies: Report of the ILAE Commission on Classification and Terminology, 2005–2009. *Epilepsia*. 2010;51:676–685.

Blume WT, Luders H, Mizrahi E, et al. Glossary of descriptive terminology for ictal semiology: Report of the ILAE Task Force on Classification and Terminology. *Epilepsia*. 2001;42:1212–1218.

Chadwick D. Starting and stopping treatment for seizures and epilepsy. *Epilepsia*. 2006;47(Suppl 1):58–61.

Engel J. ILAE Classification of epilepsy syndromes. *Epilepsy Res*. 2006;70S:S5–S10.

Fisher RS, Acevedo C, Arzimanoglou A, et al. ILAE official report: A practical clinical definition of epilepsy. *Epilepsia*. 2014;55(4):475–482.

Fisher RS, Cross JH, D'Souza C, et al. Instruction manual for the ILAE 2017 operational classification of seizure types. *Epilepsia*. 2017;58(4):531–542.

Fisher RS, Cross JH, French JA, et al. Operational classification of seizure types by the International League Against Epilepsy: Position Paper of the ILAE Commission for Classification and Terminology. *Epilepsia*. 2017;58(4):522–530.

Hauser WA. The natural history of seizures. In Wyllie E, ed., *The Treatment of Epilepsy: Principles and Practice*, 4th ed. Philadelphia: Lippincott Williams & Wilkins; 2006:117–124.

Hauser WA, Rich SS, Lee JRJ, et al. Risk of recurrent seizures after two unprovoked seizures. *N Engl J Med*. 1998;338:429–434.

Hirtz D, Thurman DJ, Gwinn-Hardy K, et al. How common are the "common" neurologic disorders? *Neurology*. 2007;68(5):326–337.

Kotsopoulos IA, van Merode T, Kessels FG, et al. Systematic review and meta-analysis of incidence studies of epilepsy and unprovoked seizures. *Epilepsia*. 2002;43(11):1402–1409.

Kwan P, Arzimanoglou A, Berg AT, et al. Definition of drug resistant epilepsy: Consensus proposal by the ad hoc Task Force of the ILAE Commission on Therapeutic Strategies. *Epilepsia*. 2010;51(6):1069–1077.

Shorvon S, Luciano AL. Prognosis of chronic and newly diagnosed epilepsy: Revisiting temporal aspects. *Curr Opin Neurol.* 2007;20:208–212.

Shorvon SD. The etiologic classification of epilepsy. *Epilepsia.* 2011;52(6):1052–1057.

Specchio LM, Tramacere L, LaNeve A, Beghi E. Discontinuing antiepileptic drugs in patients who are seizure free on monotherapy. *J Neurol Neurosurg Psychiatry.* 2002;72:22–25.

Wong S, Mani R, Danish S. Comparison and selection of current implantable anti-epileptic devices. *Neurotherapeutics.* 2019;16(2):369–380.

Chapter 2

Antiseizure Medications Dosage Forms and Administration Guidelines

In this chapter, dosage forms, starting dose, titration schedule, maintenance dose, dose limits, and discontinuation schedule of various antiseizure medications (ASMs) are discussed separately. In addition, significant administration guidelines, contraindications, precautions, and information for patients are discussed briefly. Indications for each of ASMs are discussed in Chapter 5. Please note that some doses describe here exceed guidelines set by the US Food and Drug Administration (FDA) or the European Medicines Agency (EMA); these higher doses are often used in clinical practice and reflect the experience of the authors.

Key Points for Prescribing Antiseizure Medications

- Choose an ASM that is appropriate for the seizure type and epilepsy syndrome. Because there often are several good options, choose the specific agent based on the patient's profile (i.e., gender, age, job), comorbidity, potential adverse effects, drug interactions, and other pharmacological properties.
- When beginning therapy with an ASM, first target the lower end of the therapeutic range or dose. Use higher doses only when lower ones have failed. This approach lessens the incidence of adverse effects.
- Titrate doses gradually when initiating therapy to improve drug tolerability and reduce adverse effects. Controlled studies show evidence of efficacy during drug titration, even though full therapeutic levels may not yet be achieved.
- If needed for immediate seizure control, carbamazepine, clobazam, brivaracetam, levetiracetam, lacosamide, oxcarbazepine, phenytoin, rufinamide, topiramate, and valproate can be rapidly titrated.
- Tailor dosing schedules to provide maximum protection (peak levels) when seizures are apt to occur. For example, if seizures typically occur in the morning after awakening (as in juvenile myoclonic epilepsy), dose the medication at bedtime so that maximal levels are present on awakening. If divided doses are used, prescribe the larger amount shortly before seizures are likely to occur (i.e., at the time of greatest vulnerability).

- If dividing a daily dose leads to unequal amounts at different dosing times, prescribe the larger dose either shortly before seizures are most likely to occur or at bedtime; bedtime dosing is often preferred when seizures occur randomly at any time because peak concentration adverse effects are less likely to be noticed when asleep. For example, if phenytoin 300 mg is the total daily dose, prescribe 100 mg to be taken in the morning and 200 mg to be taken at night.
- It is preferable to prescribe medications that can be taken once or twice daily. Patient adherence to a medication regimen is highest with once- or twice-daily dosing regimens.
- Observe closely for adverse effects. Development of adverse effects is a common reason for poor adherence (compliance) to a prescribed regimen. Because patients are often unaware of cognitive or behavioral adverse effects, question family members and close friends about adverse effects as well.
- The goal of treatment is to prevent seizures and avoid adverse effects. Assess whether these goals have been met. If not, adjust therapy accordingly. If the first drug fails, convert the patient to monotherapy on a new agent. If a second drug fails, either convert to monotherapy with a new agent or consider adding a second drug to the existing agent. (There are no data to support superiority of one course of action over another.)
- When converting from monotherapy from one drug to another, the following procedure can be used: titrate the new ASM to a therapeutic dose, lowering the dose of the first drug modestly (10–25%) to avoid adverse effects. One should maintain reasonably therapeutic levels of the original ASM while titrating the new agent to avoid seizure exacerbation. Should adverse effects appear during titration of the new agent, first try to reduce the dose of the original drug since many adverse effects are likely due to transient polypharmacy rather than an effect of the new drug. Should adverse effects persist, however, they may be caused by the new agent, and this may need to be discontinued. Once the new ASM is at a therapeutic dose or level without significant untoward adverse effects, then taper the original drug over 6 weeks or so (longer if a barbiturate or benzodiazepine).
- Once two appropriate drugs prescribed either singly or in combination have failed, consider epilepsy surgery after confirming the diagnosis of epilepsy.
- If epilepsy surgery cannot be performed, consider alternative therapies such as trials of other ASMs, neurostimulation devices (i.e., vagal nerve stimulation [VNS], responsive neurostimulation [RNS], deep brain stimulation [DBS]), ketogenic diet, or investigational therapies (see Chapter 1 for more details).

Antiseizure Medications

For an explanation of the contraindications and precautions of each drug, please go to the appropriate chapter. For example, for the explanation of *marked hepatic disease* as a relative contraindication for prescribing *acetazolamide*, see Chapter 13.

Acetazolamide

Brand Name: Diamox
Dosage Forms: Tablets 125 mg, 250 mg
Note: The extended-release preparation is not recommended for use as an ASM.

Dosage

Starting Dose:
Adults and children: 4–8 mg/kg/day, given in two divided doses. When given in combination with other ASMs, the recommended starting dosage in adults is 250 mg twice daily. *Elderly*: Consider dosage reduction.

Maintenance Dose: The usual maintenance dose is 375–1,500 mg/day or 8–30 mg/kg/day. An elderly patient with an age-related renal impairment is more likely to develop hyperchloremic metabolic acidosis; therefore, use lower doses.

Maximum Dosage Limit: *In all age groups*: 1,500 mg/day.

Discontinuation Schedule: A dosage reduction of 50% per two weeks is safe at the time of discontinuation.

Administration Guidelines

May be taken with or without food. To prepare an PO liquid for patients who are unable to take tablets, crush tablets and suspend in any highly flavored carbohydrate syrup (e.g., cherry or chocolate). Up to 500 mg may be suspended in 5 mL of syrup; however, concentrations of 250 mg/5 mL are more palatable. The resultant suspensions are stable for about 1 week.

Patient Education

1. If you miss a dose, take it as soon as you can. If it is almost time for your next dose, take only that dose. Do not take double or extra doses.
2. Adverse effects that you should report to your physician as soon as possible include
    - Blood in urine, pain or difficulty passing urine
    - Black tarry stools
    - Dark yellow or brown urine, pale stools, yellowing of the eyes or skin
    - confusion or depression
    - Difficulty breathing, shortness of breath
    - Dry mouth or increased thirst
    - Fatigue or severe lack of energy
    - Fever, sore throat
    - Lower back pain
    - Muscle weakness
    - Ringing in the ears
    - Seizures
    - Skin rash, itching
    - Unusual bleeding or bruising
    - Irregular heartbeat

Box 2.1 Relative Contraindications to Use of Acetazolamide

- Adrenal insufficiency
- Renal diseases
- Anuria
- Renal failure
- Marked hepatic disease
- Hyperchloremic metabolic acidosis
- Electrolyte imbalances
- Hypokalemia
- Hyponatremia
- Acetazolamide hypersensitivity

See Chapters 12, 13, and 14.

Box 2.2 Acetazolamide Precautions

- Breastfeeding
- Pregnancy
- Elderly
- Pulmonary diseases
- Hematological diseases
- Sulfonamide hypersensitivity
- Sunlight or ultraviolet exposure

See Chapters 9, 10, 11, 18, and 26.

3. Do not stop taking acetazolamide suddenly. Your physician may want you to reduce your dose gradually.
4. You may get drowsy. Do not drive, use machinery, or do anything that needs mental alertness until you know how acetazolamide affects you.
5. Drink several glasses of water a day. This will help to reduce possible kidney problems.
6. If you are diabetic, monitor blood and urine sugar and ketones regularly. Acetazolamide can increase sugar levels. Report to your physician if you notice any changes.

Clonazepam

Brand Names: Ceberclon, Klonopin

Dosage Forms: Tablets 0.5 mg, 1 mg, 2 mg; wafers (orally disintegrating tablets) 0.125 mg, 0.25 mg, 0.5 mg, 1 mg, 2 mg

Dosage

Starting Dose:

Adults and adolescents (weight ≥30 kg or 10 years of age or older): 0.5–1.0 mg/day, divided in two equal doses or just at bedtime.

Elderly and debilitated adult patients: May require lower initial dosages.

Children and infants (weight <30 kg or up to 10 years of age): 0.01–0.03 mg/kg/day (not to exceed 0.05 mg/kg/day), given orally in two or three equally divided doses.

Titration and Maintenance Dose: In adults and adolescents, dosage may be increased by 0.5–1 mg every 3–7 days until seizures are controlled or adverse reactions limit further increase. The typical maintenance dose range is 2–8 mg/day. In elderly and debilitated adult patients, slower dosage titration is recommended. In children and infants, increase dosage by not more than 0.25–0.5 mg every 3 days to a maximum maintenance dosage of 0.1–0.2 mg/kg/day administered in 2–3 divided doses until seizures are controlled or adverse reactions limit further increase. Sometimes bedtime dosing alone is sufficient.

Maximum Dosage Limits:

Adults and adolescents (weight ≥30 kg): 20 mg/day
Children and infants (weight <30 kg): 0.2 mg/kg/day

Discontinuation Schedule: A dosage reduction of 0.04 mg/kg per month is safe at the time of discontinuation.

Administration Guidelines

Clonazepam may be administered orally without regard to meals.
Conventional PO tablets: Should be swallowed whole with a glass of water.
Disintegrating tablet (ODT): Make sure hands are dry before touching the tablet. Peel foil back from blister package. Do not push tablet through the foil. Place tablet in mouth and tablet should melt quickly. You may drink some water after tablet melts.

Adults and adolescents: 1–3 mg PO 1–2 times per day for a seizure cluster. In general, we prefer using clonazepam ODT to diazepam for seizure clusters if an PO preparation can be taken rather than diazepam because of its longer duration of anticonvulsant action in the central nervous system and lack of need for a source of drinking water.

Patient Education

1. If you miss a dose and remember within an hour, take it as soon as you can. If it is more than an hour since you missed a dose, skip that dose and go back to your regular schedule. Do not take double or extra doses.
2. Adverse effects that you should report to your physician as soon as possible include
   Confusion or drowsiness
   Unusual behavior or thoughts of hurting yourself
   Worsening seizures

Box 2.3 Relative Contraindications to Use of Clonazepam

- Abrupt discontinuation
- Benzodiazepine hypersensitivity
- Ethanol intoxication
- Acute respiratory insufficiency

Box 2.4 Clonazepam Precautions

- Bipolar disorder
- Depression
- Psychosis
- Suicidal ideation
- Benzodiazepine dependence
- Substance abuse
- Elderly
- Pregnancy
- Obstetric delivery
- Breastfeeding
- Central nervous system depression and coma
- Dementia
- Chronic pulmonary diseases
- Sleep apnea
- Neuromuscular diseases (e.g., myasthenia gravis)
- Parkinson's disease
- Hepatic diseases
- Renal impairment
- Shock

See Chapters 9–13, 22, and 23.

Double vision or abnormal eye movements
Hallucinations (seeing and hearing things that are not really there)
Lightheadedness or fainting spells
Mood changes, depression, excitability, or aggressive behavior
Movement difficulty, staggering or jerky movements
Muscle cramps
Restlessness
Tremors
Weakness or tiredness

3. Your body may become dependent on clonazepam. If you have been taking clonazepam regularly for some time, do not suddenly stop taking it. You must gradually reduce the dose or you may get severe adverse effects.
4. You may get drowsy or dizzy. Do not drive, use machinery, or do anything that needs mental alertness until you know how clonazepam affects you. To reduce the risk of dizzy and fainting spells, do not sit or stand up quickly. Alcohol may increase dizziness and drowsiness. Avoid alcoholic drinks.
5. Do not treat yourself for coughs, colds, or allergies without asking your physician for advice. Some ingredients can increase possible adverse effects.
6. If you are going to have surgery, tell your physician that you are taking clonazepam.

Diazepam

Brand Names: Diastat AcuDial, Dizac, Valicot, Valium, Diazepam Intensol, Valtoco (diazepam intranasal)

Dosage Forms: Tablets 2 mg, 5 mg, 10 mg; solution 1 mg/mL, 5 mg/mL; injection 5 mg/mL; rectal gel Diastat 5 mg/mL, Diastat AcuDial 10 mg (delivers set doses of 5 mg, 7.5 mg, and 10 mg), Diastat AcuDial 20 mg (delivers set doses of 10 mg, 12.5 mg, 15 mg, 17.5 mg, and 20 mg); intranasal spray: 5 mg/0.1 mL, 7.5 mg/0.1 mL, 10 mg/0.1 mL

Dosage

IV Dosage for Treatment of Status Epilepticus:

Adults and adolescents: 10–20 mg IV over 2–5 minutes; may be repeated at 10–15 minute intervals (usually for two doses), to a maximum dosage of 30 mg.

Children >5 years: 0.1–0.3 mg/kg IV over 3–5 minutes; could be given every 10–15 minutes (usually for two doses), to a maximum total dose of 15 mg.

Children and infants 1 month–5 years: 0.1–0.3 mg/kg IV over 3–5 minutes; could be repeated every 2–5 minutes (usually for two doses), to a maximum dose of 5 mg.

Neonates: 0.1–0.3 mg/kg IV over 3–5 minutes; could be given every 15–30 minutes (usually for two doses), to a maximum total dose of 2 mg.

Note: Not recommended as a first-line agent in neonates due to sodium benzoate and benzoic acid in the injection. Serious adverse reactions including fatal reactions and gasping syndrome may occur in premature neonates and low-birth-weight infants who receive drugs containing benzyl alcohol as a preservative (also available in diazepam intranasal).

Note: Many clinicians now prefer IV lorazepam to IV diazepam for the acute treatment of seizures.

Intranasal Dosage for Treatment of Seizure Clusters and Prolonged Seizures:

Adolescents and adults: 0.2 mg per kg

14–27 kg: 5 mg (one 5-mg device); 1 spray in 1 nostril
28–50 kg: 10 mg (one 10-mg device); 1 spray in 1 nostril
51–75 kg: 15 mg (two 7.5-mg devices); 1 spray in each nostril
≥76 kg: 20 mg (two 10-mg devices); 1 spray in each nostril

Children 6–11 years: 0.3 mg per kg

10–18 kg: 5 mg (one 5-mg device); 1 spray in 1 nostril
19–37 kg: 10 mg (one 10-mg device); 1 spray in 1 nostril
38–55 kg: 15 mg (two 7.5-mg devices); 1 spray in each nostril
56–74 kg: 20 mg (two 10-mg devices); 1 spray in each nostril

Second Dose: When required, may be administered after at least 4 hours after the initial dose; if the second dose is to be administered, use a new blister pack of diazepam intranasal.

Maximum Dosage Limit: Not to exceed two doses to treat a single episode.

Treatment Frequency: Do not use for more than one episode every 5 days and no more than five episodes per month.

Note: Use with caution in elderly and in patients with compromised respiratory function related to a concurrent disease process (e.g., asthma, pneumonia, or neurological disease).

PO Dosage for Adjunctive Treatment of Seizures and Intermittent Use:

(In cycles lasting 3 weeks.) Use of diazepam to control clusters or bouts of increased seizure activity in drug-resistant focal or generalized epilepsies:

Children and infants ≥ 6 months: 1–2.5 mg PO 3–4 times per day (0.5–0.75 mg/kg/day). The dose may be increased as needed and tolerated.

Adults and adolescents: 2–10 mg PO 2–4 times per day only during a seizure cluster. In general, we prefer using lorazepam for seizure clusters if an PO preparation can be taken rather than diazepam. We advise against using diazepam as adjunctive therapy and prefer it only for treating seizure clusters.

Elderly: 2–2.5 mg PO 1–2 times per day for seizure clusters. Increase the dose according to response and patient tolerability.

Note: For febrile seizure prophylaxis in children and infants 6 months–5 years, PO diazepam 0.33 mg/kg is given every 8 hours (1 mg/kg/day) during each episode of fever until the child is afebrile for at least 24 hours.

Rectal (PR) Dosage in Acute Repetitive Seizures:

Children 2–5 years: 0.5 mg/kg PR. Doses should be rounded upward to the next available dosage strength. If needed, a second dose may be given 4–12 hours after the first dose.

Children 6–11 years: 0.3 mg/kg PR. Doses should be rounded upward to the next available dosage strength. If needed, a second dose may be given 4–12 hours after the first dose.

Adults and adolescents: 0.2 mg/kg (usually 10–20 mg) PR. Doses should be rounded upward to the next available dosage strength. If needed, a second dose may be given 4–12 hours after the first dose.

Elderly and debilitated patients: 0.2 mg/kg PR. Doses should be rounded downward to reduce the adverse effects. If needed, a second dose may be given 4–12 hours after the first dose.

Note: It is recommended that rectal diazepam be used to treat no more than five episodes per month and no more than one episode every 5 days.

Note: A 2.5-mg dose may also be used as a partial replacement dose for patients who expel a portion of the first dose.

Maximum Dosage Limit: This must be individualized; generally not more than 20 mg as a single dose.

Administration Guidelines

Following parenteral administration, patient should be kept under close observation for a period of 3–8 hours or longer based on the patient's clinical response and rate of recovery.

Replace parenteral therapy with PO therapy as soon as possible.

IM injection is not recommended due to slow and erratic absorption.

For *IV injection,* do not administer rapidly because respiratory depression or hypotension may develop. In adults, inject IV slowly at a rate not exceeding 5 mg/min. In infants and children, inject IV at a rate not exceeding 1–2 mg/min. Monitor heart rate, respiratory rate, and blood pressure. A large vein should be used to avoid thrombosis. If a large vein is not available, inject into the tubing of a flowing IV solution as close as possible to the vein insertion. Do not add diazepam emulsified injection to infusion sets containing PVC.

Lorazepam

Brand Names: Ativan, Lorazepam Intensol

Dosage Forms: Tablets 0.5 mg, 1 mg, 2 mg; injection 2 mg/mL, 4 mg/mL; PO solution (Lorazepam Intensol) 2 mg/mL

Dosage

Dosage for Treatment of Status Epilepticus:

Adults: 0.1 mg/kg IV given at a rate of approximately 2 mg/min, ceasing infusion when seizures stop. A second dose of 0.05 mg/kg may be given after 10–15 minutes if needed. If this is ineffective, additional doses may be given, but we generally advise adding a second agent after failure of 0.15 mg/kg of IV lorazepam.

Adolescents: 0.07 mg/kg IV given slowly over 2–5 minutes (no more than 2 mg/min). A second dose of 0.05 mg/kg may be given after 10–15 minutes if needed.

Children and infants: 0.1 mg/kg (maximum 4 mg) IV given slowly over 2–5 minutes. A second dose of 0.05 mg/kg IV may be repeated after 10–15 minutes if needed.

Neonates: 0.05 mg/kg IV slowly over 2–5 minutes. Second dose may be given after 10–15 minutes if needed.

Note: IM administration is not a preferred route for status epilepticus since therapeutic levels may not be reached as quickly as IV administration. However, if the IV route is unavailable, then the IM route can be utilized. Lorazepam injection, undiluted, should be injected deep into the muscle mass when given IM. However, intranasal or rectal diazepam is preferred if an IV route is not available.

Note: Lorazepam injection contains benzyl alcohol, which may be toxic to neonates in high doses.

PO (PO) Dosage for Adjunctive Treatment of Seizures and Intermittent Use:

(In cycles lasting 3 weeks.) Use of lorazepam to control clusters or bouts of increased seizure activity in drug-resistant focal or generalized epilepsies

Adults and adolescents: 1–3 mg PO 1–2 times per day only during a seizure cluster. In general, we often use lorazepam for seizure clusters if an PO preparation can be taken rather than diazepam, because of its longer duration of anticonvulsant action in the central nervous system.

Administration Guidelines

Do not administer lorazepam injection by intra-arterial injection because arteriospasm can occur, which may cause tissue damage.

Rate of injection should not exceed 2 mg/min. Dilute IV dose with equal volume of compatible diluents (D5W, NS, SWI). Direct IV injection should be made with repeated aspiration to ensure that none of the drug is injected intra-arterially and that perivascular extravasation does not occur.

For *continuous IV infusion,* when PVC containers or administration sets are used to administer lorazepam, significant drug losses occur due to sorption. Use of glass or polyolefin containers is recommended.

Midazolam

Brand Names: Versed; Nayzilam (midazolam intranasal)

Dosage Forms: Injection 1 mg/mL, 5 mg/mL; syrup 2 mg/mL; intranasal: 5 mg/0.1 mL per single-dose spray

Dosage

Dosage for Treatment of Refractory Status Epilepticus:

Adults (for mechanically ventilated patients only): 0.2 mg/kg IV bolus followed by a continuous infusion of 0.75 µg/kg/min IV. Dose should be titrated upward every 5 minutes until seizures are controlled (up to 10 µg/kg/min IV). The infusion is maintained for 12 hours and slowly tapered during continuous EEG monitoring. If seizure activity returns, the infusion is restarted for another 12 hours. Tolerance may develop, and doses up to 20 µg/kg/min IV are sometimes required.

Children and infants >2 months (for mechanically ventilated patients only): 0.15 mg/kg (0.1–0.3 mg/kg) IV bolus followed by a continuous infusion of 1 µg/kg/min IV. Dose should be titrated upward every 5 minutes until seizures are controlled (up to 5 µg/kg/min IV). The infusion is maintained for 12 hours and slowly tapered during continuous EEG monitoring. If seizure activity returns, the infusion is restarted for another 12 hours. Occasionally, several days of high-dose (up to 20 µg/kg/min IV) therapy is required. In neonates, doses of 0.1–0.4 mg/kg/hour are used in patients refractory to high doses of phenobarbital.

Intranasal Dosage for Treatment of Seizure Clusters and Acute Repetitive Seizures:

First dose (≥12 years): 5 mg (1 spray) into 1 nostril.

Second dose (if needed): An additional 5 mg (1 spray) into the opposite nostril may be administered after 10 minutes if the patient has not responded to the first dose.

Do not administer the second dose if the patient has breathing difficulty or if excessive sedation occurs.

Maximum Dose and Frequency: Do not use more than two doses per single seizure episode and do not treat more than one episode every 3 days and no more than five episodes per month.

Administration Guidelines

IM and buccal midazolam (10 mg in adults and 0.2 mg/kg in children) routes are useful in acute repetitive seizures and febrile seizures in children. For buccal route, dilute 10 mg midazolam with peppermint, swirl in the mouth for 4–5 minutes, and then spit out.

Nitrazepam

Dosage Forms: Tablet 5 mg, PO suspension 2.5 mg/5 mL

This drug is often used in children (e.g., in myoclonic seizures from Lennox-Gastaut syndrome)

Dosage

Starting Dose:

Children and inf ants (weight <30 kg): 0.25 mg/kg/day in 2–3 divided doses.

Titration and Maintenance Dose:

In children and infants, increase dosage 0.25 mg/kg/day every 2 weeks, until seizures are controlled or adverse reactions limit further increase.

Maximum Dosage Limit: *Children and infants (weight <30 kg)*: 3 mg/kg/day.

Discontinuation Schedule: As with all benzodiazepines, abrupt withdrawal may precipitate seizures.

Note: In case of prolonged therapy, for all benzodiazepines, a dosage reduction of 20–25% per month is safe at the time of discontinuation.

Clobazam

Brand Names: Frisium, Onfi

Dosage Forms: Tablets 10 mg and 20 mg; PO suspension: 2.5 mg/mL

Dosage

Starting Dose:

Adults and adolescents: 5–10 mg/day, in 1–2 doses.

Elderly and debilitated adult patients: Lower initial doses.

Children and infants (weight <30 kg): 0.25 mg/kg/day in two divided doses.

Titration and Maintenance Dose: In adults and adolescents, dosage may be increased by 5–15 mg every 5 days until seizures are controlled or adverse reactions limit further increase. The typical maintenance dose range is 20–40 mg/day. In elderly and debilitated adult patients, slower dosage titration is recommended. In children and infants, increase dosage gradually every 5 days, until seizures are controlled or adverse reactions limit further increase.

Maximum Dosage Limit:

Adults and adolescents (weight >30 kg): 80 mg/day.
Children and infants (weight <30 kg): 1 mg/kg/day.

Discontinuation Schedule: As with all benzodiazepines, abrupt withdrawal may precipitate seizures.
Note: In case of prolonged therapy, for all benzodiazepines, a dosage reduction of 20–25% per month is safe at the time of discontinuation.

Brivaracetam

Brand Name: Briviact

Dosage Forms: Tablet: 10 mg, 25 mg, 50 mg, 75 mg, 100 mg; PO solution: 10 mg/mL; injection for IV use, solution: 50 mg/5 mL single-dose vial

Dosage

Starting Dose:
Adults and adolescents: 50 mg PO/IV twice daily.
Patients 4 to <16 years of age:

11 to <20 kg: 0.5–1.25 mg/kg PO BID (1–2.5 mg/kg/day)
20 to <50 kg: 0.5–1 mg/kg PO BID (1–2 mg/kg/day)

Titration and Maintenance Dose: *Adults and adolescents >16 years*: Based on patient tolerability and therapeutic response, adjust dose between 25 and 100 mg PO/IV BID (50–200 mg/day). Injection may be used for patients when PO administration is temporarily not feasible (at the same dosage and same frequency as tablets or PO solution).
Children 4–16 years:

11 to <20 kg: Based on patient tolerability and therapeutic response, adjust dose between 0.5 and 2.5 mg/kg PO BID (1–5 mg/kg/day).
20 to <50 kg: Based on patient tolerability and therapeutic response, adjust dose between 0.5 and 2 mg/kg PO BID (1–4 mg/kg/day).

Maximum Dosage Limit: *Adults and adolescents >16 years*: 150 mg PO/IV BID (300 mg/day).
Children 4–16 years:

11 to <20 kg: 2.5 mg/kg PO BID (5 mg/kg/day).
20 to <50 kg: 2 mg/kg PO BID (4 mg/kg/day).

Discontinuation Schedule: A dosage reduction of 25% per 1–2 weeks is a safe discontinuation regimen.

Administration Guidelines

May take with or without food. Swallow the whole tablet and do not chew or crush.

For PO solution, use a calibrated measuring device to deliver the prescribed dose accurately; no dilution is necessary; PO solution may also be administered using a nasogastric (NG) tube.

Infuse IV solution over 2–15 minutes.

Patient Education

1. If you miss a dose, take it as soon as you can. If it is almost time for your next dose, take only that dose. Do not take double or extra doses.
2. Adverse effects that you should report to your physician as soon as possible include
   - Thoughts about suicide or dying
   - New or worse depression
   - Feeling agitated or restless
   - Trouble sleeping (insomnia)
   - Acting aggressive, feeling angry, or being violent
   - An extreme increase in activity and talking (mania)
   - New or worse anxiety
   - Other unusual changes in behavior or mood
3. You may get drowsy, tired, dizzy, and have problems with your balance and coordination. Do not drive, use machinery, or do anything that needs mental alertness until you know how brivaracetam affects you. Alcohol can increase drowsiness and dizziness. Avoid alcoholic drinks.
4. If you are going to have surgery, tell your physician that you are taking brivaracetam.

Contraindications to Use: Hypersensitivity to brivaracetam.
Brivaracetam Precautions: Suicidal behavior and ideation.

Cannabidiol

Brand Name: Epidiolex
Dosage Form: PO solution: 100 mg/mL

Dosage

Cannabidiol is indicated for the treatment of seizures associated with Lennox-Gastaut

syndrome or Dravet syndrome in patients 2 years of age and older. Obtain serum transaminases (ALT and AST) and total bilirubin levels in all patients prior to starting the treatment.

Cannabidiol is administered orally; the recommended starting dosage is 2.5 mg/kg taken twice daily (5 mg/kg/day). After 1 week, the dosage can be increased to a maintenance dosage of 5 mg/kg twice daily (10 mg/kg/day). Based on clinical response and tolerability, cannabidiol can be increased up to a maximum recommended maintenance dosage of 10 mg/kg twice daily (20 mg/kg/day).

Discontinuation Schedule: If cannabidiol is to be discontinued, the dosage should be gradually reduced.

Administration Guidelines

Food may affect cannabidiol levels.

Patient Education

1. If you miss a dose, take it as soon as you can. If it is almost time for your next dose, take only that dose. Do not take double or extra doses.
2. Adverse effects that you should report to your physician as soon as possible include
   - Loss of appetite, nausea, vomiting
   - Fever, feeling unwell, unusual tiredness
   - Yellowing of the skin or the whites of the eyes (jaundice)
   - Itching
   - Unusual darkening of the urine
   - Right upper stomach area pain or discomfort
   - Thoughts about suicide or dying
   - New or worse depression
   - New or worse anxiety
   - Feeling agitated or restless
   - Panic attacks
   - Trouble sleeping (insomnia)
   - New or worse irritability
   - Acting aggressively, being angry, or violent
   - Acting on dangerous impulses
   - An extreme increase in activity and talking (mania)
   - Other unusual changes in behavior or mood
3. You may get drowsy, dizzy, or have blurred vision. Do not drive, use machinery, or do anything that needs mental alertness until you know how cannabidiol affects you. Alcohol can increase drowsiness and dizziness. Avoid alcoholic drinks.
4. If you are going to have surgery, tell your physician that you are taking cannabidiol.

Contraindications to Use: Hypersensitivity to cannabidiol.
Cannabidiol Precautions: Hepatocellular injury.

Carbamazepine

Brand Names: Carbatrol, Epitol, Equetro, Tegretol, Tegretol-XR

Dosage Forms:

Carbamazepine (Tegretol): Tablets 200 mg; chewable tablets 100 mg; PO suspension 100 mg/5 mL.

Epitol: Tablet 200 mg.

Tegretol-XR: Tablets 100 mg, 200 mg, 400 mg.

Carbatrol: Capsule-XR 100 mg, 200 mg, 300 mg.

Dosage

Starting Dose: *Adults and adolescents*: 100–200 mg twice daily.

Children 6–12 years: 100 mg twice daily (or 50 mg four times per day of suspension) or 10 mg/kg/day given in two divided doses for tablets, or four divided doses for the suspension.

Children <6 years: 10 mg/kg/day divided in 2–3 daily doses for tablets, or four divided doses for the suspension.

Titration and Maintenance Dose: *Adults and adolescents*: Increase 200 mg/day every 5–7 days; give daily dose in two divided doses for extended-release preparation and 2–4 divided doses for the regular preparation. Effective range is generally 400–1,200 mg/day (7–15 mg/kg/day), although higher doses can be used if serum levels remain low.

Children 6–12 years: Increase by 100 mg/day at 5–7 day intervals; give daily dose in two divided doses for the extended-release preparation and 2–4 divided doses for the regular preparation. Dose should be adjusted to the minimum effective level. The usual maintenance dosage range is 15–30 mg/kg/day.

Children <6 years: Increase weekly as needed; most patients will respond to doses lower than 35 mg/kg/day. If satisfactory response is not achieved, plasma drug concentrations should be checked to ensure adequate plasma levels. The safety of doses higher than 40 mg/kg/day has not been established.

Note: Extended-release tablets (Tegretol-XR) are not recommended in children younger than 6 years of age by manufacturers, but this is because testing has not been done and it may be difficult for young children to swallow a tablet rather than use the chewable 100-mg pill or the suspension. Children younger than 12 years who receive greater than or equal to 400 mg/day of carbamazepine may be converted to extended-release formulations using the same total daily dosage divided twice daily.

Note: A loading dose is not generally recommended.

Maximum Dosage Limit: These depend on serum level, and, because of autoinduction of hepatic microsomal enzymes, dosage guidelines vary from one patient to the next.

Adults and elderly: 1,600 mg/day (higher doses can be used depending on serum levels)
Adolescents >15 years: 1,200 mg/day (higher doses can be used depending on serum levels)
Children and adolescents 6–15 years: 1,000 mg/day (depending on serum level)
Children <6 years: 40 mg/kg/day

Discontinuation Schedule: A dosage reduction of 20–25% per 1–2 weeks is a safe discontinuation regimen.

Administration Guidelines

Administer with meals or with a large amount of water to minimize gastrointestinal adverse effects. May need to split doses to avoid GI upset.

For administration of suspension via nasogastric or enteral feeding tubes: To minimize any interaction that might occur with enteral feedings, turn off feedings at least 15 minutes before and hold for 15 minutes after a dose. Flush the tube with 15–30 mL (in adults) of water, D_5W, or NS prior to administration. To minimize the loss of drug, dilute the suspension with an equal volume of water prior to administration. Follow dose administration with flushing the tube with an additional 15–30 mL (in adults) of water, D_5W, or NS. Do not administer carbamazepine suspension with any other liquid medications or diluents since combination with other suspensions may form precipitants with loss of bioavailability.

For conversion from PO tablets/capsules to PO suspension: Patients should be converted to the suspension from the PO tablets or capsules by administering the same number of milligrams per day in smaller, more frequent doses (e.g., changing from twice per day for tablets to four times per day for the suspension).

Patient Education

1. If you miss a dose, take it as soon as you can. If it is almost time for your next dose, take only that dose. Do not take double or extra doses.
2. Adverse effects that you should report to your physician as soon as possible include
   Blurred or double vision, uncontrollable eye movements
   Chest pain or tightness
   Difficulty breathing or shortness of breath, wheezing
   Fainting spells
   Fast or irregular heartbeat (palpitations)
   Dark yellow or brown urine
   Pain or difficulty passing urine
   Increased thirst

Mouth ulcers
Fever or chills, sore throat
Redness, blistering, peeling, or loosening of the skin, including inside the mouth
Skin rash, hives, itching
Seizures
Stomach pain
Vomiting
Yellowing of the eyes or skin
Swollen joints or muscle/joint aches and pains
Unusual bleeding or bruising
Ringing in the ears
Confusion
Lightheadedness
Mood changes, nervousness, or hostility
Unusual tiredness or weakness

3. Do not change brands or dosage forms of carbamazepine without discussing the change with your physician.
4. You may get drowsy, dizzy, or have blurred vision. Do not drive, use machinery, or do anything that needs mental alertness until you know how carbamazepine affects you. To reduce dizzy or fainting spells, do not sit or stand up quickly. Alcohol can increase drowsiness and dizziness. Avoid alcoholic drinks.
5. If you are female and are taking birth control pills or other hormonal birth control methods (like injections), you should know that the birth control might not work as well while you are taking carbamazepine. Discuss this issue with your physician.
6. Carbamazepine may make your skin more sensitive to the sun or ultraviolet light. Keep out of the sun, or wear protective clothing outdoors and use a sunscreen (at least SPF 15). Do not use sun lamps or sun tanning beds or booths.
7. If you are going to have surgery, tell your physician that you are taking carbamazepine.

Box 2.5 Relative Contraindications to Use of Carbamazepine

- Bone marrow suppression
- Atrioventricular block or bundle-branch block
- Carbamazepine hypersensitivity
- Tricyclic antidepressant hypersensitivity
- Monoamine oxidase inhibitor therapy

See Chapters 17 and 18.

Box 2.6 Carbamazepine Precautions

- Atonic seizures
- Absence seizure
- Myoclonic seizures
- Barbiturate hypersensitivity
- Hydantoin hypersensitivity
- Breastfeeding
- Pregnancy
- Neonates
- Elderly
- Abrupt discontinuation
- Psychosis
- Alcoholism
- Glaucoma and increased intraocular pressure
- Hepatic diseases
- Hypercholesterolemia
- Hyponatremia
- Artery diseases
- Renal diseases
- Sunlight or ultraviolet exposure

See Chapters 7, 9–15, 17, 18, and 26.

Cenobamate

Brand Name: Xcopri
Dosage Forms: Tablets: 12.5 mg, 25 mg, 50 mg, 100 mg, 150 mg, and 200 mg

Dosage

Cenobamate is indicated for the treatment of focal-onset seizures in adult patients. The recommended initial dosage of cenobamate is 12.5 mg once daily (weeks 1 and 2), titrated to the recommended maintenance dosage of 200 mg once daily (week 3 and 4, 25 mg once daily; week 5 and 6, 50 mg once daily; week 7 and 8, 100 mg once daily, week 9 and 10, 150 mg once daily; week 11 and thereafter, 200 mg once daily). Dosing is preferred at bedtime. Dose may be further increased in 50 mg increments every 2 weeks. If side effects occur, the drug may be dosed twice daily.

The maximum dosage is 400 mg once daily.

Discontinuation Schedule: If cenobamate is to be discontinued, the dosage should be gradually reduced over a period of at least 2 weeks, unless safety concerns require abrupt withdrawal.

Administration Guidelines

Cenobamate may be taken any time with or without food. Cenobamate tablets should be swallowed whole with liquid and not chewed or crushed.

Patient Education

1. If you miss a dose, take it as soon as you can. If it is almost time for your next dose, take only that dose. Do not take double or extra doses.

2. Adverse effects that you should report to your physician as soon as possible include
   Swelling of your face, eyes, lips, or tongue
   Painful sores in the mouth or around your eyes
   Trouble swallowing or breathing
   Yellowing of your skin or eyes
   Skin rash
   Unusual bruising or bleeding
   Hives
   Severe fatigue or weakness
   Fever, swollen glands, or sore throat that does not go away or comes and goes
   Severe muscle pain
   Frequent infections that do not go away
   Thoughts about suicide or dying
   Trouble sleeping (insomnia)
   New or worse irritability
   New or worse depression
   Acting aggressive, being angry, or violent
   New or worse anxiety
   Acting on dangerous impulses
   Feeling agitated or restless
   Extreme increase in activity and talking (mania)
   Panic attacks
   Other unusual changes in behavior or mood
3. You may get drowsy, dizzy, or have blurred vision. Do not drive, use machinery, or do anything that needs mental alertness until you know how cenobamate affects you. To reduce dizzy or fainting spells, do not sit or stand up quickly. Alcohol can increase drowsiness and dizziness. Avoid alcoholic drinks.
4. If you are female and are taking birth control pills or other hormonal birth control methods (like injections), you should know that the birth control might not work as well while you are taking cenobamate. Discuss this issue with your physician.
5. If you are going to have surgery, tell your physician that you are taking cenobamate.

Contraindications to Use:

Hypersensitivity to cenobamate
Familial short QT syndrome

Cenobamate Precautions: Use caution when administering with other drugs that shorten the QT interval. DRESS syndrome (drug rash with eosinophilia and systemic symptoms) has been reported with cenobamate and immediate investigation is required should any symptoms such as rash or fever develop.

Corticotropin, ACTH

Brand Names: Acthar, HP Acthar

Dosage Forms: Repository corticotrophin injection: 80 units/mL (in 5-mL multidose vials)

Dosage

Infants with infantile spasm: Various regimens have been used. Low-doses of 5–40 units/day IM for 1–6 weeks have been recommended by some neurologists, while others recommend larger doses of 40–160 units/day IM for 3–12 months. The usual dosage range is 20–40 units/day (50–100 IU/m^2) IM or 5–8 units/kg/day IM in two divided doses for 1–3 weeks. If response is complete, taper ACTH over 1–4 months. If response is observed but is incomplete, increase the dose to 60–80 IU/day (150–200 IU/m^2) for 2 weeks. If spasms and hypsarrhythmia resolve, ACTH should be tapered over 1–4 months. If relapse occurs during tapering, the dose may be increased to the previously effective dose for 2 weeks and then another tapering begun. If therapy at these doses is not successful, ACTH should be rapidly tapered and another medication should be tried.

Administration Guidelines

Dissolve 25 or 40 units of ACTH in 1 or 2 mL of NS injection or sterile water for injection. The solution is stable for 24 hours at room temperature or for 1 week under refrigeration.

If using the repository suspension, warm to room temperature before administration. Shake thoroughly prior to administration.

Using a 22-gauge needle, inject deeply into a large muscle mass (IM). Aspirate prior to injection to avoid injection into a blood vessel. Massage area following administration. Rotate sites of injection.

Patient Education

1. Adverse effects that you should report to your physician as soon as possible include
    - Bloody or black, tarry stools
    - Nausea, vomiting
    - Stomach pain
    - Rounding out of face
    - Weight gain, increased thirst
    - Frequent passing of urine
    - Fever, sore throat, sneezing, cough, or other signs of infection
    - Wounds that will not heal
    - Confusion, excitement, restlessness
    - Depression, mood swings
    - Irregular heartbeat
    - Pain in hips, back, ribs, arms, shoulders, or legs
    - Pain, redness, swelling, signs of allergy, or scarring at the injection site
    - Skin problems, acne, thin and shiny skin
    - Swelling of feet or lower legs

Unusual bruising, pinpoint red spots on the skin
Unusual tiredness or weakness

2. Avoid contact with people who have an infection. You will have an increased risk of infection while receiving corticotropin. Do not receive any vaccinations because you may get a strong reaction. Avoid people who have recently taken the PO polio vaccine. Tell your physician if you are exposed to anyone with measles or chickenpox, or if you develop sores or blisters that do not heal properly.
3. If you are going to have surgery, tell your physician that you have received corticotropin within the last 12 months.

Box 2.7 Relative Contraindications to Use of Corticotropin (ACTH)

- Adrenal insufficiency
- Cushing syndrome
- Hypercortisolism
- Heart failure
- Herpes infection
- Ocular infections
- Porcine protein hypersensitivity
- Scleroderma
- Surgery

Box 2.8 Corticotropin (ACTH) Precautions

- Corticosteroid hypersensitivity
- Diabetes mellitus
- Hypothyroidism
- Hepatic diseases
- Hypernatremia
- Hypertension
- Hypokalemia
- Renal diseases
- Infections
- Myasthenia gravis
- Thromboembolic diseases

See Chapters 12–14.

Eslicarbazepine Acetate

Brand Name: Aptiom

Dosage Forms: Tablets 200, 400, 600, 800 mg

Dosage

Starting Dose: 400 mg orally once daily for 1 week.

Maintenance Dose: The usual maintenance dose is 800 mg once daily.

Maximum Dosage Limit: 1,200 mg/day.

Discontinuation Schedule: A dosage reduction of 20–25% per 1–2 weeks is a safe discontinuation regimen.

Administration Guidelines

May be taken with or without food. The Aptiom tablet may be crushed or swallowed whole.

Patient Education

1. If you miss a dose, take it as soon as you can. If it is almost time for your next dose, take only that dose. Do not take double or extra doses.
2. Adverse effects that you should report to your physician as soon as possible include
   Suicidal behavior and ideation
   New or worse depression, anxiety, irritability or changes in behavior or mood
   Hives; difficult breathing; swelling of your face, lips, tongue, or throat
   Nausea
   Lack of energy, feeling tired or irritable, severe weakness
   Muscle pain
   Confusion, vision changes, thinking problems,
   Trouble with walking or coordination
   Upper stomach pain, loss of appetite, dark urine, jaundice
3. Do not stop taking your medicine suddenly. Your physician may want you to reduce your dose gradually.
4. You may get drowsy. Do not drive, use machinery, or do anything that requires mental alertness until you know how this drug affects you.
5. Report to your physician if you notice any changes.
6. If you are female and are taking birth-control pills, you should know that the birth control might not work as well while you are taking eslicarbazepine. Discuss this issue with your physician.

Box 2.9 Contraindications to Use of Eslicarbazepine Acetate

- Hypersensitivity to eslicarbazepine acetate or oxcarbazepine

Box 2.10 Eslicarbazepine Acetate Precautions

- Breastfeeding
- Pregnancy
- Elderly
- Kidney diseases
- Severe liver diseases

See Chapters 9–13.

Ethosuximide

Brand Name: Zarontin

Dosage Forms: Capsules 250 mg; syrup 250 mg/5 mL

Dosage

Starting Dose:

Adults and children >6 years: 250 mg PO 1–3 times daily.

Children 3–6 years: 10–15 mg/kg/day (maximum initial dose 250 mg/day), given in 1–3 divided doses.

Titration and Maintenance Dose: *Adults and children >6 years*: May increase dosage by 250 mg/day at 4- to 7-day intervals, until seizure control is achieved, or to a maximum dose of 1.5 g/day. The usual maintenance dose is 20–40 mg/kg/day (750–1,500 mg/day), given in 2–3 divided doses.

Children 3–6 years: Increase every 4–7 days; usual maintenance dose is 15–40 mg/kg/day, given in 2–3 divided doses.

Maximum Dosage Limit: Dosages exceeding 1.5 g daily should be administered only under strict supervision.

Discontinuation Schedule: A gradual reduction over 4 weeks is recommended (or 50% per week). If necessary, abrupt discontinuation of ethosuximide is probably safe because of its long half-life.

Administration Guidelines

Take with food or after meals to avoid stomach upset

Contraindications to Use: Succinimide hypersensitivity

Patient Education

1. If you miss a dose, take it as soon as possible. However, if it is within 4 hours of your next dose, skip the missed dose and go back to your regular dosing schedule. Do not use double doses.
2. Adverse effects that you should report to your physician as soon as possible include
   - Chest pain or tightness
   - Shortness of breath, or wheezing
   - Fever, sore throat
   - Mouth ulcers
   - Mood changes, nervousness, or hostility
   - Muscle aches
   - Unusual tiredness or weakness
   - Redness, blistering, peeling or loosening of the skin, including inside the mouth
   - Skin rash and itching
   - Unusual bleeding or bruising

3. You may get drowsy, dizzy, or have blurred vision. Do not drive, use machinery, or do anything that requires mental alertness until you know how ethosuximide affects you. To reduce dizzy or fainting spells, do not sit or stand up quickly. Alcohol can increase drowsiness and dizziness. Avoid alcoholic drinks.
4. If you are going to have surgery, tell your physician that you are taking ethosuximide.

Box 2.11 Ethosuximide Precautions

- Abrupt discontinuation
- Bone marrow suppression
- Breastfeeding
- Pregnancy
- Infants
- Porphyria
- Hematological diseases
- Renal diseases
- Hepatic diseases

See Chapters 9, 10, 12, 13, and 18.

Methsuximide

Brand Name: Celontin

Dosage Forms: Capsules 150, 300 mg

Dosage

Adults: 300–600 mg/day in 2–3 divided doses for the first week; may increase by 300 mg/day at weekly intervals up to 1.5 g/day in three divided doses; an initial maintenance dose of 900 mg/day is advised.

Children: 10–15 mg/kg/day in three divided doses; increase weekly up to a maximum of 30 mg/kg/day.

Ezogabine

Brand Name: Potiga (This drug is no longer available in the United States.)

Other Names: Retigabine (generic); Trobalt (brand) in Europe

Dosage Forms: Tablets 50 mg, 100 mg, 200 mg, 300 mg, and 400 mg

Dosage

Starting Dose:

Adults (>18 years): 300 mg/day in three divided doses.

Elderly (>65 years): 150 mg/day in three divided doses.

Titration and Maintenance Dose: *Adults*: Titrate by 150 mg increase per week. Usual maintenance dose is 200–300 mg three times a day

(600–900 mg/day). May increase to 1,200 mg/day, in three divided doses, based on efficacy and tolerability. At 1,200 mg/day, the incidence of dose-related adverse effects may significantly affect patient tolerance. Because ezogabine may cause retinal abnormalities with long-term use, patients who fail to show substantial clinical benefit after adequate titration should be discontinued from ezogabine.

Maximum Dosage Limits:

Adults: 1,200 mg/day.

Elderly (>65 years): 750 mg/day in three divided doses.

Children and adolescents <18 years: Safe and effective use has not been established.

Discontinuation Schedule: If ezogabine dose is reduced, discontinued, or substituted with an alternative medication, the dosage should be gradually reduced over a period of at least 3 weeks, unless safety concerns require abrupt withdrawal.

Administration Guidelines

Should be given orally in 3 equally divided doses daily, with or without food. Tablets should be swallowed whole.

Relative Contraindication: Hypersensitivity to ezogabine.

Patient Education

1. If you miss a dose, take it as soon as you can. If it is almost time for your next dose, take only that dose. Do not take double or extra doses.
2. You should have a complete eye exam if you are currently taking ezogabine or before starting treatment, and then every 6 months while taking ezogabine.
3. Adverse effects that you should report to your physician as soon as possible include
   Inability to start urinating
   Trouble emptying your bladder
   Pain with urination
   Suicidal thinking and behavior
   Hallucinations

Box 2.12 Ezogabine Precautions

- Breastfeeding
- Pregnancy
- Elderly
- Hepatic impairment
- Renal impairment
- Heart diseases
- Ocular diseases (e.g., retinal abnormalities)

See Chapters 9–12, 16, 17, and 27.

New or worse depression, anxiety, irritability or changes in behavior or mood
Loss of coordination
Vision changes
Fast, slow, or pounding heartbeat
Any changes in color to your body
Rash, itching, swelling, severe dizziness, or trouble breathing.

4. You may get drowsy or dizzy while using ezogabine. Do not drive, use machinery, or do anything that requires mental alertness until you know how ezogabine affects you. Alcohol can increase drowsiness and dizziness. Avoid alcoholic drinks.
5. Do not stop taking ezogabine suddenly.

Felbamate

Brand Names: Felbamyl, Felbatol, Taloxa

Dosage Forms: Tablets 400 mg, 600 mg; suspension 600 mg/5 mL.

Dosage

Starting Dose:

Adults and adolescents >14 years: 1,200 mg/day in three divided doses for monotherapy or adjunctive therapy for the first 2 weeks.

Adolescents and children 2–14 years of age: 15 mg/kg/day in three divided doses only as adjunctive therapy for the first 2 weeks.

Titration and Maintenance Dose: *Adults and adolescents >14 years*: For monotherapy increase 600 mg every 2 weeks under close clinical supervision to 2,400 mg/day. Thereafter, increase up to 3,600 mg/day based on clinical response. For adjunctive therapy, follow these two steps:

While starting felbamate, reduce the dosage of present ASMs (phenytoin, phenobarbital, valproic acid, and carbamazepine) by 20%.
Increase the dosage of felbamate by 1,200 mg/day every week up to 3,600 mg/day. Further reduction of concomitant ASMs dosage may be necessary.

Adolescents and children 2–14 years of age: For adjunctive therapy, follow these two steps:

While starting felbamate, reduce the dosage of present ASMs (phenytoin, phenobarbital, valproic acid, and carbamazepine) by 20%.
Increase the dosage of felbamate by 15 mg/kg/day every week up to 45 mg/kg/day. Further reduction of concomitant ASM dosage may be necessary.

Note: For conversion to monotherapy in adults and adolescents above 14 years of age, follow these four steps:

1. Initiate felbamate at 1,200 mg/day in 3–4 divided doses.
2. Reduce the dosage of concomitant ASMs by one-third.

3. At week 2, increase felbamate dosage to 2,400 mg/day and reduce the dosage of concomitant ASMs by an additional one third of the original doses.
4. At week 3, increase felbamate dosage to 3,600 mg/day and reduce the dosage or discontinue other ASMs as clinically indicated.

Note: Loading dose is not recommended.

Note: The elderly may require lower initial doses of felbamate and slower dose titration.

Maximum Dosage Limit: *Adults and adolescents >14 years*: 5,400 mg/day (doses >3,600 mg/day may be associated with greater risk of aplastic anemia and liver failure).

Adolescents and children 2–14 years of age: 45 mg/kg/day.

Discontinuation Schedule: A dosage reduction of 20–25% per 2 weeks is safe at the time of discontinuation.

Administration Guidelines

Administer with meals to minimize gastrointestinal adverse effects.

Patient Education

1. If you miss a dose, take it as soon as you can. If it is almost time for your next dose, take only that dose. Do not take double or extra doses.
2. Adverse effects that you should report to your physician immediately include
   Fainting
   Fast or irregular heartbeat
   Wheezing or trouble breathing
   Skin rash, hives, or itching
   Swelling in face, throat, or lips
   Unusual bleeding or bruising
   Yellow eyes or skin
   Loss of seizure control
   Unusual tiredness or weakness
3. Adverse effects that you should report to your physician as soon as possible include
   Constipation
   Loss of appetite, nausea, or vomiting
   Fever
   Drowsiness or dizziness
   Headache
   Trouble sleeping, nervousness
4. Taking felbamate has led to a few cases of a serious blood disorder called aplastic anemia and a few cases of liver failure. Talk to your physician about these risks.
5. Make sure your doctor knows if you have liver or kidney disease or a history of blood problems.

6. You may get drowsy, dizzy, or have blurred vision. Do not drive, use machinery, or do anything that requires mental alertness until you know how felbamate affects you. To reduce dizzy or fainting spells, do not sit or stand up quickly. Alcohol can increase drowsiness and dizziness. Avoid alcoholic drinks.
7. Felbamate may make your skin more sensitive to the sun or ultraviolet light. Keep out of the sun, or wear protective clothing outdoors and use a sunscreen (at least SPF 15). Do not use sun lamps or sun tanning beds or booths.

Box 2.13 Relative Contraindications to Use of Felbamate

- Blood disorders
- Hepatic impairment
- Hypersensitivity to felbamate
- Hypersensitivity to methocarbamol or meprobamate

See Chapters 13 and 18.

Box 2.14 Felbamate Precautions

- Renal impairment
- Breastfeeding
- Pregnancy
- Elderly
- Abrupt discontinuation
- Sunlight or ultraviolet exposure

See Chapters 9–12 and 26.

Gabapentin

Brand Names: Gabarone, Neurontin

Dosage Forms:

Gabarone: Tablets 100 mg, 300 mg, 400 mg

Gabapentin (Neurontin): Tablets 600 mg, 800 mg; capsule 100 mg, 300 mg, 400 mg; PO solution 250 mg/5 mL

Dosage

Starting Dose:

Adolescents, adults, and elderly: 300 mg one or two times per day.
Children 3–12 years: 10–15 mg/kg/day PO in three divided doses.

Titration and Maintenance Dose: *Adolescents, adults, and elderly*: May increase rapidly using 300 mg at bedtime on day one, 300 mg twice daily on day 2, and then 300 mg three times daily starting on day 3. Usual maintenance dose is 900–1,800 mg/day; however, doses up to 3,600 mg/day have been used. Do not give doses less frequently than every 12 hours. Dosage adjustments of other anticonvulsants are not necessary. Doses for the elderly are often lower and can be based on creatinine clearance (CrCl).

Children 3–12 years: Titrate upward to effective dose over a period of 3 days. If >5 years, the effective dose is 25–35 mg/kg/day PO, given in three divided doses. If 3–4 years of age, the effective dose is 40 mg/kg/day PO, given in three divided doses. Do not give doses less frequently than every 12 hours. Depending on the clinical response, titration may continue as needed up to 50 mg/kg/day. Doses higher than 50 mg/kg/day have occasionally been used.

Children <3 years: Safety is not established. However, experts administer it to their patients whenever benefits outweigh the risks.

Note: Loading dose is not suggested.

Maximum Dosage Limits: *Adults, elderly, and adolescents*: 3,600 mg/day PO (higher doses have been used, but are probably not more effective).

Children 3–12 years: 50 mg/kg/day PO suggested; higher dosages occasionally have been used in refractory patients.

Discontinuation Schedule: If gabapentin dose is reduced or discontinued, this should be done gradually over a minimum of 1 week. A dosage reduction of 25% per 2 weeks is safe at the time of discontinuation.

Administration Guidelines

May be administered without regard to meals; however, administration with meals may minimize adverse gastrointestinal effects.

In patients with difficulty in swallowing, gabapentin capsules may be opened and the contents mixed with drinks (e.g., orange juice) or foods (e.g., applesauce). Scored tablets may be cut in half for dosage titration or ease of swallowing. If the scored 600- or 800-mg tablets are split, the extra half-tablet should be used for the next dose. If the extra half-tablet is not used within 3 days, it should be thrown away.

Contraindications to Use: Gabapentin hypersensitivity.

Box 2.15 Gabapentin Precautions

- Abrupt discontinuation
- Absence seizure
- Breastfeeding
- Pregnancy
- Infants
- Children
- Elderly
- Renal impairment

See Chapters 7 and 9–12.

Patient Education

1. If you miss a dose, take it as soon as you can. However, if it is less than 4 hours until your next dose, do not take the missed dose and return to your regular dosing schedule. Do not take double or extra doses.
2. Adverse effects that you should report to your physician as soon as possible include
   Difficulty breathing or tightening of the throat
   Swelling of lips or tongue
   Rash
   Fever
   Hyperactivity
   Hostile or aggressive behavior
   Mood changes or changes in behavior
   Difficulty concentrating
3. You may get drowsy, dizzy, or have blurred vision. Do not drive, use machinery, or do anything that requires mental alertness until you know how gabapentin affects you. To reduce dizzy or fainting spells, do not sit or stand up quickly. Alcohol can increase drowsiness and dizziness. Avoid alcoholic drinks.
4. If you are going to have surgery, tell your physician that you are taking gabapentin.

Lacosamide

Brand Name: Vimpat

Dosage Forms: Tablets 50 mg, 100 mg, 150 mg, 200 mg, syrup 10 mg/mL, 200 mg/20 mL injection

Dosage

Starting Dose:

Adolescents >17 years, adults: 100 mg/day in two divided doses.

Titration and Maintenance Dose: *Adolescents >17 years, adults*: Titrate by 100 mg per week. Usual maintenance dose is 200–400 mg per day in two divided doses. May increase to 600 mg/day, in two divided doses, based on efficacy and tolerability. In clinical trials, the 600 mg daily dose was not more effective than the 400 mg daily dose and was associated with a substantially higher rate of adverse reactions.

Maximum Dosage Limits: 600 mg/day.

Children <17 years: Safe and effective use has not been established. However, experts administer it to their patients, whenever benefits outweigh the risks.

Discontinuation Schedule: If lacosamide dose is reduced, discontinued, or substituted with an alternative medication, this should be done gradually over a minimum interval of 1 week.

Administration Guidelines

May be administered without regard to meals.

Note: Lacosamide injection for IV use is indicated when PO administration is temporarily not feasible. In this situation, the initial total daily IV dosage should be equivalent to the total daily dosage and frequency of PO lacosamide and should be infused intravenously over a period of 30–60 minutes. At the end of the IV treatment period, the patient may be switched to lacosamide PO administration at the equivalent daily dosage and frequency of the IV administration.

Relative Contraindication to Use: Hypersensitivity to lacosamide.

Patient Education

1. If you miss a dose, take it as soon as you can. If it is almost time for your next dose, take only that dose. Do not take double or extra doses.
2. Adverse effects that you should report to your physician as soon as possible include
   Fast, slow, or pounding heartbeat
   Shortness of breath
   Feel lightheaded
   Fainted
   Suicidal behavior and ideation
   New or worse depression, anxiety, irritability or changes in behavior or mood
   Rash, itching, swelling, severe dizziness, or trouble breathing
3. You may get drowsy or dizzy while using lacosamide. Do not drive, use machinery, or do anything that needs mental alertness until you know how lacosamide affects you.
4. Do not stop taking lacosamide suddenly. This medication may cause dependence, especially if it has been used regularly for an extended period of time or if it has been used in high doses. In such cases, if you suddenly stop this drug, withdrawal reactions may occur.

Box 2.16 Lacosamide Precautions

- Suicidal behavior and ideation
- Cardiac rhythm and conduction abnormalities
- Syncope
- Phenylketonuria
- Pregnancy
- Breastfeeding
- Renal impairment
- Hepatic impairment

See Chapters 9, 10, 12–14, 17, and 22.

Lamotrigine

Brand Name: Lamictal

Dosage Forms:

Lamotrigine (Lamictal): Tablets 25 mg, 100 mg, 150 mg, 200 mg

Lamotrigine XR (Lamictal) (extended-release tablets): 25 mg, 50 mg, 100 mg, 200 mg, 250 mg, 300 mg

Lamotrigine (Lamictal) chewable dispersible: Chewable tablets 2 mg, 5 mg, 25 mg

Dosage

In patients not receiving valproic acid or enzyme-inducing ASMs (e.g., carbamazepine, phenobarbital primidone, phenytoin):

Starting Dose:

Adults and adolescents >12 years of age: 25 mg daily for the first 2 weeks.

Children and adolescents 2–12 years of age: 0.3 mg/kg/day in 1–2 divided doses given for the first 2 weeks (rounded down to the nearest whole tablet).

Titration and Maintenance Dose:

Adults and adolescents >12 years of age: 25 mg twice daily (50 mg/day) for weeks 3–4; then the dose may be increased by up to 50 mg daily every 1–2 weeks until the maintenance dosage is achieved. The usual maintenance dose is 200–400 mg/day, given in 1–2 divided doses.

Children and adolescents 2–12 years of age: 0.6 mg/kg/day given in two divided doses for weeks 3–4. Round the dose down to the nearest whole tablet. Thereafter, the dose should be increased every 1–2 weeks as follows: calculate 0.6 mg/kg/day, round this amount down to the nearest whole tablet, and add this amount to the previously administered daily dose. The usual maintenance dose is 4.5–7.5 mg/kg/day (maximum 300 mg/day in two divided doses). Maintenance dose in patients less than 30 kg may need to be increased by as much as 50%, based on clinical response.

In patients currently receiving treatment with an enzyme-inducing ASM (e.g., carbamazepine, phenobarbital, primidone, phenytoin):

Starting Dose:

Adults and adolescents >12 years: 50 mg daily for the first 2 weeks.

Children 2–12 years of age: 0.6 mg/kg/day in two divided doses given for the first 2 weeks.

Titration and Maintenance Dose:

Adults and adolescents >12 years: 100 mg daily is given in two divided doses for weeks 3–4. Thereafter, doses may be increased by 100 mg/day every 1–2 weeks until the maintenance dosage is achieved. The usual maintenance dose is 300–500 mg/day given in two divided doses (maximum 700 mg/day in these patients). Conversion to monotherapy, if desired, requires two transitional steps. First, the patient is titrated to the targeted dose of lamotrigine while maintaining the dose of the enzyme-inducing ASM at a fixed level. The recommended target maintenance dose for monotherapy conversion is 150–200 mg twice daily (total 300–400 mg daily, although lower doses may be effective). Second, after achieving the targeted lamotrigine dose, the enzyme-inducing ASM is gradually withdrawn over a period of 6–12 weeks. If adverse effects appear after stopping the enzyme-inducing ASM, the lamotrigine dose may need to be lowered because its level will rise as hepatic enzyme activity returns to normal.

Children and adolescents 2–12 years of age: 1.2 mg/kg/day given in two divided doses for weeks 3–4. Round the dose down to the nearest whole tablet. After week 4, the usual maintenance dose range is 5–15 mg/kg/day (maximum 400 mg/day) given in two divided doses for adjunctive therapy. To achieve the usual maintenance dose, the dose may be increased every 1–2 weeks by about 1.2 mg/kg/day (round this amount down to the nearest whole tablet and add this amount to the previously administered daily dose). Maintenance doses in patients weighing <30 kg may need to be increased by as much as 50% based on clinical response. It may take several weeks to months to achieve an individualized maintenance dose.

In patients currently receiving valproic acid with or without enzyme-inducing ASMs or other ASMs concomitantly:

Starting Dose:

Adults and adolescents >12 years of age: 25 mg every other day for the first 2 weeks.

Children and adolescents 2–12 years of age: 0.15 mg/kg/day in 1–2 divided doses given for the first 2 weeks (rounded down to the nearest whole tablet).

Titration and Maintenance Dose:

Adults and adolescents >12 years of age: 25 mg daily for weeks 3–4; then, the dose may be increased by 25–50 mg daily every 2 weeks until the maintenance dosage is achieved. The usual maintenance dose is 100–400 mg/day, given in 1–2 divided doses. The usual maintenance dose range for patients who add lamotrigine to valproic acid alone is 100–200 mg/day.

Children and adolescents 2–12 years of age: 0.3 mg/kg/day given in 1–2 divided doses for weeks 3–4. Round the dose down to the nearest whole tablet. After week 4, the usual maintenance dose range is from 1–5 mg/kg/day (maximum 200 mg/day) given in 1–2 divided doses. To achieve the usual maintenance dose, doses may be increased every 1–2 weeks by 0.3 mg/kg/day (round this amount down to the nearest whole tablet and add this amount to the previously administered daily dose). Maintenance doses in patients weighing less than 30 kg may need to be increased by as much as 50%, based on clinical response. The usual maintenance dose range in patients adding lamotrigine to valproic acid alone is 1–3 mg/kg/day.

Note: Conversion to lamotrigine monotherapy from combined lamotrigine and valproate therapy in adults requires 4 steps:

1. The patient should be stabilized on a current maintenance dose of valproate and a target dose of lamotrigine 150–200 mg/day while taking valproate. If the patient is not currently at lamotrigine 150–200 mg/day, the dose may be increased by 25–50 mg/day every 1–2 weeks to reach that dose.
2. While maintaining lamotrigine dose at 150–200 mg/day, decrease valproate dose to 500 mg/day by decrements of 250–500 mg/day per week and maintain valproate dose of 500 mg/day for 1 week.
3. Increase lamotrigine dose to 300 mg/day while simultaneously decreasing valproate dose to 250 mg/day and maintain for 1 week.
4. Finally, discontinue valproate completely and increase lamotrigine dose as needed for seizure control.

Note: Lamotrigine should be initiated at a low-dose, with gradual increase. This may minimize the occurrence of skin rash.

Note: Avoid use in children weighing <6.7 kg because therapy cannot be initiated using the dosing guidelines and currently available chewable tablet strengths.

Note: If the decision is made to restart a patient who has discontinued lamotrigine for a period of more than 5 half-lives, it is recommended that initial dosing recommendations and guidelines be followed.

Maximum Dosage Limits: Individualize the maximum dosage limits to the patient's age, weight, indication, concurrent medication, and clinical response.

Discontinuation Schedule: Discontinuation of lamotrigine should be done in a stepwise fashion over 2–6 weeks (approximately 50% dosage reduction per week) unless safety concerns warrant a more rapid withdrawal.

Administration Guidelines

May be administered without regard to meals. Lamotrigine XR extended-release tablets are taken once daily, with or without food. Tablets must be swallowed whole and must not be chewed, crushed, or divided.

Note: The lowest available tablet strength is a 2-mg chewable dispersible tablet, and all doses should be rounded down to the nearest 2-mg dose. Only whole dispersible tablets should be administered; do not cut in half.

Contraindication to Use: Hypersensitivity to lamotrigine.

Box 2.17 Lamotrigine Precautions

- Hypersensitivity to other antiseizure medications
- Abrupt discontinuation
- Suicidal ideation
- Pregnancy
- Labor and delivery
- Breastfeeding
- Children
- Elderly
- Hepatic diseases
- Renal impairment

See Chapters 9–13, 22, and 26.

Patient Education

1. If you take regular Lamictal tablets, swallow the tablets with a drink of water. Do not chew these tablets as they have a bitter taste. If lamotrigine upsets your stomach, take it with food or milk.
2. Lamictal chewable dispersible tablets may be swallowed whole, chewed, mixed in water, or mixed in diluted fruit juice to aid swallowing. To mix the tablets in water or juice, add the tablets to a small amount of liquid in a glass or spoon. The tablets will dissolve in about 1 minute. Once dissolved, mix or swirl the liquid, and take the entire solution immediately. It is important that you swallow all of the liquid used to prepare the dose so that the full prescribed dose is given.
3. If you miss a dose, take it as soon as you can. If it is almost time for your next dose, take only that dose. Do not take double or extra doses.
4. Adverse effects that you should report to your physician immediately include
   Fever
   Painful sores in the mouth, eyes, or nose
   Redness, blistering, peeling or loosening of the skin, including inside the mouth
   Skin rash of any type, itching
   Swelling of the face, lips or tongue
   Swollen lymph glands
5. Adverse effects you should report to your physician as soon as possible include
   Blurred or double vision
   Hand tremor
   Somnolence, cognitive difficulties
   Uncontrollable eye movements
   Changes in seizure type or frequency
   Depression or mood changes
   Difficulty walking or controlling muscle movements
   Unusual weakness or tiredness

6. You may get drowsy or dizzy or have blurred vision. Do not drive, use machinery, or do anything that requires mental alertness until you know how lamotrigine affects you. To reduce dizzy or fainting spells, do not sit or stand up quickly. Alcohol can increase drowsiness and dizziness. Avoid alcoholic drinks or medicines containing alcohol.
7. If you are female and are taking hormonal birth control methods (e.g., birth control pills), you should know that the birth control might not work as well while you are taking lamotrigine. Discuss this issue with your physician.
8. If you are going to have surgery, tell your physician that you are taking lamotrigine.

Levetiracetam

Brand Name: Keppra

Dosage Forms: Tablets 250 mg, 500 mg, 750 mg, 1,000 mg; PO solution 100 mg/mL; injection 500 mg/5 mL.

Dosage

Starting Dose:

Adults and adolescents >16 years: 250–500 mg twice daily.
Adolescents and children 4–15 years: 10 mg/kg twice daily (20 mg/kg/day).
Children <4 years: Safe and effective use has not been established. However, experts administer it to their patients whenever benefits outweigh the risks.

Titration and Maintenance Dose: *Adults and adolescents >16 years*: Usual maintenance dose is 500–750 mg twice daily. May be titrated as needed by 1,000 mg/day every 2 weeks until achievement of good clinical response (not to exceed 3,000 mg/day), in two divided doses. For conversions between PO and IV administration, use equivalent total daily dosages and frequencies. Doses >3,000 mg/day may not provide additional benefit.

Adolescents and children 4–15 years: Increase the daily dose every 2 weeks by increments of 20 mg/kg/day to the recommended dose of 60 mg/kg/day PO twice daily. If a patient cannot tolerate a total daily dose of 60 mg/kg, the daily dose may be reduced. If body weight <20 kg, administer PO solution; if body weight >20 kg, administer either solution or tablets.

Note: Treatment may be initiated with either IV or PO therapy.

Note: Loading dose is not necessary.

Note: Minimum known effective dosage is 1,000 mg/day in adults. Lower doses have not been fully tested.

Note: The total daily dose should be the same when switching from PO to IV formulations.

Maximum Dosage Limit:

Adolescents >16 years, adults and elderly: 3,000 mg/day PO or IV.
Adolescents <16 years and children: 60 mg/kg/day PO for the treatment of focal onset seizures (maximum 3,000 mg/day); 3,000 mg/day PO for the treatment of myoclonic seizures; IV administration not recommended.
Children 4–11 years: 60 mg/kg/day PO.

Discontinuation Schedule: A dosage reduction of 25% per 2 weeks is safe at the time of discontinuation.

Administration Guidelines

PO administration:

May be administered without regard to meals.
Tablets are crushable but have a bitter taste.

IV administration:

Dilute the total dose in 100 mL of compatible diluent (0.9% sodium chloride injection, lactated Ringer's injection, or dextrose 5% injection) and infuse over 15 minutes.
Diluted preparation is stable for at least 24 hours when stored in polyvinyl chloride bags at controlled room temperature of 15–30°C (59–86°F).
Diluted preparation is physically compatible with lorazepam, diazepam, and valproate sodium.

Contraindications to Use: Hypersensitivity to levetiracetam.

Patient Education

1. If you miss a dose, take it as soon as you can. If it is almost time for your next dose, take only that dose. Do not take double or extra doses.
2. Adverse effects that you should report to your physician immediately include
   Difficulty breathing or tightening of the throat
   Rash
   Swelling of lips or tongue

Box 2.18 Levetiracetam Precautions

- Abrupt discontinuation
- Breastfeeding
- Pregnancy
- Children
- Elderly
- Depression
- Psychosis
- Renal diseases
- Renal failure

See Chapters 9–12 and 22.

3. Adverse effects you should report to your physician as soon as possible include
   Agitation, restlessness, irritability, or other changes in mood
   Changes in seizure type or frequency
   Difficulty walking or controlling muscle movements
   Unusual weakness or tiredness
4. You may get drowsy or dizzy. Do not drive, use machinery, or do anything that requires mental alertness until you know how levetiracetam affects you. To reduce dizzy spells, do not sit or stand up quickly. Alcohol can increase drowsiness and dizziness. Avoid alcoholic drinks or medicines containing alcohol.
5. If you are going to have surgery, tell your physician that you are taking levetiracetam.

Oxcarbazepine

Brand Names: Trileptal, Oxtellar XR (extended-release)

Dosage Forms: Tablets 150 mg, 300 mg, 600 mg; extended-release tablets (Oxtellar XR) 150 mg, 300 mg, 600 mg; PO suspension 300 mg/5 mL

Dosage

Starting Dose:

Adults and adolescents >16 years: 150–300 mg twice daily; Oxtellar XR: 600 mg once per day.

Adolescents and children 2–16 years: 8–10 mg/kg/day in two divided doses. For patients <20 kg, a starting dose of 16–20 mg/kg may be considered. Oxtellar XR (age 6–17 years): 8–10 mg/kg PO once daily; not to exceed 600 mg/day in the first week.

Titration and Maintenance Dose: *Adults and adolescents >16 years*: Oxcarbazepine should be titrated upward by 300–600 mg/day every week over 2–4 weeks to achieve the recommended dose of 900–2,400 mg/day. *Oxtellar XR*: May increase at weekly intervals by 600 mg/day increments to target dosage range of 1,200–2,400 mg once daily.

Adolescents and children 2–16 years: Increase the dose by 5 mg/kg/day every 3 days to the recommended daily maintenance dosage as follows:

- 30–50 mg/kg/day in children 2–4 years of age
- 600–900 mg/day for those 20–24.9 kg
- 900–1,200 mg/day for those 25–34.9 kg
- 900–1,500 mg/day for those 35–44.9 kg
- 1,200–1,500 mg/day for those 45–49.9 kg

- 1,200–1,800 mg/day for those 50–59.9 kg
- 1,200–2,100 mg/day for those 60–69.9 kg
- 1,500–2,100 mg/day for those ≥ 70 kg

Target Maintenance Dose for Oxtellar XR (Age 6–17 Years): May titrate to higher dose at weekly intervals in 8–10 mg/kg/day increments (not to exceed 600 mg) to reach the following target maintenance dosage ranges:

- 20–29 kg: 900 mg PO once daily
- >29–39 kg: 1,200 mg PO once daily
- >39 kg: 1,800 mg PO once daily

Children and infants <2 years: Safe and effective use has not been established. However, experts administer it to their patients whenever benefits outweigh the risks.

Note: Loading dose is not studied.

Note: When converting from immediate-release oxcarbazepine to Oxtellar XR, higher doses of Oxtellar XR may be required.

Note: When converting to oxcarbazepine from other ASMs, initiate at 300 mg twice daily while beginning to reduce the dose of other ASMs. The dosage of concurrent ASMs should be completely withdrawn over 3–6 weeks as tolerated.

Note: For adjunct treatment of focal onset seizures, maintenance dose is usually up to 1,200 mg/day. Dosages higher than 1,200 mg/day are considered more effective; however, many patients withdraw due to intolerable CNS adverse-effects from combined ASM therapy.

For conversion of patients from carbamazepine to oxcarbazepine:

Individualize the dosage. The usual daily maintenance dose of oxcarbazepine is approximately 1.5 times that of carbamazepine in adults and 1.2 times that of carbamazepine in the elderly.

Maximum Dosage Limit:

- *Adolescents >16 years, adults and elderly*: 2,400 mg/day.
- *Adolescents and children 4–16 years*: Age- and weight-dependent.
- *Children 2 to <4 years*: 60 mg/kg/day (in two divided doses).

Discontinuation Schedule: A dosage reduction of 25% per 2 weeks is safe at the time of discontinuation.

Administration Guidelines

May be taken without regard to meals.

PO suspension: Shake well before each use. To ensure accurate dosage, use calibrated PO syringe provided. Dosage may be mixed in a small glass of water prior to administration if desired. Use within 7 weeks of first opening the bottle.

Contraindications to Use: Hypersensitivity to oxcarbazepine.

Patient Education

1. If you miss a dose, take it as soon as you can. If it is almost time for your next dose, take only that dose. Do not take double or extra doses.
2. Adverse effects that you should report to your physician as soon as possible include
   Fever, rash, muscle aches or pain, hives, or difficulty breathing
   Redness, blistering, peeling or loosening of the skin, including inside the mouth
   Swelling of the legs and ankles
   Vision changes
   Infection
   Unusual bruising or bleeding
   Nausea or vomiting
   Confusion
   Difficulty speaking or walking
   Dizziness
   Muscle incoordination
   Unexplained tiredness or weakness.
3. You may get drowsy or dizzy when you first start taking this medicine. Do not drive, use machinery, or do anything that requires mental alertness until you know how oxcarbazepine affects you. Alcohol can increase drowsiness and dizziness. Avoid alcoholic drinks.
4. If you are female and are taking birth control pills or using other hormonal birth control methods (like injections), you should know that the birth control might not work as well while you are taking this drug. Talk to your physician about alternatives or use of additional birth control methods while taking this drug.
5. If you are going to have surgery, tell your physician that you are taking oxcarbazepine.

Box 2.19 Oxcarbazepine Precautions

- Carbamazepine hypersensitivity
- Breastfeeding
- Pregnancy
- Infants
- Elderly
- Abrupt discontinuation
- Ethanol intoxication
- Hyponatremia
- Heart failure
- Cardiac conduction disturbances
- Renal impairment

See Chapters 9–12, 14, and 26.

Perampanel

Brand Name: Fycompa

Dosage Forms: Tablets 2 mg, 4 mg, 6 mg, 8 mg, 10 mg, 12 mg

Dosage

Starting Dose:

Children >12 years and adults: 2 mg once daily at bedtime in patients not on enzyme-inducing ASMs and 4 mg in patients on enzyme-inducing ASMs.

Titration and Maintenance Dose: *Children >12 years and adults*: May increase based on clinical response and tolerability by a maximum of 2 mg once daily at bedtime in weekly increments to a dose of 4 mg to 12 mg once daily at bedtime. A dose of 12 mg once daily resulted in somewhat greater reductions in seizure rates than the dose of 8 mg once daily but with a substantial increase in adverse reactions. For elderly, maximum frequency for dosage increases is every 2 weeks. In patients with mild and moderate hepatic impairment, maximum recommended daily dose is 6 mg and 4 mg once daily at bedtime, respectively; maximum frequency for dosage increases is every 2 weeks.

Maximum Dosage Limits:

Children >12 years and adults: 12 mg/day.

Children <12 years: Safe and effective use has not been established.

Discontinuation Schedule: If perampanel dose is reduced, discontinued, or substituted with an alternative medication, this should be done gradually, but if withdrawal is a response to adverse events, prompt withdrawal can be considered.

Administration Guidelines

May be administered without regard to meals.

Relative Contraindications to Use: Hypersensitivity to perampanel.

Patient Education

1. Perampanel is usually taken 1 time a day at bedtime.
2. If you miss a dose, resume dosing the following day at your prescribed daily dose. Do not take double or extra doses.
3. Side effects that you should report to your physician as soon as possible include
    - Suicidal thinking and behavior
    - New or worse depression, anxiety, irritability or changes in behavior or mood
    - Dizziness
    - Gait disturbance
    - Loss of coordination
    - Falls
    - Somnolence and fatigue
    - Rash, itching, swelling, severe dizziness, or trouble breathing.
4. You may get drowsy or dizzy while using perampanel. Do not drive, use machinery, or do anything that requires mental alertness until you know how perampanel affects you. Alcohol can increase drowsiness and dizziness. Avoid alcoholic drinks.

Box 2.20 Perampanel Precautions

- Breastfeeding
- Pregnancy
- Suicidal behavior and ideation
- Elderly
- Central nervous system depression
- Ethanol intoxication
- Hepatic impairment
- Renal impairment

See Chapters 9–13 and 22.

5. Do not stop taking perampanel suddenly.
6. If you are female and are taking birth control pills, you should know that the birth control might not work as well while you are taking perampanel. Discuss this issue with your physician.

Phenobarbital

Brand Name: Luminal

Dosage Forms: Tablets 15 mg, 30 mg, 32 mg, 60 mg, 90 mg, 100 mg; capsules 16 mg (Solfoton); elixir 15 mg/5 mL, 20 mg/5 mL; injection 30 mg/mL, 60 mg/mL, 65 mg/mL, 130 mg/mL

Dosage

For Treatment of Status Epilepticus:

Loading dose (adults, children, and infants): 10–20 mg/kg IV (not to exceed 100 mg/min or 2 mg/kg/min in children). In the absence of mechanical ventilation, a dose of 10 mg/kg IV should be administered initially and followed by an additional 5 mg/kg IV approximately 30–60 minutes after the first dose. An additional 5 mg/kg may be given for refractory seizures. The usual maximum total loading dose is 25–30 mg/kg. A post-distribution serum concentration can be obtained 1–2 hours after completion of the loading infusion to assess the adequacy of the dose.

Maintenance Dose: Initiate maintenance dose 12–24 hours after the loading dose. Adverse reactions (e.g., apnea, hypotension) may complicate acute seizure management when phenobarbital is given after benzodiazepines (e.g., lorazepam or diazepam). Phenobarbital is usually only used when benzodiazepines and phenytoin fail to abort status epilepticus.

Neonates: Initially, a loading dose of 15–20 mg/kg IV in single or divided doses. In the absence of mechanical ventilation, a smaller dose (10 mg/kg) should be administered initially and followed by an additional dose approximately 30–60 minutes after the first dose. Total loading doses up to 40 mg/kg have been used.

For Treatment of All Types of Epileptic Seizures, Including Focal, Clonic, Myoclonic, Tonic, or Tonic-Clonic Seizures Not Responding to Other ASMs:

PO maintenance dosage (also may be given IM or IV if needed):

Adults and adolescents: Start at 0.5 mg/kg/day (30 mg at bedtime for typical adult) and titrate in 30 mg increments per 1–2 weeks to total of 1.5–4 mg/kg/day in 1–2 divided doses. Because phenobarbital is sedating and has a long half-life, a single daily dose administered at bedtime is recommended. If morning sedation occurs, then twice daily dosing can be used, with the larger dose at bedtime.

Children 5–12 years: Start at 1–2 mg/kg/day and titrate to 3–6 mg/kg/day PO in 1–2 divided doses.

Children 1–5 years: Start at 1–2 mg/kg/day and titrate to 6–8 mg/kg/day PO in 1–2 divided doses.

Infants: Start at 2 mg/kg/day and titrate to 5–6 mg/kg/day PO in 1–2 divided doses.

Neonates: 1–4 mg/kg PO once daily. May increase to 5 mg/kg/day PO if serum concentrations are inadequate.

Note: Phenobarbital should be titrated upward gradually over several weeks or more to allow patients to develop tolerance to sedative effect. The dosage should be adjusted, as necessary, to achieve a therapeutic phenobarbital concentration (usually 15–40 μg/mL). IV administration should be used only in patients unable to take PO medication.

Note: PO loading dose is possible as 10–20 mg/kg divided into equal doses and given over 24–48 hours.

Maximum Dosage Limit:

Adolescents, adults, and elderly: 300 mg/day PO, provided not sedated at lower doses. *Children and infants*: Individualized dosage.

Discontinuation Schedule: A dosage reduction of 25% per month is safe at the time of discontinuation.

Administration Guidelines

PO administration:

- All dosage forms may be given with food.
- For patients with difficulty swallowing, tablets may be crushed and mixed with food or fluids.
- Administer undiluted or mixed PO solution with water, milk, or fruit juice. Administer using a calibrated measuring device for accurate measurement of the dose.

Parenteral administration:

- Phenobarbital is administered IM or IV. IV administration is for hospitalized patients only.
- Never inject intra-arterially.

- Protect injection from light.
- Phenobarbital sodium injection is incompatible with many other injectable medications.

IM injection:

- Inject deeply into the gluteal muscle to minimize tissue irritation. Do not inject >5 mL into any one site. Aspirate prior to injection to avoid injection into a blood vessel.

Slow IV injection:

- IV injection should only be used in emergency situations or when other routes are not feasible.
- Avoid extravasation.
- In adult patients, the maximum rate of slow IV injection is 60 mg/min in less acute situations and a maximum of 100 mg/min for status epilepticus, but hypotension or the need for assisted ventilation may occur when the drug is administered at these rates. If hypotension occurs, the administration rate should be reduced by 50%. During injection, blood pressure, respiration, and cardiac function should be maintained; vital signs monitored; and equipment for resuscitation and artificial ventilation should be readily available.
- In pediatric patients, phenobarbital should be diluted with at least an equal volume of a compatible fluid and slowly injected at a rate no greater than 2 mg/kg/min in infants and usually no more than 30 mg/min in older children. If hypotension occurs, the administration rate should be reduced by 50%.

Patient Education

1. Try not to miss doses. If you are on a regular schedule and miss a dose, take it as soon as you can. If it is almost time for your next dose, take only that dose. Do not take double or extra doses.
2. Adverse effects that you should report to your physician as soon as possible include
   Bone tenderness
   Changes in the frequency or severity of seizures
   Confusion, agitation
   Changes in behavior, mood, or mental ability
   Hallucinations (seeing and hearing things that are not really there)
   Difficulty breathing or shortness of breath
   Eye problems
   Fever, sore throat
   Lightheadedness or fainting spells
   Redness, blistering, peeling or loosening of the skin, including inside the mouth
   Skin rash, itching, hives
   Slow heartbeat
   Swelling of the face or lips
   Unusual bleeding or bruising, pinpoint red spots on the skin

Weight loss
Yellowing of skin or eyes
Unusual tiredness or weakness

3. After receiving phenobarbital, you may get drowsy or dizzy. Do not drive, use machinery, or do anything that requires mental alertness until you know how phenobarbital affects you. To reduce dizzy or fainting spells, do not sit or stand up quickly. Alcohol can increase possible unpleasant effects. Avoid alcoholic drinks.
4. Phenobarbital can reduce the effectiveness of birth control pills or other hormonal birth control drugs. Talk to your physician about alternatives or use of additional birth control methods while taking this drug.
5. If you are going to have surgery, tell your physician that you are taking phenobarbital.

Box 2.21 Relative Contraindications to Use of Phenobarbital

- Agranulocytosis
- Barbiturate hypersensitivity
- Ethanol intoxication
- Hepatic encephalopathy
- Intra-arterial administration
- Porphyria
- Subcutaneous administration

See Chapters 2, 13, and 18.

Box 2.22 Phenobarbital Precautions

- IV administration
- Carbamazepine hypersensitivity
- Hydantoin hypersensitivity
- Breastfeeding
- Pregnancy
- Labor
- Neonates
- Elderly
- Central nervous system depression and mental status changes
- Depression
- Suicidal ideation
- Substance abuse
- Alcoholism
- Pain
- Osteomalacia/osteoporosis
- Cardiac diseases
- Hypotension
- Anticoagulant therapy
- Hepatic diseases
- Pulmonary diseases
- Sleep apnea
- Renal impairment
- Anuria
- Shock
- Exfoliative dermatitis
- Abrupt discontinuation

See Chapters 2, 6, 9–13, 17, 22, 26, and 29.

Phenytoin

Brand Names: Dilantin, Di-Phen, Phenytek

Dosage Forms: Chewable tablet 50 mg; capsule 100 mg; XR capsule 30 mg, 100 mg, 200 mg, 300 mg; PO suspension 125 mg/5 mL; injection 50 mg/mL

Note: IV phenytoin solutions contain phenytoin sodium, which is 92% phenytoin. Phenytoin capsules contain phenytoin sodium, which is 92% phenytoin. Chewable tablets and suspensions contain 100% phenytoin. Different phenytoin dosage forms are not directly interchangeable.

Dosage

IV Loading Dosage (in Status Epilepticus):

Adults, adolescents, children, and infants: Loading dose of 18–20 mg/kg via slow IV push or via IV infusion in NS in patients with unknown or undetectable phenytoin concentrations. In patients with detectable serum phenytoin, reduce loading dose correspondingly. If seizures are not terminated after the initial loading dose, consider additional ASMs. The full antiseizure effect of phenytoin is not immediate; IV benzodiazepines (e.g., lorazepam or diazepam) should be given initially or concurrently. Some experts advocate an additional phenytoin dose of 5–10 mg/kg IV if the initial loading dose fails to terminate seizures (but not in neonates). Total loading dose should not exceed 30 mg/kg. Ideally, begin maintenance dose within 8 hours.
Note: In patients currently receiving phenytoin with suboptimal serum concentrations, calculate the required loading dose as follows:

Loading dose = 0.8 × weight ×
(desired serum level − current serum level)

Loading Dose in Non-Emergent Situations:
PO non-emergent loading dosage (suspension, chewable tablets, or non-sustained release capsules):

Adults and children: 15–20 mg/kg PO for non-emergent loading doses in a patient not currently on phenytoin. The loading dose can be divided into two doses separated by 2 hours, but it may be given at once in a single dose. Do not use the PO loading dose in emergent situations. Although loading doses of phenytoin have been administered successfully via the PO route, this approach requires several hours to achieve a therapeutic concentration. Sustained-release capsules should not be used for loading doses. In patients with detectable but subtherapeutic serum phenytoin levels, reduce the loading dose correspondingly. Following the completion of PO loading, begin maintenance dose within 12–24 hours.

Note: There is one report of PO phenytoin loading with a single dose of 18 mg/kg capsules or suspension in 44 patients. The drug was well-tolerated and mean serum phenytoin level was 15.1 mg/L after 16–24 hours (Osborn et al., 1987).

IV Non-Emergent Loading Dose: *Adults and children*: If the patient cannot take PO doses, IV phenytoin injection could be used following a similar dosing strategy as for PO non-emergent treatment to raise phenytoin serum concentrations. Follow IV administration guidelines.

Titration and Maintenance Dose:

Adults: 4.5–7 mg/kg/day PO (may be given IV if needed) is appropriate for most patients. Give phenytoin injection in multiple daily doses, at regular intervals. If sustained-release capsules are used, the dose can be given as a single daily PO dose in many patients once dosage is stabilized. If chewable tablets, PO suspension, or non–sustained-release capsules are used, the daily dosage should be divided into 2–3 divided doses per day. Multiple daily doses should be given at regular intervals. Dosage adjustment for phenytoin is complex due to nonlinear kinetics. If plasma concentration at steady state is <8 μg/mL, the daily dose can be increased by 100 mg/day in adults. If plasma concentration at steady state is >7 and <12 μg/mL, the daily dose can be increased by 50 mg/day if an increase in level is needed. If plasma concentration at steady state is >11 μg/mL, the daily dose can be increased by 25–30 mg/day in adults if further increase in level is needed.

Adolescents, children, infants, and neonates: Initially, 5 mg/kg/day PO (IV if needed) in two divided doses and adjust to clinical effect and serum drug concentrations. Usual doses range as follows:

- 5–8 mg/kg/day in neonates
- 8–10 mg/kg/day in children 6 months–3 years
- 7.5–9 mg/kg/day in children 4–6 years
- 7–8 mg/kg/day in children 7–9 years
- 6–7 mg/kg/day children 10–16 years

Dosing frequency may be variable in children due to fast drug clearance. Some neonates may require phenytoin every 8 hours.

Note: Monitor phenytoin serum concentrations during chronic therapy.

For Seizure Prophylaxis Due to Specific Conditions:

During Neurosurgery: *Adults, adolescents, and children*: The loading dose is 18–20 mg/kg via IV infusion in NS. Typical initial maintenance dose is 4.5–7 mg/kg/day IV, divided into 2 or more doses as long as needed.

In Women with Pregnancy-Induced Hypertension: *Adult females*: 18 mg/kg IV infusion loading dose then daily maintenance as long as needed (delayed-release capsules). Magnesium sulfate is the preferred agent in these patients.

For Prophylaxis and Treatment of Seizures Secondary to Eclampsia: *Adult females*: 18 mg/kg IV loading dose followed by daily maintenance as long as needed. Magnesium sulfate is the preferred agent in these patients. In addition, maternal and neonatal morbidity are lower with magnesium.

Maximum Dosage Limit: None. Phenytoin dosage must be individualized.

Discontinuation Schedule: A dosage reduction of 25% per 1–2 weeks is safe at the time of discontinuation.

Administration Guidelines

- Shake PO suspension well prior to each dose. Administer using a calibrated measuring device. If given via an enteral tube, adsorption to the tubing can be minimized by diluting the suspension with a compatible diluent (e.g., at least 20 mL of NS or sterile water for administration to adults) before administering. After administration, flush the tube with at least 20 mL of the diluent (in adults). Continuous enteral feedings interfere with phenytoin absorption and lower serum phenytoin concentrations by up to 80% in some patients. Tube feedings should generally be discontinued for 1–2 hours before and after administration of each phenytoin dose.
- For patients with difficulty swallowing, the prompt-release capsules may be opened and the contents mixed with food or fluids. To prevent direct contact with the PO mucosa, the patient should drink a liquid first, followed by the drug mixture, and then followed with a full glass of water or milk.
- Administer extended-release capsules intact. Do not crush, cut, or chew. While food does not affect the absorption of Dilantin Kapseals, some generic products exhibit reduced absorption in the presence of a high-fat meal. It may be best to administer generic extended-release phenytoin capsules on an empty stomach or in a consistent manner in relation to food to avoid bioavailability problems.
- Do not administer phenytoin by IM injection. IM phenytoin absorption is unreliable and phenytoin may cause tissue injury, necrosis, or aseptic abscess.
- Prior to IV administration, the patient should preferably have good IV access. The vein utilized should be free from injury or thrombophlebitis.
- Continuous monitoring of the electrocardiogram, blood pressure, and respiration is essential during loading dose administration, and the patient should be observed throughout the period when maximal serum phenytoin concentrations occur, up to 1 hour after the end of a loading dose infusion. In the case of parenteral administration of maintenance doses, continuous clinical cardiac monitoring (rate, rhythm, blood pressure) and close clinical observation are recommended during dose administration.

- Phenytoin IV injections or infusions should be administered through a free-flowing IV of NS or other non–dextrose-containing saline IV solution.
- Avoid extravasation; phenytoin is irritating to tissues and may cause injury.
- The rate of administration of IV phenytoin is critically important. Do not exceed recommended infusion rates:
    - *Adults*: Inject IV at a rate not to exceed 50 mg/min. Consider slower infusion rates in those with concurrent cardiac disease.
    - *Elderly or debilitated adults*: Inject IV at a rate not to exceed 25–50 mg/min.
    - *Children*: Inject IV at a rate of 0.5–1 mg/kg/min, not to exceed 50 mg/min. However, the higher infusion rate may be indicated in selected circumstances.
    - *Infants and neonates*: Inject IV at a rate not to exceed 0.5–1 mg/kg/min. Due to their small veins, infants may be more at risk of thrombophlebitis or other tissue injury from the use of phenytoin IV. Do not infuse via scalp veins.
- For intermittent IV infusion, dilute phenytoin in NS to a final concentration of ≥6.7 mg/mL. For example: A dosage of 1,000 mg would be diluted with NS to a minimum volume of 150 mL.
- Phenytoin injection is poorly soluble; complete infusion administration within 1 hour of infusion preparation.
- Flush the IV line or catheter with NS for injection before and after dose to reduce risk of local vein irritation.

Patient Education

1. Try not to miss a scheduled dosage, especially if you are taking phenytoin extended-release capsules just once per day. If you miss a dose, take it as soon as you can. If it is less than 4 hours to your next dose, take only that dose. If you only take a dose once a day and do not remember until the next day, skip the missed dose and resume your normal schedule. Do not take double or extra doses.
2. Adverse effects that you should report to your physician as soon as possible include

    Chest pain or tightness
    Fast or irregular heartbeat
    Fainting spells or lightheadedness
    Difficulty breathing, wheezing or shortness of breath
    Confusion, nervousness, hostility, or other behavioral changes
    Headache
    Loss of seizure control
    Poor control of body movements or difficulty walking
    Dark yellow or brown urine

Vomiting
Yellowing of the eyes or skin
Double vision or uncontrollable and rapid eye movement
Fever, sore throat
Mouth ulcers
Redness, blistering, peeling or loosening of the skin or inside the mouth
Skin rash, itching
Stomach pain
Swollen or painful lymph glands (nodes)
Unusual bleeding or bruising, pinpoint red spots on skin
Sexual problems (painful erections, loss of sexual desire)
Unusual tiredness or weakness

3. Do not change brands or dosage forms of phenytoin without discussing the change with your physician.
4. You may feel dizzy or drowsy. Do not drive, use machinery, or do anything that requires mental alertness until you know how phenytoin affects you. To reduce the risk of dizzy or fainting spells, do not sit or stand up quickly. Alcohol can make you dizzier. Avoid alcoholic drinks.
5. Birth control pills or other hormonal birth control drugs may not work properly while you are taking phenytoin; talk with your physician about the use of other methods of birth control.
6. Phenytoin can cause unusual growth of gum tissue. Visit your dentist regularly. Problems can arise if you need dental work and in the daily care of your teeth. Try to avoid damage to your teeth and gums when you brush or floss your teeth.
7. Do not take antacids at the same time as phenytoin. If you get an upset stomach and want to take an antacid or medicine for diarrhea, make sure there is an interval of 2–3 hours before or after you take phenytoin.
8. If you are going to have surgery, tell your physician that you are taking phenytoin.

Box 2.23 Relative Contraindications to Use of Phenytoin

- Adams-Stokes syndrome
- Atrioventricular block or bundle-branch block
- Bradycardia
- Bone marrow suppression
- Hydantoin hypersensitivity
- IM administration
- Jaundice
- Methemoglobinemia

See Chapters 2, 13, 17, and 18.

Box 2.24 Phenytoin Precautions

- IV administration
- Abrupt discontinuation
- Barbiturate hypersensitivity
- Carbamazepine hypersensitivity
- Absence seizures
- Myoclonic seizures
- Breastfeeding
- Pregnancy
- Obstetric delivery
- Neonates
- Elderly
- Psychosis
- Alcoholism
- Dental diseases
- Encephalopathy
- Fever
- Hemolytic anemia
- Lymphoma
- Hodgkin disease
- Cardiac arrhythmias
- Coronary artery disease
- Heart failure
- Hypotension
- Hepatic diseases
- Vitamin K deficiency
- Renal diseases
- Diabetes mellitus
- Thyroid diseases
- Hypoglycemia
- Hyponatremia
- Myasthenia gravis
- Osteomalacia/osteoporosis
- Porphyria
- Radiation therapy
- Systemic lupus erythematosus

See Chapters 2, 7, 9–18, 22, 26, and 29.

Fosphenytoin Sodium

Brand Name: Cerebyx

Dosage Forms: 150 mg/2 mL (100 mg phenytoin sodium equivalent), 750 mg/10 mL (500 mg phenytoin sodium equivalent)

Dosage

Phenytoin Equivalent (PE):

Status Epilepticus: The loading dose of 18–20 mg PE/kg administered at 100–150 mg PE/min.

Non-Emergent and Maintenance Dosing:

Loading dose: 15–20 mg PE/kg given IV or IM. Max IV infusion rate is 150 mg PE/minute. In children, rates of infusion should be 1–3 PE/kg/minute. *Maintenance dose*: 4–6 mg PE/kg/day.

Administration Guidelines

The dose, concentration, and infusion rate of IV fosphenytoin are expressed as phenytoin sodium equivalent (PE). Dilute fosphenytoin in 5% dextrose or 0.9% saline solution for injection to a concentration range of 1.5–25 mg PE/mL. IM administration may be given as a single daily dose.

Pregabalin

Brand Name: Lyrica

Dosage Forms: Capsules 25 mg, 50 mg, 75 mg, 100 mg, 150 mg, 200 mg, 225 mg, 300 mg

Dosage

Starting Dose:

Children >12 years, adults, and the elderly (CrCl >60 mL/min): 150 mg/day in 2–3 divided doses.

Titration and Maintenance Dose: *Children >12 years, adults, and the elderly (CrCl >60 mL/min)*: Titrate by 75 mg to 150 mg per week. Usual maintenance dose is 150 mg twice daily. May increase to 600 mg/day, in 2–3 divided doses, based on efficacy and tolerability. At 600 mg/day, the incidence of dose-related adverse effects (dizziness, drowsiness, and blurred vision) may significantly affect patient tolerance.

Note: Loading dose is not studied.

Maximum Dosage Limit:

Children >12 years, adults, and the elderly: 600 mg/day.

Children <12 years: Safe and effective use has not been established.

Discontinuation Schedule: If pregabalin dose is reduced, discontinued, or substituted with an alternative medication, this should be done gradually over a minimum interval of 1 week.

Administration Guidelines

May be administered without regard to meals.

Relative Contraindication to Use: Hypersensitivity to pregabalin.

Patient Education

1. Swallow the capsules with a drink of water. If pregabalin upsets your stomach, take it with food or milk.
2. If you miss a dose, take it as soon as you can. If it is almost time for your next dose, take only that dose. Do not take double or extra doses.
3. Adverse effects that you should report to your physician as soon as possible include
    - Change in amount of urine
    - Slow or irregular heartbeat
    - Difficulty speaking
    - Loss of coordination
    - Mental or mood changes
    - Uncontrolled movements (e.g., tremor, twitching)
    - Vision changes
    - Muscle pain/tenderness/weakness (especially, if you are tired or have a fever)
    - Stomach/abdominal pain

Unusual bleeding or bruising
Rash, itching, swelling, severe dizziness, or trouble breathing

4. You may get drowsy or dizzy while using pregabalin. Do not drive, use machinery, or do anything that requires mental alertness until you know how pregabalin affects you. To reduce dizzy or fainting spells, do not sit or stand up quickly. Alcohol can increase drowsiness and dizziness. Avoid alcoholic drinks.
5. If you have a heart condition, such as congestive heart failure, and notice that you are retaining water (edema) and have swelling in your hands or feet, contact your physician immediately.
6. Do not stop taking pregabalin suddenly. This medication may cause dependence, especially if it has been used regularly for an extended period of time, or if it has been used in high doses. In such cases, if you suddenly stop this drug, withdrawal reactions may occur.
7. If you are going to have surgery, tell your physician that you are taking pregabalin.

Box 2.25 Pregabalin Precautions

- Breastfeeding
- Pregnancy
- Infants and children
- Elderly
- Central nervous system depression
- Ethanol intoxication
- Substance abuse
- Heart failure
- Myopathy
- Ocular diseases (e.g., glaucoma)
- Diabetes mellitus
- Renal impairment

See Chapters 9–12, 16, 17, and 27.

Primidone

Brand Name: Mysoline

Dosage Forms: Tablets 50 mg, 250 mg; PO suspension 250 mg/5 mL

Dosage

Starting Dose:

Adults, adolescents, and children >8 years: 62.5–250 mg/day once daily at bedtime or divided into two doses.

Children <8 years and infants: 50 mg/day at bedtime or divided into two doses.

Titration and Maintenance Dose:

Adults, adolescents, and children >8 years: Increase dose by 100–125 mg/day every 3–7 days. The usual dose is 750–1,500 mg/day in 3–4 divided doses.

Children <8 years and infants: Increase dose by 50 mg/day every 3–7 days. Usual doses range from 10–25 mg/kg/day in 3–4 divided doses.

Neonates: 12–25 mg/kg/day in 2–4 divided doses. Start at lower doses and titrate.

Maximum Dosage Limit:

Children >8 years, adolescents, adults and elderly: 2,000 mg/day.

Infants and children <8 years: 25 mg/kg/day (or up to a maximum dosage 1,000 mg/day).

Neonates: 25 mg/kg/day.

Discontinuation Schedule: A dosage reduction of 25% per month is safe at the time of discontinuation.

Administration Guidelines

Primidone is administered orally with meals to minimize indigestion or gastrointestinal irritation.

Contraindications/Precautions with Use:

Because primidone is metabolized to phenobarbital, it shares all the contraindications/precautions of this drug.

Primidone is not commonly used as an anticonvulsant in young children and infants. Due to immature hepatic and renal function (particularly in the first few weeks of life), neonates (especially those with prematurity) must be carefully monitored during primidone use via serum concentrations and clinical status. Children are more likely than adults to react with paradoxical excitement to primidone or have drug intolerance.

Patient Education

1. If you miss a dose, take it as soon as you can if it is more than an hour until your next dose. If it is almost time for your next dose, take only that dose. Do not take double or extra doses.
2. Adverse effects that you should report to your physician as soon as possible include
    - Blurred or double vision, uncontrollable rolling or movements of the eyes
    - Irritability or mood changes
    - Unusual excitement or restlessness (more likely in children and the elderly)
    - Lightheadedness or fainting spells
    - Shortness of breath or difficulty breathing
    - Redness, blistering, peeling or loosening of the skin, including inside the mouth
    - Skin rash, or itching
    - Unusual weakness or tiredness or sedation.
3. After taking primidone you may get drowsy or dizzy. Do not drive, use machinery, or do anything that requires mental alertness until you know how primidone affects you. To reduce dizzy or fainting

spells, do not sit or stand up quickly. Alcohol can increase possible unpleasant effects. Avoid alcoholic drinks.

4. Primidone can reduce the effectiveness of birth control pills or other hormonal birth control drugs. Talk to your physician about alternatives or use of additional birth control methods while taking this drug.
5. If you are going to have surgery, tell your physician that you are taking primidone.

Rufinamide

Brand Name: Banzel

Dosage Forms: Tablets 100 mg, 200 mg, 400 mg, PO suspension 40 mg/mL

Dosage

Starting Dose:

Children >4 years: 10 mg/kg/day administered in 2 equally divided doses.

Adults: 400–800 mg/day administered in 2 equally divided doses.

Note: The safety and effectiveness in patients with Lennox-Gastaut syndrome have not been established in children younger than 4 years.

Note: Patients on valproate should begin rufinamide at a dose lower than 10 mg/kg/day (children) or 400 mg/day (adults).

Titration and Maintenance Dose:

Children >4 years: Titrate by 10 mg/kg increments every other day to a target dose of 45 mg/kg/day or 3,200 mg/day, whichever is less.

Adults: The dose should be increased by 400–800 mg every other day until a maximum dose of 3200 mg/day.

Maximum Dosage Limit:

Children >4 years: 45 mg/kg/day or 3200 mg/day, whichever is less.

Adults: 3,200 mg/day.

Box 2.26 Rufinamide Precautions

- Breastfeeding
- Pregnancy
- Hepatic impairment
- Elderly
- Heart diseases

See Chapters 9–11, 13, and 17.

Discontinuation Schedule: If rufinamide dose is reduced, discontinued, or substituted with an alternative medication, this should be done gradually (25% every 2 days).

Administration Guidelines

Should be given with food. Tablets can be administered whole, as half tablets, or crushed.

Contraindications to Use: Patients with familial short QT syndrome.

Patient Education

1. If you miss a dose, take it as soon as you can. If it is almost time for your next dose, take only that dose. Do not take double or extra doses.
2. Adverse effects that you should report to your physician as soon as possible include
   Loss of coordination
   Suicidal thinking and behavior
   Severe muscle pain
   Unusual bleeding or bruising
   Rash, itching, swelling, fever, severe dizziness, or trouble breathing
3. You may get drowsy or dizzy while using rufinamide. Do not drive, use machinery, or do anything that needs mental alertness until you know how rufinamide affects you. Alcohol can increase drowsiness and dizziness. Avoid alcoholic drinks.
4. Do not stop taking rufinamide suddenly.
5. If you are female and are taking birth control pills, you should know that the birth control might not work as well while you are taking rufinamide. Discuss this issue with your physician.

Tiagabine

Brand Name: Gabitril

Dosage Forms: Tablets 2 mg, 4 mg, 12 mg, 16 mg

Box 2.27 Tiagabine Precautions

- Abrupt discontinuation
- Pregnancy
- Breastfeeding
- Children
- Status epilepticus
- Bipolar disorder or mania
- Hepatic diseases

See Chapters 9, 10, 13, and 22.

Dosage

Starting Dose:

Adults and adolescents 12–18 years of age who are already taking enzyme-inducing ASMs: 4 mg twice daily for 1 week.

Children 2–11 years: 0.1 mg/kg/day for 2 weeks.

Titration and Maintenance Dose:

Adults who are already taking enzyme-inducing ASMs: After 1 week, increase by 4–8 mg/day at weekly intervals until clinical response is achieved, or up to 56 mg per day. The usual adult maintenance dose is 24–56 mg/day in 2–4 divided doses. If tiagabine is used in a patient who is not taking an enzyme-inducing ASM (e.g., patients receiving valproate monotherapy), lower doses (12–22 mg/day) or a slower dose titration schedules are used.

Adolescents 12–18 years of age who are already taking enzyme-inducing ASMs: Increase by 4 mg at the beginning of week 2. Thereafter, may increase by 4–8 mg/day at weekly intervals. The daily dosage should be given in 2–4 divided doses. Doses >32 mg/day have been tolerated rarely.

Children 2–11 years: Increase every 2 weeks by 0.1 mg/kg/day up to a target dosage of 0.4–0.6 mg/kg/day in patients not currently taking enzyme-inducing ASMs. In children taking at least one concomitant enzyme-inducing ASM, upward titration may occur every 1–2 weeks, with a higher target dosage of 0.7–1 mg/kg/day.

Note: Dosage adjustment of tiagabine should be considered whenever a change in patient's enzyme-inducing status occurs as a result of the addition, discontinuation, or dose change of the enzyme-inducing agent.

Note: Loading dose is not necessary.

Maximum Dosage Limits:

Adults and elderly: 56 mg/day, dependent on concomitant drug therapy.

Adolescents 12–18 years of age: 32 mg/day, dependent on concomitant drug therapy.

Children 2–11 years: 0.6–1 mg/kg/day, dependent on concomitant drug therapy.

Discontinuation Schedule: A dosage reduction of 25% per 2 weeks is safe at the time of discontinuation.

Administration Guidelines

Tiagabine should be taken with food.

Contraindications for Use: Hypersensitivity to tiagabine.

Patient Education

1. If you miss a dose, take it as soon as you can. If it is almost time for your next dose, take only that dose. Do not take double or extra doses.
2. Adverse effects that you should report to your physician as soon as possible include

Confusion
Depression
Difficulty remembering things
Difficulty speaking
Difficulty with movements or with walking
Tingling of the hands or feet
Seizures, whether new or a change in previous seizure pattern
Redness, blistering, peeling or loosening of the skin, including inside the mouth
Skin rash or itching
Sore throat or pain on swallowing
Vomiting
Weakness

3. You may get drowsy or dizzy when you first start taking this medicine. Do not drive, use machinery, or do anything that requires mental alertness until you know how tiagabine affects you. To reduce dizzy or fainting spells, do not sit or stand up quickly. Alcohol can increase drowsiness and dizziness. Avoid alcoholic drinks.
4. If you are going to have surgery, tell your physician that you are taking tiagabine.

Topiramate

Brand Names: Topamax, Trokendi XR (topiramate) extended-release capsules

Dosage Forms: Tablets 25 mg, 50 mg 100 mg, 200 mg; capsule, sprinkle 15 mg, 25 mg; extended-release capsules: 25 mg, 50 mg, 100 mg, and 200 mg

Dosage

Starting Dose for Initial Monotherapy:

Adults, adolescents, and children >10 years: 25 mg nightly for 1 week; 50 mg once daily for Trokendi XR.

Children 2–10 years of age: 0.5–1 mg/kg/day for 1–2 weeks. Trokendi XR for children 6–9 years of age: the initial dose is 25 mg/day nightly for the first week.

Titration and Maintenance Dose: *Adults, adolescents, and children >10 years*: During weeks 2–4 increase gradually (weekly) by 25 mg/day, administered in two daily divided doses, up to 100 mg daily. Initial maintenance dose is 50 mg twice daily. If further increases are needed, increase the daily dose in 50 milligram increments on a weekly basis, and dose twice daily. If urgent seizure control is needed, more rapid titration of drug can be performed, starting at 50 mg twice daily. *Trokendi XR*: Week 2, 100 mg once daily; week 3, 150 mg once daily; week 4, 200 mg once daily; week 5, 300 mg once daily; week 6, 400 mg once daily. The recommended dose for Trokendi XR in adults and in children 10 years of age and older is 400 mg orally once daily.

Children 2–10 years of age: Increase gradually by 0.5–1 mg/kg/day every 1–2 weeks. Recommended maintenance dose is 3–6 mg/kg/day. *Trokendi XR for children 6–9 years of age*: Target total daily maintenance dosing is as follows:

Weight (kg)	Minimum maintenance dose (mg/day)	Maximum maintenance dose (mg/day)
Up to 11	150	250
12–22	200	300
23–31	200	350
32–38	250	350
>38	250	400

Reprinted with permission, www.trokendixr.com/assets/TrokendiXRPrescribingInformation.pdf/accessed

Starting Dose for Adjunctive Therapy:

Adults and adolescents >17 years: 25 mg/day for 1 week; 25 to 50 mg once daily for Trokendi XR.

Children and adolescents 2–16 years: 1−3 mg/kg/day (maximum initial dose 25 mg/day) for 1 week; the same for Trokendi XR.

Titration and Maintenance Dose:

Adults and adolescents >17 years: Gradually increase by 25 mg weekly until 100 mg total daily dose is reached, administering the drug in two daily divided doses. The recommended initial target dose is 150–200 mg/day administered in two divided doses. Higher doses may be used, but doses greater than 400 mg/day rarely will improve responses. Daily doses higher than 1,600 mg have not been studied.

Children and adolescents 2–16 years: The dose may be increased every 1–2 weeks by increments of no more than 1–3 mg/kg/day. The recommended final daily dose is approximately 5−9 mg/kg/day administered in two divided doses. Dose must be individualized. In clinical trials of patients with Lennox-Gastaut syndrome, doses of topiramate up to 1,000 mg/day (approximately 18 mg/kg/day) are used for adjunctive treatment.

Infants and children <2 years: Doses up to 7.7 mg/kg/day, in divided doses, was efficacious and well-tolerated.

Note: For the adjunctive treatment of refractory epileptic spasms associated with West syndrome in children, use an initial dosage of 25 mg once daily adding to the current ASMs regimen. Dosage is increased by 25 mg every 2–3 days until spasms are controlled, or a maximum dosage of 24 mg/kg/day PO given in divided doses is achieved. More than half of the treated children may achieve monotherapy with topiramate after slow reduction of their other ASMs.

Note: It is not necessary to monitor plasma concentrations of topiramate to optimize therapy.

Note: Loading dose is not studied.

Maximum Dosage Limits:

Adolescents >16 years, adults, and elderly: More than 600 mg/day is rarely needed, may increase up to 1,600 mg/day.

Adolescents <16 years: 9 mg/kg/day for focal-onset or generalized seizures; up to 18 mg/kg/day for Lennox-Gastaut syndrome.

Children >2 years: 9 mg/kg/day for focal-onset or generalized seizures; up to 18 mg/kg/day for Lennox-Gastaut syndrome; higher dosages have occasionally been used in refractory seizure types.

Children <2 years: Safe and effective dose is not established. However, experts administer it to their patients whenever the benefits outweigh the risks.

Discontinuation Schedule: A dosage reduction of 25% per 2 weeks is safe at the time of discontinuation.

Administration Guidelines

Topiramate may be given orally without regard to meals. Because of the bitter taste, the tablets should not be broken.

The contents of the capsules may be sprinkled on a small amount of soft food (e.g., applesauce, ice cream, or yogurt) for administration. Prepare entire dose and swallow immediately after preparation. Do not chew. Drink fluids to ensure entire dose is swallowed. Do not store any sprinkle/food mixture for use at a later time. Alternatively, you may swallow the whole capsule.

Relative Contraindications to Use: Hypersensitivity to topiramate; metabolic acidosis

Contraindications for Trokendi XR: With recent alcohol use (i.e., within 6 hours prior to and 6 hours after Trokendi XR).

Patient Education

1. If you miss a dose, take it as soon as you can. If it is almost time for your next dose, take only that dose. Do not take double or extra doses.
2. Adverse effects that you should report to your physician as soon as possible include
   - Agitation, restlessness, irritability, depression, or other changes in mood
   - Difficulty speaking
   - Tingling, pain, or numbness in the hands or feet
   - Difficulty walking or controlling muscle movements
   - Decreased sweating and/or rise in body temperature

Difficulty breathing; fast or irregular breathing patterns
Eye pain, redness, or swelling
Vision problems, like blurred vision
Hearing impairment
Kidney stones (severe pain in the side or back or on urination)
Nosebleeds
Redness, blistering, peeling or loosening of the skin, including inside the mouth
Skin rash, itching
Stomach pain with nausea or vomiting
Swelling of the face, lips, or tongue
Yellowing of the skin or eyes
Unusual weakness or tiredness.

3. You should drink plenty of fluids while taking topiramate. If you have had kidney stones in the past, this will help to reduce your chances of forming kidney stones.
4. You may get drowsy, dizzy, or have blurred vision. Do not drive, use machinery, or do anything that requires mental alertness until you know how topiramate affects you. To reduce dizziness, do not sit or stand up quickly. Alcohol can increase drowsiness and dizziness. Avoid alcoholic drinks.
5. If you take birth control pills, topiramate may reduce their effectiveness at preventing pregnancy. Talk with your physician about the use of other methods of birth control.
6. If you are going to have surgery, tell your physician that you are taking topiramate.

Box 2.28 Topiramate Precautions

- Abrupt discontinuation
- Breastfeeding
- Pregnancy
- Infants and children
- Elderly
- Status epilepticus
- Closed-angle glaucoma and increased intraocular pressure
- Visual disturbances
- Ambient temperature increase
- Chronic obstructive pulmonary disease
- Emphysema
- Biliary cirrhosis
- Hepatic diseases
- Inborn errors of metabolism
- Diarrhea
- Renal diseases
- Renal impairment
- Nephrolithiasis
- Depression
- Suicidal ideation
- Status asthmaticus
- Surgery

See Chapters 9–14, 18, 22, and 27.

Valproic Acid, Valproate, Divalproex Sodium

Brand Names: Depacon, Depakene, Depakote, Depakote-ER, Depakote Sprinkle

Dosage Forms:

Valproic acid (Depakene): Capsules 250 mg; syrup 250 mg/5 mL as sodium salt

Divalproex (Depakote): Tablets 125 mg, 250 mg, and 500 mg (enteric-coated delayed-release tablets); extended-release tablets 250 mg, 500 mg; capsules 125 mg (Sprinkle). This is a dimer of valproic acid and sodium valproate (1:1).

Valproate sodium (Depacon): 500 mg/5 mL

Dosage

Starting Dose:

Adults and children ≥2 years: 7–10 mg/kg/day PO, 3–4 times daily for non-enteric-coated capsules or syrup; twice daily is recommended for delayed-release tablets and once daily for the extended-release preparation. A typical adult starting dose is 500 mg/day.

Children <2 years: Not recommended. This population is more at risk for fatal hepatotoxicity from valproic acid. However, experts administer it to their patients whenever the benefits outweigh the risks.

Titration and Maintenance Dose: *Adults and children >10 years*: Increase by 5 mg/kg/day at weekly intervals as tolerated and necessary. For most patients not taking enzyme-inducing drugs, optimal clinical response is achieved at doses lower than 15–20 mg/kg/day. For patients who do not respond, measure plasma concentrations to determine whether they are within the usual accepted range (50–100 µg/mL).

Children 2–9 years: Younger children, especially those receiving concomitant enzyme-inducing ASMs, may need larger (sometimes >100 mg/kg/day) maintenance doses to attain target total and unbound serum valproic acid concentrations compared to adults. The extended-release valproic acid is difficult to titrate, and the immediate-release product may be a better choice in young children.

Note: For elderly, use reduced initial dosage and slower dose titration. Dose reductions or discontinuation should be considered in elderly patients with decreased food or fluid intake and in patients with excessive somnolence.

Note: When converting to valproic acid monotherapy from other ASMs, the dosage of the concomitant ASM can usually be reduced by 25% every 2 weeks. This reduction can begin at the initiation of valproic acid therapy or be delayed for 1–2 weeks to avoid rebound seizures.

Note: When converting from divalproex delayed-release tablets (Depakote) to divalproex extended-release tablets (Depakote-ER), the dosage of Depakote-ER should be given once daily at a dose 8–20%

higher than the total daily dose of Depakote. Based on strength, if the Depakote dose cannot be directly converted to Depakote-ER, consider increasing the Depakote total daily dose to the next higher dosage before converting to a daily dose of Depakote-ER.

Starting Dose for Initiation of IV Treatment in Patients Unable to Tolerate or Receive PO Therapy: *Adults and children >2 years*: Initially, 10–15 mg/kg/day IV at 20 mg/min.

Note: For conversion to IV dosing in patients who are currently receiving PO valproic acid therapy from an established dosage regimen, give the normal PO daily dosage by the IV route in an equivalent daily dosage in divided doses every 6 hours.

Note: Patients should be switched from IV to PO products as soon as possible. The use of IV administration has not been studied in periods longer than 14 days.

For Treatment of Status Epilepticus:

Rectal Dosage (Valproic Acid):

Adults: 400–600 mg PR either as an enema or in a wax base suppository.

Children: 20 mg/kg/dose PR.

IV route: Initial loading dose of 20 mg/kg at 20 mg/min, followed by 1 mg/kg/hour with close monitoring; or, alternatively, 30 mg/kg at 50 mg/min, followed by 10 mg/kg every 6 hours.

Maximum Dosage Limits:

Children >10 years, adults, and elderly: 60 mg/kg/day PO or IV or 3,000 mg/day.

Children 2–9 years: Maximum dosages are not well established; use of Depakote-ER not recommended.

Children <2 years: Use is not recommended. However, experts administer it to their patients whenever the benefits outweigh the risks.

Discontinuation Schedule: A dosage reduction of 25% per week is safe at the time of discontinuation.

Administration Guidelines

PO administration:

- May be administered with food or with a large amount of water to minimize gastrointestinal irritation. May also split doses to minimize GI upset.
- To prevent local irritation to the mouth and throat, capsules should be swallowed whole and not chewed or crushed.
- Do not mix PO solution with carbonated beverages because valproic acid will be liberated and may cause an unpleasant taste as well as local irritation to the mouth and throat.
- Sprinkle capsules may be swallowed intact. Alternatively, the capsule contents are sprinkled on a small amount (roughly 5 mL) of

semisolid food (e.g., applesauce, pudding) immediately before administration. Do not crush or chew the mixture containing the coated particles. Use any food–drug mixture immediately after preparation; do not store for future use.

- Delayed-release tablets are enteric-coated and should be swallowed whole. Do not cut, chew, or crush.
- Extended-release tablets are not bioequivalent to Depakote delayed-release tablets. Tablets should be swallowed whole. Do not cut, chew, or crush.

IV administration:

- The total daily dose of PO and IV dosages are equivalent. If the total daily dose exceeds 250 mg, the IV dosage should be given in a divided regimen.
- Patients receiving doses near the maximum recommended daily dose of 60 mg/kg/day IV, particularly those not receiving enzyme-inducing drugs, should be monitored more closely.
- Dilute prescribed dose with at least 50 mL of a compatible sterile diluent (D_5W, NS, or lactated Ringer's) for IV administration.
- Administer dosage as an IV infusion over 60 minutes. The recommended infusion rate is generally 20 mg/min. It has also been administered as rapid infusion over 5–10 min (1.5–3 mg/kg/min) (not per label; rapid infusion has been associated with increased adverse effects risk but in limited studies was well-tolerated).

Rectal administration:

- Valproic acid syrup may be diluted 1:1 with water for use as a retention enema.

Patient Education

1. Swallow valproic acid capsules whole with a drink of water. If valproic acid upsets your stomach, take it with food or milk; do not take it with carbonated drinks.
2. Try not to miss a scheduled dosage. If you take only one dose each day and miss the dose, take it as soon as you remember. If you do not remember until the next day, skip the missed dose and go on with your regular schedule. Do not take double or extra doses. If you take more than one dose a day and miss a dose, take it if you remember within 6 hours. Space the other doses for that day at regular intervals; do not take two doses at once.
3. Adverse effects that you should report to your physician as soon as possible include

   Agitation, restlessness, irritability, or other changes in mood
   Blurred or double vision; uncontrollable eye movements
   Trembling of hands or arms

Changes in the frequency or severity of seizures
Redness, blistering, peeling or loosening of the skin, including
Inside the mouth
Skin rash or itching
Stomach pain or cramps
Yellowing of skin or eyes
Unusual bleeding or bruising or pinpoint red spots on the skin
Unusual swelling of the arms or legs
Unusual tiredness or weakness.

4. Do not change brands or dosage forms of valproic acid without discussing the change with your physician.
5. You may get drowsy, dizzy, or have blurred vision. Do not drive, use machinery, or do anything that needs mental alertness until you know how valproic acid affects you. To reduce dizzy or fainting spells, do not sit or stand up quickly. Alcohol can increase drowsiness and dizziness. Avoid alcoholic drinks.
6. Valproic acid can cause blood problems. This can mean slow healing and a risk of infection. Problems can arise if you need dental work and in the day-to-day care of your teeth. Try to avoid damage to your teeth and gums when you brush or floss your teeth.
7. If you are going to have surgery, tell your physician that you are taking valproic acid.

Box 2.29 Relative Contraindications to Use of Valproate

- Encephalopathy
- Hepatic diseases
- Pancreatitis
- Urea cycle disorders
- Hypersensitivity to valproate
- Porphyria

See Chapters 13 and 14.

Box 2.30 Valproate Precautions

- Pregnancy
- Breastfeeding
- Neonates
- Infants
- Elderly
- Hypoalbuminemia
- HIV infection/AIDS
- Acute head injury
- Renal diseases
- Coagulopathy
- Thrombocytopenia
- Abrupt discontinuation
- Systemic lupus erythematosus
- Diabetes mellitus

See Chapters 9–13, 16, 18, and 30.

Vigabatrin

Brand Name: Sabril

Dosage Forms: Tablet 500 mg

Dosage

Adults: 500 mg PO every 12 hours; may increase by 500 mg/day gradually to a maximum of 4 g/day. Lower doses should be used in patients with renal dysfunction.

Children: Doses range from 40–150 mg/kg/day twice a day.

Discontinuation Schedule: A dosage reduction of 500 mg every fifth day is safe at the time of discontinuation.

Patient Education

1. If you miss a dose of this medicine, take it as soon as possible. However, if it is almost time for your next dose, skip the missed dose and go back to your regular dosing schedule. Do not double the doses.
2. Adverse effects that you should report to your physician immediately include
   - Amnesia
   - Blue-yellow color blindness
   - Decreased vision or other vision changes
   - Eye pain
   - Increase in seizures
   - Uncontrolled rolling eye movements.
3. If you are taking this medicine for a long time, it is very important that your eye doctor check you approximately every 3 months for any visual problems.
4. You may get drowsy, dizzy, or become less alert. Make sure you know how you react to this medicine before you drive, use machines, or do anything else that could be dangerous if you are dizzy, drowsy, or not alert.

Zonisamide

Brand Name: Zonegran

Dosage Forms: PO capsules 25 mg, 50 mg, and 100 mg

Dosage

Starting Dose:

Adults and adolescents >16 years: 50–100 mg/day, once or twice (divided doses) daily, for 2 weeks.

Adolescents and children <16 years: Safe and effective use has not been established. However, experts suggest an initial dose of 2–4 mg/kg/day once or twice (divided doses) daily.

Titration and Maintenance Dose: *Adults and adolescents >16 years*: After 2 weeks, the dose may be increased to 200 mg/day once or twice (divided doses) daily for at least 2 weeks. The dose can then be increased to 300 mg once daily and 400 mg once daily every 2 weeks. Usual maintenance dose is 200–400 mg/day. Higher doses are of uncertain benefit. There is little experience with doses greater than 600 mg/day.

Adolescents and children <16 years: Titration is usually slow, with increments of 1–2 mg/kg/day every 1–2 week. The target dosage is 4–8 mg/kg/day.

Note: Loading dose is not studied.

Maximum Dosage Limit:

Adolescents >16 years, adults, and elderly: 600 mg/day.
Adolescents <16 years and children: 12 mg/kg/day.

Discontinuation Schedule: A dosage reduction of 25% per 2 weeks is safe at the time of discontinuation.

Administration Guidelines

Zonisamide may be taken with or without food.

Relative Contraindications to Use: Sulfonamide hypersensitivity.

Patient Education

1. Swallow the capsules whole with a drink of water. Do not bite into or break open the capsule.
2. If you miss a dose, take it as soon as you can. If it is almost time for your next dose, take only that dose. Do not take double or extra doses.
3. Adverse effects that you should report to your physician immediately include
   Changes in seizure type or frequency
   Decreased sweating or a rise in body temperature
   Depression

Box 2.31 Zonisamide Precautions

- Abrupt discontinuation
- Ambient temperature increase
- Dehydration
- Anticholinergic medications
- Pregnancy
- Breastfeeding
- Children
- Hepatic diseases
- Nephrolithiasis
- Renal diseases

See Chapters 9, 10, and 12–14.

Seeing or hearing things or people that are not really there
Unusual thoughts
Severe drowsiness, difficulty concentrating, or coordination problems
Speech or language problems
Difficulty breathing or tightening of the throat
Fever, sore throat, sores in your mouth, or easy bruising
Redness, blistering, peeling or loosening of the skin, including inside the mouth
Skin rash or itching
Swelling of lips or tongue
Sudden back pain, abdominal pain, pain when urinating, bloody or dark urine
Vomiting

4. Drink 6–8 glasses of water a day. This may help to prevent kidney stones.
5. You may get drowsy or dizzy or have coordination problems. Do not drive, use machinery, or do anything that requires mental alertness until you know how zonisamide affects you. To reduce dizzy spells, do not sit or stand up quickly. Alcohol can increase drowsiness and dizziness. Avoid alcoholic drinks or medicines containing alcohol.
6. If you are going to have surgery, tell your physician that you are taking zonisamide.

Suggested Reading

American Society of Health System Pharmacists. *AHFS Drug Information 2006*. Bethesda, MD: Author; 2006.

Abbott Laboratories. Depacon package insert. Lake Forest, IL: Author; 2006.

Facts and Comparisons. *Drug Facts and Comparisons*. St. Louis: Wolters Kluwer Health; 2007.

E-epilepsy. Information on anti-epilepsy drugs. http://www.e-epilepsy. org.uk/pages/spc/

Jarrar RG, Buchhalter JR. Therapeutics in pediatric epilepsy, part 1: The new antiepileptic drugs and the ketogenic diet. *Mayo Clinic Proc.* 2003;78:359–370.

Lacy CF, Armstrong LL, Goldman MP, et al. *Drug Information Handbook 2007*. Hudson, OH: Lexi-Comp; 2007.

Mayo Clinic. Medical information and tools for healthy living. http://www.mayoclinic.com/health/drug-information

Osborn HH, Zisfein J, Sparano R. Single-dose oral phenytoin loading. *Ann Emerg Med.* 1987;16:407–412.

Privitera MD, Cavitt J, Ficker DM, Szaflarski JP, Welty TE, Kaplan MJ. *Clinician's Guide to Antiepileptic Drugs*. Philadelphia: Lippincott Williams & Wilkins; 2006.

RxList. Internet drug index for prescription drugs and medications. http://www.rxlist.com

Tomson T. Drug selection for the newly diagnosed patient: When is a new generation antiepileptic drug indicated? *J Neurol*. 2004;251:1043–1049.

Wyllie E, Gupta A, Lachhwani DK. *The Treatment of Epilepsy: Principles and Practice*, 4th ed. Philadelphia: Lippincott Williams & Wilkins; 2006.

Online Resources

Brivaracetam (Briviact). www.briviact.com/2020

Cannabidiol (Epidiolex). www.epidiolex.com/2020

Cenobamate. https://reference.medscape.com/drug/xcopri-cenobamate-1000328/2020

Diazepam. https://reference.medscape.com/drug/valtoco-diazepam-intranasal-1000326/2020

Eslicarbazine acetate (Aptiom). www.aptiom.com/2014

Ezogabine (Potiga). www.potiga.com/2014

Lacosamide (Vimpat). www.vimpat.com/2014

Midazolam. https://reference.medscape.com/drug/nayzilam-midazolam-intranasal-1000286/2020

Oxcarbazepine (Oxtella). www.oxtellarxr.com/2020

Perampanel (Fycompa). us.eisai.com/wps/wcm/connect/Eisai/Home/Our.../FYCOMPA/2014

Rufinamide (Banzel). www.banzel.com/2014

Topiramate(Trokendi).www.trokendixr.com/assets/TrokendiXRPrescribingInformation.pdf/2020

Valproic acid. https://reference.medscape.com/drug/depakene-stavzor-valproic-acid-343024#11/2020

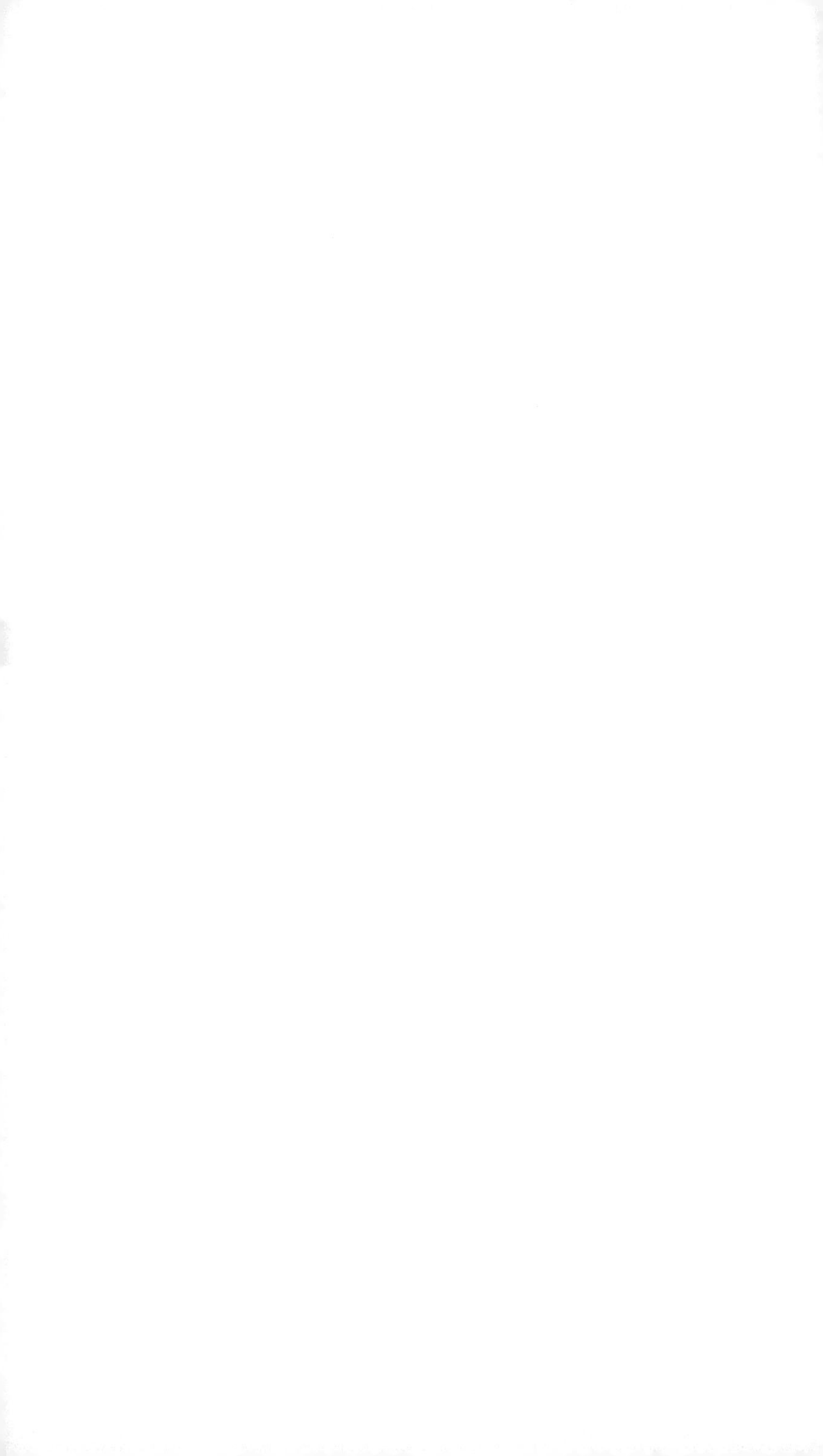

Chapter 3

Mechanisms of Action and Pharmacokinetic Properties of Antiseizure Medications

Mechanisms of Action of Antiseizure Medications

At the molecular level, the majority of antiseizure medications (ASMs) modulate excitatory and inhibitory neural transmission. ASMs probably exert their anticonvulsant effects at both the cell membrane and intracellularly. The major targets of anticonvulsant drugs include the following:

- Sodium channels
- Calcium channels
- γ-Aminobutyric acid $(GABA)_A$ and $GABA_B$ receptors
- Potassium channels
- Glutamate
- Glutamate receptors including *N*-methyl-D-aspartate (NMDA) receptors, non-NMDA receptors (α-amino-3-hydroxy-5-methylisoxazole [AMPA] and kainic acid [KA] receptors), and metabotropic glutamate receptors
- Synaptic vesicle proteins

How the various drugs prevent or attenuate seizures is not fully understood, and the mechanisms listed here only summarize some of the known potential effects of these agents on the neurons and glia. In an ideal world, the specific defect(s) would be identified that underlie epilepsy in individual patients, and therapy would then be targeted to correct the dysfunctional mechanism. In reality, identification of the specific defect is rarely possible, and empiric therapy must be planned. The mechanisms listed here are offered to enhance fundamental understanding of the various agents, so that the reader gains further insight into the drugs (Facts and Comparisons, 2007; Johannessen and Tomson, 2006; Levy et al., 2002; White et al., 2007; see also Online Resources list at end of References).

Acetazolamide

The anticonvulsant activity of acetazolamide may depend on a direct inhibition of carbonic anhydrase in the central nervous system (CNS), which reduces intracellular bicarbonate levels and may thereby reduce depolarizing

GABA responses. It also may alter potassium conductance that induces membrane hyperpolarization.

Benzodiazepines

Benzodiazepines exert their effects through enhancement of the GABA-benzodiazepine receptor complex. They bind at the $\alpha1$, $\alpha2$, $\alpha3$, or $\alpha5$ subunit in combination with a γ subunit of $GABA_A$ receptors. Three types of benzodiazepine (BNZ) receptors are located in the CNS and other tissues. The BNZ_1 receptors are located in the cerebellum and cerebral cortex, the BNZ_2 receptors are located in the cerebral cortex and spinal cord, and the BNZ_3 receptors are located in peripheral tissues. Allosteric (structural) modification of the receptors exerts anticonvulsant activity. Benzodiazepines bind nonspecifically to BNZ_2 receptors (as well as BNZ_1), which ultimately enhance the effects of GABA by increasing GABA affinity for the GABA receptor. Binding of GABA to the site opens the chloride channel, resulting in hyperpolarization of the cell membrane that prevents further excitation of the cell.

Brivaracetam

The precise mechanism by which brivaracetam exerts its anticonvulsant activity is not known. Brivaracetam displays a high and selective affinity for synaptic vesicle protein 2A (SV2A) in the brain (like levetiracetam. but with 20-fold greater affinity), which may contribute to its anticonvulsant effects.

Cannabidiol

The precise mechanisms by which cannabidiol exerts its anticonvulsant effects in humans are unknown. Cannabidiol does not appear to exert its anticonvulsant effects through interaction with cannabinoid receptors. Cannabidiol possesses affinity for multiple targets, across a range of target classes, resulting in functional modulation of neuronal excitability (Gray and Whalley, 2020).

Carbamazepine

Carbamazepine blocks use- and voltage-dependent sodium channels, inhibiting sustained repetitive firing of action potentials. Like phenytoin, carbamazepine reduces post-tetanic potentiation of synaptic transmission in the spinal cord. This effect may explain its ability to limit the spread of seizures. At therapeutic concentrations, it may block NMDA receptors as well.

Cenobamate

The precise mechanism by which cenobamate exerts its therapeutic effects is unknown. Cenobamate has been demonstrated to reduce repetitive neuronal firing by inhibiting voltage-gated sodium currents. It is also a positive allosteric modulator of the $GABA_A$ ion channel.

Eslicarbazepine Acetate

The precise mechanism(s) by which eslicarbazepine exerts anticonvulsant activity is unknown, but it probably involves inhibition of voltage-gated sodium channels.

Ethosuximide

Ethosuximide reduces the current in the T-type calcium channel found on primary afferent neurons. Activation of the T-channel causes low-threshold calcium spikes in thalamic relay neurons, which are believed to play a role in the spike-and-wave pattern observed during absence seizures.

Ezogabine

The precise mechanism(s) by which ezogabine exerts anticonvulsant activity is unknown. In vitro studies indicate that ezogabine enhances transmembrane potassium currents mediated by the KCNQ ion channels. By activating KCNQ channels, ezogabine probably stabilizes the resting membrane potential and reduces brain excitability. In vitro studies also suggest that ezogabine may exert therapeutic effects through augmentation of GABA-mediated currents.

Felbamate

Felbamate may be an antagonist at the strychnine-insensitive glycine-recognition site of the NMDA receptor-ionophore complex. Antagonism of the NMDA receptor glycine binding site may block the effects of the excitatory amino acids and suppress seizure activity. Felbamate has also direct interaction with voltage-dependent sodium channels and voltage-sensitive calcium currents and enhances GABA-evoked chloride currents. Felbamate may increase the seizure threshold by attenuating neuronal excitability and may decrease seizure spread.

Gabapentin

Recent studies suggest that gabapentin has a selective inhibitory effect on voltage-gated calcium channels containing the $\alpha 2\delta 1$ subunit, reducing neurotransmitter release from neurons. It may also potentiate adenosine triphosphate (ATP)-activated inward rectifying potassium channels. In animal studies, gabapentin has increased GABA responses at nonsynaptic sites in neuronal tissues and has reduced the release of monoamine neurotransmitters. In humans, nuclear magnetic resonance (NMR) spectroscopy has indicated that gabapentin may increase GABA synthesis.

Lacosamide

The precise mechanism(s) by which lacosamide exerts anticonvulsant activity is unknown. In vitro studies have shown that lacosamide selectively enhances slow inactivation of voltage-gated sodium channels, resulting in stabilization of hyperexcitable neuronal membranes and inhibition of repetitive neuronal firing.

Lamotrigine

Lamotrigine may stabilize neuronal membranes by acting at voltage-sensitive sodium channels. The blocking of sodium channels can decrease the presynaptic release of glutamate and aspartate, resulting in decreased seizure frequency. This mechanism is similar to that of carbamazepine and phenytoin. Lamotrigine is also a weak dihydrofolate reductase inhibitor in vitro and in animal studies. In clinical studies, however, no effect of lamotrigine on folate concentrations has been noted, although it is possible that folate concentrations may decrease during gestation. Lamotrigine has also been found to modulate neurotransmitter release through an interaction with N- and P-type voltage-gated calcium channels.

Levetiracetam

This agent appears to act via the involvement of a novel binding site, the synaptic vesicle protein, SV2A. This protein is involved in exocytosis and neurotransmitter release. Levetiracetam also interferes with release of intracellular Ca^{2+} initiated by Gq-coupled receptor activation.

Oxcarbazepine

The primary antiepileptic activity of oxcarbazepine is attributed to its 10-monohydroxy (MHD) metabolite. Studies indicate that voltage-sensitive sodium channels are blocked, thereby stabilizing neural membranes, inhibiting repetitive neuronal firing, and diminishing synaptic impulse activity. Modulation of potassium and calcium channels may also be involved. GABA receptors are not affected by oxcarbazepine or MHD with clinical relevance.

Perampanel

The precise mechanism(s) by which perampanel exerts anticonvulsant activity is unknown. Perampanel is a noncompetitive antagonist of the ionotropic α-amino-3-hydroxy-5-methyl- 4-isoxazolepropionic acid (AMPA) glutamate receptor on postsynaptic neurons.

Phenobarbital

Phenobarbital and other barbiturates augment GABA responses by promoting the binding of GABA to the receptor and increasing the length of time that chloride channels are open. Phenobarbital also may reduce the effects of glutamate and inhibit neurotransmitter release from nerve terminals, an effect mediated by depression of voltage-dependent calcium channels. Phenobarbital inhibits the spread of seizure activity in the cortex, thalamus, and limbic system and increases the threshold for electrical stimulation of the motor cortex. There is a decrease in both presynaptic and postsynaptic excitability. All actions result in a hyperpolarized cell membrane that prevents further excitation of the cell.

Phenytoin

Phenytoin exerts its anticonvulsant effect mainly by limiting the spread of seizure activity and reducing seizure propagation. Because phenytoin does not elevate the seizure threshold, it is less effective against drug-induced or electroconvulsive-induced seizures. The primary site of action of phenytoin appears to be the motor cortex, where the spread of seizure activity is inhibited. Phenytoin also reduces the maximal activity of brainstem centers responsible for the tonic phase of grand mal seizures. Phenytoin exerts its anticonvulsant effects with less CNS sedation than does phenobarbital. In toxic concentrations, phenytoin is excitatory and can induce seizures.

Mechanisms of Action

1. Major action occurs at therapeutic doses in which drug appears to bind with axonal Na^+ channels in the activated or inactivated state (but not the resting state). Phenytoin prolongs the inactivation state of the Na^+ channel by preventing the opening of the inactivation gate (located in proximity to the cytoplasmic side).
2. Higher doses inhibit Ca^{2+} influx across the cell membrane through voltage-gated Ca^{2+} channels (N-type). The latter effect may explain the ability of phenytoin to inhibit neurotransmitter release of serotonin and norepinephrine.

Pregabalin

Pregabalin is a structural analogue of GABA. Pregabalin is structurally related to gabapentin, but pregabalin has shown greater potency than gabapentin in seizure disorders (3–10 times more potent in animal studies). Pregabalin does not show direct GABA-mimetic effects and has no effect on GABAergic mechanisms. Pregabalin reduces neuronal calcium currents by binding to the $\alpha 2\delta$ subunit of calcium channels, and this particular mechanism may be responsible for reduced excitatory neurotransmitter release.

Primidone

The anticonvulsant activities of primidone are attributed to both the parent drug and to the active metabolites. Primidone is metabolized to phenobarbital; therefore, it shares all the actions of phenobarbital (i.e., raises the seizure threshold and inhibits spread from a seizure focus). Phenylethylmalonamide (PEMA) is the major metabolite of primidone. This is a less potent anticonvulsant than phenobarbital, but it may potentiate the effects of phenobarbital. PEMA is more toxic than primidone.

Rufinamide

The precise mechanism(s) by which rufinamide exerts anticonvulsant activity is unknown. The results of in vitro studies suggest that the main mechanism of action of rufinamide is modulation of the activity of sodium channels and, in particular, prolongation of the inactive state of the channel.

Tiagabine

Tiagabine inhibits neuronal and glial reuptake of GABA by binding to recognition sites associated with the GABA uptake carrier. Tiagabine inhibits the reuptake of GABA, while vigabatrin inhibits enzymatic metabolism of GABA. By blocking GABA reuptake into presynaptic neurons, tiagabine permits more GABA to be available for receptor binding on postsynaptic cells. Unlike tiagabine and vigabatrin, the mechanisms of action of other ASMs indicated for adjunctive treatment of partial seizures are not primarily mediated through GABA transmission.

Topiramate

Topiramate blocks voltage-sensitive sodium channels. Topiramate also enhances the activity of GABA at $GABA_A$ receptors by increasing the frequency at which GABA activates $GABA_A$ receptors. In addition, topiramate inhibits excitatory transmission by antagonizing some types of glutamate receptors. Specifically, topiramate antagonizes the ability of kainate to activate the kainate/AMPA (non-NMDA) subtype of excitatory amino acid (glutamate) receptor. It may also potentiate ATP-activated inward rectifying potassium channels. Topiramate is also a weak carbonic anhydrase inhibitor, which reduces intracellular bicarbonate levels and may thereby reduce depolarizing GABA responses; however, this mechanism is unlikely to contribute to its antiepileptic effects.

Valproic Acid, Valproate, Divalproex Sodium

Valproate has a broad preclinical and clinical profile. Several effects possibly related to mechanisms of action include the following:

- Valproate inhibits Ca^{2+} influx through low threshold T-type channels reducing Ca^{2+} currents, similar to ethosuximide.
- Valproate inhibits sustained high-frequency repetitive firing of neurons by inhibiting Na^+ ion influx through its specific voltage-gated ion channel (similar to phenytoin).
- It is believed that valproate increases brain concentrations of GABA. A number of mechanisms have been proposed, including inhibition of GABA-T action, activation of GABA synthesis via increased GAD activity, and increased release of GABA into the synapse.

Vigabatrin

Vigabatrin potentiates GABA by irreversibly inhibiting GABA-transaminase, the enzyme responsible for degradation of GABA. Anticonvulsant actions appear to be a result of increased GABA concentrations in the midbrain.

Zonisamide

The exact mechanisms of action are unknown. It appears that zonisamide exhibits a dual mechanism of action; it stops the spread of seizures and also suppresses the seizure focus. In vitro pharmacological studies suggest that zonisamide blocks voltage-sensitive sodium channels and reduces voltage-dependent, transient inward currents (T-type calcium currents), thereby stabilizing neuronal membranes and suppressing neuronal hyper-synchronization. Zonisamide also has weak carbonic anhydrase inhibiting activity, but this effect is not thought to be an important contributing factor in the anticonvulsant activity of zonisamide. In animal models, zonisamide has a profile of activity similar to carbamazepine and phenytoin and is more active against the tonic phase than the clonic phase of convulsion.

Pharmacokinetic Properties of Antiseizure Medications

For more details, the reader is referred to several excellent texts (*Facts and Comparisons*, 2007; IPCS INCHEM 2019; Jarrar and Buchhalter, 2003; Johannessen and Tomson, 2006; Landmark CJ et al., 2020; Levy et al.,

2002; Perucca et al., 2020) and the Online Resources list at the end of the References section.

Acetazolamide

Absorption: Rapid.

Peak Serum Concentrations: 2–4 hours.

Protein Binding: Approximately 90%.

Half-Life: 6–9 hours.

Elimination: Renal.

Benzodiazepines

Clonazepam

Absorption: Rapid.

Onset of Action: 20–60 minutes.

Duration of action: Up to 6–8 hours in children and up to 12 hours in adults.

Protein Binding: Approximately 85%.

Half-Life: Approximately 22–33 hours in children and 19–50 hours in adults.

Metabolism: Hepatic.

Elimination: Renal.

Clobazam

Absorption: Rapid.

Peak Serum Concentrations: 1–4 hours.

Protein Binding: Approximately 85%.

Half-Life: 11–77 hours.

Metabolism: Hepatic.

Elimination: Renal.

Diazepam

Absorption: Rapid.

Peak Serum Concentrations (PO dosing): 30 minutes to 2 hours. With the parenteral (IV) or rectal forms, peak blood levels are reached within 15 minutes after administration and are of the same magnitude as after PO administration.

Protein Binding: Approximately 98%.

Half-Life: 20–50 hours.

Metabolism: Hepatic.

Elimination: Renal.

Lorazepam

Absorption: Rapid.

Peak Serum Concentrations: 2 hours.

Protein Binding: Approximately 90%.

Half-Life: 10–20 hours.

Metabolism: Hepatic.

Elimination: Renal.

Midazolam (Intranasal)

Absorption: Rapid; the mean absolute bioavailability is approximately 44%.

Peak Serum Concentrations: 8–28 minutes.

Protein Binding: 97%.

Half-Life: 2–6 hours.

Metabolism: Liver and intestinal cytochrome P450 3A4.

Elimination: Renal.

Nitrazepam

Absorption: Rapid.

Peak Serum Concentrations: 2 hours.

Protein Binding: Approximately 85–90%.

Half-Life: 30 hours.

Metabolism: Hepatic.

Elimination: Renal.

Brivaracetam

Absorption: Rapid.

Peak Serum Concentrations: 1 hour.

Protein Binding: ≤20%.

Half-Life: 9 hours.

Metabolism: Hepatic and extrahepatic.

Elimination: Renal.

Cannabidiol

Peak Serum Concentrations: 2.5–5 hours.

Protein Binding: > 94%.

Half-Life: 56–61 hours.

Metabolism: In the liver and the gut (primarily in the liver) by CYP2C19 and CYP3A4 enzymes, and uridine 5'-diphospho-glucuronosyltransferase (UGT)1A7, UGT1A9, and UGT2B7 isoforms.

Elimination: Excreted in feces, with minor renal clearance.

Carbamazepine

Absorption: Slow and variable. The suspension is absorbed faster, and the XR tablets slightly slower, than the conventional tablets.

Peak Serum Concentrations: 4–5 hours for tablet and 1.5 hours for suspension.

Protein Binding: Approximately 76%.

Half-Life: 25–65 hours initially and 12–17 hours after repeated dosing (considerably shorter in children).

Metabolism: Hepatic (>90%). Carbamazepine is a potent hepatic enzyme inducer and can induce its own metabolism. Onset of enzyme induction is at about 3 days, with maximum effect at about 30 days.

Active Metabolite: Carbamazepine 10,11-epoxide.

Elimination: Renal.

Cenobamate

Absorption: 88% orally bioavailable.

Peak Serum Concentrations: 1–4 hours.

Protein Binding: 60%.

Half-Life: 50–60 hours.

Metabolism: Hepatic.

Elimination: Renal>>Fecal.

Eslicarbazepine Acetate

Absorption: Eslicarbazepine acetate is mostly undetectable after PO administration. Eslicarbazepine, the major metabolite, is primarily responsible for the pharmacological effect of eslicarbazepine acetate. Food has no effect on the pharmacokinetics of eslicarbazepine acetate.

Peak Serum Concentrations: 1–4 hours.

Protein Binding: <40%.

Half-Life: 13–20 hours.

Metabolism: Hepatic. Eslicarbazepine has moderate inhibitory effect on CYP2C19. A mild activation of UGT1A1-mediated glucuronidation was observed in vitro. It can induce CYP3A4.

Active Metabolites: Eslicarbazepine (91%); (R)-licarbazepine 5%; oxcarbazepine 1%.

Elimination: Renal.

Ethosuximide

Absorption: Rapid.

Peak Serum Concentrations: 4 hours in adults and 3–7 hours in children.

Protein Binding: Less than 5%.

Half-Life: 60 hours in adults and 30 hours in children.

Metabolism: Hepatic (65%). The hepatic microsomal isoenzyme CYP-3A4 appears to be involved. Ethosuximide does not inhibit or induce the hepatic CYP-450 microsomal enzymes or UDP-glucuronosyltransferase.

Elimination: Renal.

Ezogabine

Absorption: Rapid.

Peak Serum Concentrations: 0.5–2 hours.

Protein Binding: Approximately 22–30%.

Half-Life: 7–11 hours. Coadministration of ezogabine with medications that are inhibitors or inducers of cytochrome P450 enzymes is unlikely to affect the pharmacokinetics of ezogabine. However, the inducers for UGTs, such as carbamazepine and phenytoin, may reduce serum levels.

Metabolism: Hepatic.

Elimination: Renal.

Felbamate

Absorption: Rapid.

Peak Serum Concentrations: 1–6 hours.

Protein Binding: Approximately 22–30%.

Half-Life: 14–23 hours in adults; lower in children. The metabolism of felbamate is enhanced by enzyme-inducing ASMs such as phenobarbital, phenytoin, primidone, and carbamazepine, resulting in an average felbamate half-life of approximately 14 hours.

Metabolism: Hepatic (60%).

Elimination: Renal.

Gabapentin

Absorption: Rapid.

Peak Serum Concentrations: 2–3 hours. In general, the concentration-to-dose ratio of gabapentin increases significantly with age. Approximately 30% larger doses would be required in younger children (<5 years) to achieve the same exposure as in older children.

Protein Binding: Less than 3%.

Half-Life: 5–9 hours.

Metabolism: Not metabolized. Gabapentin does not interact with other ASMs to any clinically significant degree.

Elimination: Renal.

Lacosamide

Absorption: Rapid.

Peak Serum Concentrations: 1–4 hours.

Protein Binding: Less than 15%.

Half-Life: 13 hours.

Metabolism: Renal.

Elimination: Renal.

Lamotrigine

Absorption: Rapid.

Peak Serum Concentrations: 1–3 hours. Peak plasma concentrations occur up to 4.8 hours after an PO dose in patients on concomitant valproic acid. A second peak may be seen 4–6 hours after administration; this may suggest entero-hepatic circulation.

Protein Binding: Approximately 55%. It does not displace other ASMs from their protein-binding sites.

Half-Life: 14–60 (mean: 24) hours in adults. After multiple dosing in normal adults, lamotrigine may induce its own metabolism, which may decrease the half-life by 25%. Carbamazepine, phenytoin, phenobarbital, and primidone can decrease lamotrigine half-life (to average 15 hours). Valproic acid increases elimination half-life (to average 60 hours) whether given with or without the other ASMs. Clearance in children is up to twofold higher than in adults.

Metabolism: Hepatic (>90%).

Elimination: Renal.

Levetiracetam

Absorption: Rapid.

Peak Serum Concentrations: 1 hour.

Protein Binding: Less than 10%.

Half-Life: 5–8 hours.

Metabolism: Not extensively metabolized. Levetiracetam does not interact with other ASMs to any clinically significant degree.

Elimination: Renal.

Oxcarbazepine

Absorption: Rapid.

Peak Serum Concentrations of MHD (monohydroxy derivative): 4–8 hours.

Protein Binding: 40% (of MHD).

Half-Life: The half-lives of oxcarbazepine and MHD are 2 and 9 hours, respectively. Children 2–6 years have a higher clearance (more than twice) and need a larger dose/kg body weight of oxcarbazepine.

Metabolism: Hepatic. Rapid reduction in the liver to MHD. Mild enzyme inducer.

Elimination: Renal.

Perampanel

Absorption: Rapid.

Peak Serum Concentrations: 0.5–2.5 hours (fasted condition); 2–3 (fed condition).

Protein Binding: About 95%.

Half-Life: 105 hours.

Metabolism: Hepatic.

Elimination: Feces and renal.

Phenobarbital

Absorption: Variable.

Onset of Action: Onset of action after IV administration is within 5 minutes, reaching a maximum in about 30 minutes. The peak brain/plasma concentration ratio occurs slowly about 20–40 minutes after an IV dose.

Peak Serum Concentrations: Peak serum concentrations are achieved 8–12 hours after PO dosing.

Protein Binding: About 20–45%.

Half-Life: In adults 50–120 hours (mean: 96 hours); in children 37–73 hours (mean: 69 hours); in infants 53–73 hours (mean: 63 hours); in neonates 45–200 hours (mean: 111 hours).

Metabolism: Hepatic (75%). Phenobarbital accelerates the clearance of other drugs metabolized via hepatic microsomal enzymes, but there is no clear evidence that phenobarbital accelerates its own metabolism.

Elimination: Renal.

Phenytoin

Absorption: Variable and slow.
Onset of Action: Brain and cerebrospinal fluid concentrations are equal to plasma concentrations 10–20 minutes following an IV administered loading dose.

Peak Serum Concentrations: Rapid-release dosage forms reach peak concentrations in 1.5–6 hours, whereas a dose of sustained-release capsules may not reach peak concentrations for 12 hours. The absorption rate is also dose dependent. Time to achieve peak concentration (T-max) may occur 1–2 hours after a 200-mg PO dose, whereas T-max may not be observed for up to 18 hours after an 800-mg dose. Because the absorption rate of phenytoin is dose dependent, PO loading doses should be administered in divided doses.

Protein Binding: About 90–95%; less in patients with renal failure or hypoproteinemia.

Note: Patients with hepatic failure can have an increase in serum bilirubin concentration, which can displace phenytoin from protein binding sites and increase the free fraction of the drug. Other hypoalbuminemic states with potential for an increased free fraction of phenytoin include major trauma, burns, nephrotic syndrome, malnutrition, or surgery. The measurement of unbound ("free") phenytoin serum concentrations may be helpful in these specific conditions.

Half-Life: Because of the saturable metabolism, it is inaccurate to report a fixed value for phenytoin half-life. It depends on dosage and various patient factors. Half-life of the drug is longer when the plasma levels are higher, and plasma levels can rise out of proportion to an increase in dose. The half-life of phenytoin in the low to mid-therapeutic range varies from 12 to 36 hours (average: 24 hours). For most patients, half-life of 20–60 hours may be found at therapeutic levels.

Note: Fever (≥101°F) for more than 24 hours can also induce hepatic oxidative enzymes and potentially decrease phenytoin serum concentrations. Liver disease can reduce the clearance of phenytoin or, paradoxically, increase its clearance if protein binding is significantly decreased.

Metabolism: Hepatic. Metabolic capacity can be saturated at therapeutic concentrations. Below the saturation point, phenytoin is eliminated in a linear, first-order process. Above the saturation point, elimination is much slower and occurs via a zero-order process. Phenytoin accelerates the clearance of other drugs metabolized via hepatic microsomal enzymes.

Note: Phenytoin dosage forms are available as either phenytoin acid (tablets and PO suspension) or phenytoin sodium (capsules and injection). Phenytoin sodium contains 8% less phenytoin than does phenytoin acid. Due to its unique metabolism, switching patients from phenytoin sodium to phenytoin acid without adjusting the dose to account for this 8% difference could lead to phenytoin toxicity.

Elimination: Renal (metabolites). Less than 5% of phenytoin is eliminated renally.

Pregabalin

Absorption: Rapid.

Peak Serum Concentrations: 1–1.5 hours.

Protein Binding: None.

Half-Life: 6 hours.

Metabolism: Negligible (<2%) hepatic metabolism. Pregabalin does not interact with other ASMs to any clinically significant degree.

Elimination: Renal.

Primidone

Absorption: Rapid, but variable.

Peak Serum Concentrations: 3–4 hours.

Protein Binding: Phenylethylmalonamide (PEMA) and primidone are bound only minimally to plasma proteins. About 20–45% of phenobarbital is plasma protein-bound.

Half-Life: Plasma half-life of primidone is 10–12 hours. Plasma half-life of PEMA is 29–36 hours. Both PEMA and phenobarbital, which has a long half-life of several days, accumulate during long-term therapy.

Metabolism: Hepatic. Primidone accelerates the clearance of other drugs metabolized via hepatic microsomal enzymes.

Active Metabolites: Phenobarbital and PEMA.

Elimination: Renal.

Rufinamide

Absorption: Slow and dose-dependent.

Peak Serum Concentrations: 4–6 hours.

Protein Binding: 34%.

Half-Life: 6–10 hours.

Metabolism: Hepatic. The metabolic route is not cytochrome P450 dependent. However, potent cytochrome P450 enzyme inducers, such as carbamazepine and phenytoin, increase the clearance of rufinamide, and valproate decreases rufinamide clearance. Rufinamide is a weak inhibitor of CYP 2E1 and a weak inducer of CYP 3A4 enzymes.

Elimination: Renal.

Tiagabine

Absorption: Rapid.

Peak Serum Concentrations: 45 minutes in the fasting state (0.5–2 hours).

Protein Binding: 96%. Valproate displaces tiagabine from its binding sites on serum proteins.

Half-Life: 4–13 (average: 7) hours. In patients who take hepatic enzyme-inducing drugs, elimination half-life is about 4–7 hours. The mean half-life of tiagabine in children is shorter (3.2 hours in those taking an inducing ASM vs. 5.7 hours in children taking valproic acid concomitantly).

Metabolism: Hepatic. Tiagabine is thought to be metabolized primarily by the hepatic cytochrome P-450 isoenzyme CYP3A4. Tiagabine does not inhibit or induce the hepatic CYP450 microsomal enzymes.

Elimination: Feces and renal.

Topiramate

Absorption: Rapid.

Peak Serum Concentrations: 1–4 (average: 2) hours. Children <11 years require much higher doses in mg/kg body weight to achieve drug concentrations comparable to adults.

Protein Binding: 13–41% (average: 15%).

Half-Life: 19–25 (mean: 21) hours.

Metabolism: Hepatic (30%).

Elimination: Renal.

Valproic Acid, Valproate, Divalproex Sodium

Absorption: Rapid.

Peak Serum Concentrations: 1–4 hours following PO administration of the sodium salt or valproic acid and within 3–5 hours for divalproex delayed-release and 4–17 hours following divalproex extended-release tablets.

Protein Binding: 90%, but protein binding decreases as the serum concentration increases.

Half-Life: 7–20 hours.

Metabolism: Hepatic. Valproic acid inhibits the activity of CYP2C9 and UGT at clinically relevant concentrations in human liver microsomes.

Elimination: Renal.

Vigabatrin

Absorption: Rapid.

Peak Serum Concentrations: 0.7–1.1 hours.

Protein Binding: None.

Half-Life: 6–8 hours.

Metabolism: Not metabolized by liver. Vigabatrin does not interact with other ASMs to any clinically significant degree.

Elimination: Renal.

Zonisamide

Absorption: Rapid.

Peak Serum Concentrations: 2–7 hours.

Protein Binding: About 40–60%. Zonisamide is extensively bound to erythrocytes, resulting in an eight-fold higher concentration of zonisamide in red blood cells than in plasma.

Half-Life: In plasma is about 63 hours (50–70 hours) and in red blood cells is approximately 105 hours. The elimination half-life of zonisamide in plasma is about 27–38 hours during combination therapy with enzyme-inducing ASMs.

Metabolism: Hepatic (70%). However, zonisamide does not inhibit or induce cytochrome P-450 enzymes or UGT.

Elimination: Renal.

References

Facts and Comparisons. *Drug Facts and Comparisons*. St. Louis: Wolters Kluwer Health/Facts & Comparisons; 2007.

Gray RA, Whalley BJ. The proposed mechanisms of action of CBD in epilepsy. *Epileptic Disord*. 2020;22(S1):10–15.

IPCS INCHEM. Chemical safety information from intergovernmental organizations. http://www.inchem.org/2019.

Jarrar RG, Buchhalter JR. Therapeutics in pediatric epilepsy, Part 1: The new antiepileptic drugs and the ketogenic diet. *Mayo Clin Proc*. 2003;78:359–370.

Johannessen SI, Tomson T. Pharmacokinetic variability of newer antiepileptic drugs. *Clin Pharmacokinet*. 2006;45:1061–1075.

Landmark CJ, Johannessen SI, Patsalos PN. Therapeutic drug monitoring of antiepileptic drugs: Current status and future prospects. *Expert Opin Drug Metab Toxicol*. 2020:16:227–238.

Levy RH, Mattson RH, Meldrum BS, Perucca E. *Antiepileptic Drugs*, 5th ed. Philadelphia: Lippincott Williams & Wilkins; 2002.

Perucca E, Brodie MJ, Kwan P, Tomson T. 30 years of second-generation antiseizure medications: Impact and future perspectives. *Lancet Neurol*. 2020;19:544–556.

White HS, Smith MD, Wilcox KS. Mechanisms of action of antiepileptic drugs. *Int Rev Neurobiol*. 2007;81:85–110.

Online Resources

Brivaracetam (Briviact). www.briviact.com/2020

Cannabidiol (Epidiolex). www.epidiolex.com/2020

Cenobamate. reference.medscape.com/drug/xcopri-cenobamate-1000328/2020

Eslicarbazine acetate (Aptiom). www.aptiom.com/2014

Ezogabine (Potiga). www.potiga.com/2014

Lacosamide (Vimpat). www.vimpat.com/2014

Midazolam (Nayzilam). www.nayzilam.com/2020

Perampanel (Fycompa). us.eisai.com/wps/wcm/connect/Eisai/Home/Our.../FYCOMPA/2014

Rufinamide (Banzel). www.banzel.com/2014

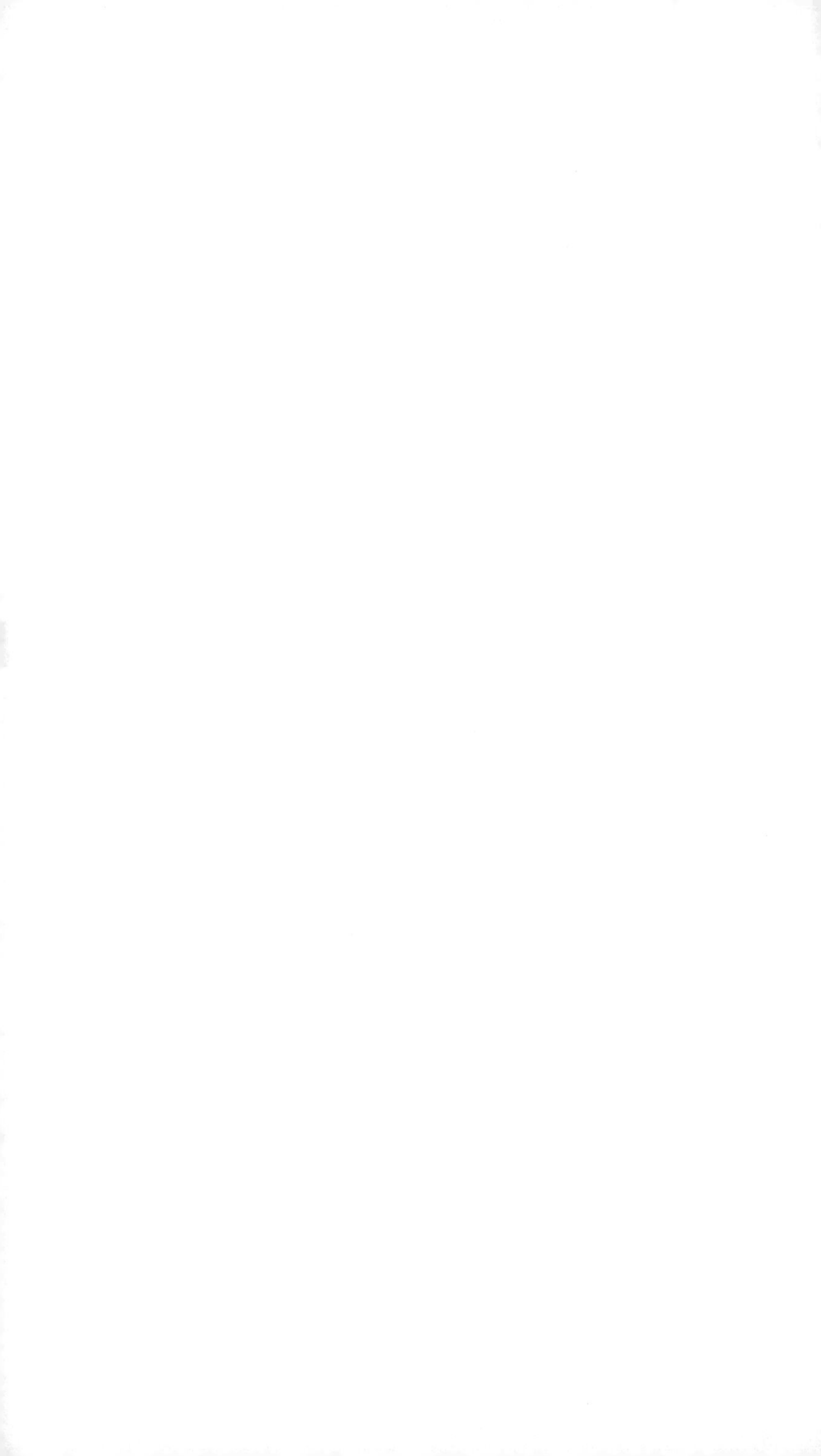

Chapter 4

Monitoring Antiseizure Medications and Their Toxicity

There is a correlation between the serum concentration of any antiseizure medication (ASM) and its therapeutic and toxic effects. Therapeutic drug monitoring seeks to optimize the desirable effects of ASMs while minimizing their undesirable properties. The role of drug monitoring is somewhat controversial because the therapeutic level varies from one patient to the next and is not certain for some ASMs. Moreover, it is not clear that higher levels are more effective than lower levels for many agents. Some clinicians hold the view that levels are irrelevant as long as patients are seizure free and do not experience adverse effects. However, ascertaining that seizures are controlled requires hoping that a seizure does not occur while time passes, and this may be unacceptable to many patients. Therefore, there may be advantage to obtaining baseline serum levels to ensure that serum concentrations are within the range generally found in patients who either respond to medication or who take a dose known to be therapeutic.

Indications for drug monitoring of ASMs include (Johannessen and Tomson, 2006; Neels et al., 2004; Reimers et al., 2018) the following:

1. *Newly diagnosed epilepsy*, to ensure that the drug is in the appropriate target range
2. *After change in drug dosage*, to assess new drug concentration
3. *If there is a lack of clinical response*, to assess patient adherence to the drug regimen
4. *In the presence of mental retardation*, to ensure that high levels, often associated with adverse effects, are not present. These individuals may not be able to voice complaints about adverse effects.
5. *In patients with renal or hepatic impairment*
6. *In pregnant patients*, who are subject to significant alterations in levels as pregnancy progresses
7. *In patients with poor compliance*, to encourage compliance with drug therapy

For ASM monitoring, blood samples should be drawn after steady-state concentrations have been achieved, which is at least 5 half-lives after the first dose and once any enzyme induction or inhibition has had an opportunity to take full effect. Sampling in the end-of-dose condition, immediately prior to taking the next dose, provides trough levels that are easily comparable (Neels et al., 2004).

No optimum serum concentration range applies to all patients. Some patients will respond to concentrations below the lower limit of the recommended range, while others will require concentrations above it. In fact, some experts have suggested that the lower limit of the therapeutic range should be disregarded, and any concentration up to the toxic limit should be considered potentially therapeutic. Furthermore, the therapeutic range can be expected to differ in patients on monotherapy compared with those on polytherapy regimens. Thus, drug monitoring is not a substitute for clinical judgment (Johannessen et al., 2003).

In addition to ASM serum-level monitoring for the listed indications, it may be useful to monitor blood or urine parameters, such as blood counts, liver enzymes, and others, for adverse effects of ASMs (Facts and Comparisons, 2007; Johannessen et al., 2003; Johannessen and Tomson, 2006; Leikin and Paloucek, 2002; Neels et al., 2004; Thomson PDR, n.d.). However, the value of regularly monitoring these parameters, although recommended by pharmaceutical manufacturers and government regulatory agencies, has never been proved to be either clinically useful nor to enhance safety. Idiosyncratic reactions are neither predictable nor necessarily aborted by medication withdrawal, so periodic monitoring for these effects is unlikely to alter the course of illness; at best, the reaction might be detected sooner. Similarly, many alterations in serum chemistry measures or blood count, such as elevations of liver enzymes in the absence of symptoms, decrease in white blood cell count, or lowering of serum sodium, in the absence of symptoms are commonly disregarded by physicians. Detection of these "abnormalities" usually has no consequence or any justifiable consequence. The patients most at risk for serious adverse effects appear to be those with concurrent illness or preexisting abnormalities in laboratory screening tests.

In view of these considerations, one might take one of several approaches, each having merit and none with proven advantage.

1. One might take the view that meaningful abnormalities of screening laboratory tests are extraordinarily rare for nearly all drugs and that routine screening is therefore unnecessary and wasteful. Moreover, the value of earlier detection of severe idiosyncratic reaction is uncertain. If only symptomatic abnormalities would result in changing therapy (ignoring asymptomatic abnormalities), then there is no value in assessing patients without symptoms. One would therefore not perform any routine screening and assess only those patients who develop symptoms suggestive of a drug complication.
2. An intermediate approach could be justified. For patients who are to be treated with an ASM known to have particular adverse effects (e.g., valproate, which rarely causes liver toxicity), one might obtain baseline liver function tests prior to initiating treatment. Should the baseline tests prove normal, then further monitoring is almost certainly unnecessary. Should the baseline tests be abnormal, then periodic monitoring may have some value because there is evidence that patients with baseline abnormalities are those mainly at risk for serious drug reactions.

3. Last, a more active approach might be employed. Routine screening of blood or urine could be performed, adhering to manufacturer recommended guidelines. This approach is tremendously wasteful of medical resources and subjects many patients to regular, unnecessary laboratory testing. Its chief justification is that relevant abnormalities might rarely be detected earlier than if routine testing was not done, perhaps avoiding some serious complications. Unfortunately, as noted earlier, there is no medical evidence that routine screening actually saves lives or prevents drug complications. Therefore, we do not favor this approach.

Acetazolamide

Therapeutic Target Range (mg/L): 10–15.

Monitoring Parameters

- Intraocular pressure
- Ophthalmologic examination
- Serum bicarbonate (if symptomatic)
- Serum chloride (if symptomatic)

Manifestations and Treatment of Overdose

Manifestations: Lethargy, metabolic acidosis, tachycardia, and tachypnea have been reported and electrolyte imbalances may be expected to occur with acute poisoning. Confusion, lethargy, metabolic acidosis, and bone marrow depression have been reported with chronic toxicity.

Treatment: Decontamination and hemodialysis.

Benzodiazepines

Monitoring Parameters

- Complete blood count (CBC) (if symptomatic)
- Liver function tests (if symptomatic)

Manifestations and Treatment of Overdose

Manifestations: Somnolence, dysarthria, diplopia, confusion, ataxia, hyperactivity, hypotension, cyanosis, and coma.

Treatment: Decontamination, supportive measures, and flumazenil (the antagonistic action of flumazenil may precipitate seizures in patients receiving benzodiazepines).

Brivaracetam

Therapeutic Target Range (mg/L): 0.2–2.

Monitoring Parameters: CBC (if symptomatic)

Manifestations and Treatment of Overdose

Manifestations: Vertigo, balance disorder, fatigue, nausea, diplopia, anxiety, and bradycardia.

Treatment: Supportive measures. Dialysis may not be effective.

Cannabidiol

Therapeutic Target Range (mg/L): Not established.

Monitoring Parameters

- Because of the risk of hepatocellular injury, obtain serum transaminases (ALT and AST) and total bilirubin levels in all patients prior to starting treatment. Serum transaminases and total bilirubin levels should also be obtained at 1 month, 3 months, and 6 months after initiation of treatment with cannabidiol and periodically thereafter or as clinically indicated. Discontinue cannabidiol in any patients with elevations of transaminase levels greater than three times the upper limit of normal and bilirubin levels greater than two times the upper limit of normal.
- CBC (if symptomatic)
- Serum creatinine (if symptomatic)

Manifestations and Treatment of Overdose

No information is available.

Carbamazepine

Carbamazepine induces its own metabolism. Several weeks of therapy may be required before the appropriate maintenance dose is achieved.

Therapeutic Target Range (mg/L): 4–12.

Toxic Concentrations (mg/L): >12.

Monitoring Parameters

- CBC (baseline and periodic)
- Serum sodium (if symptomatic)
- Serum carbamazepine concentrations
- ECG (if symptomatic)

Manifestations and Treatment of Overdose

Manifestations: Dizziness, ataxia, cognitive dysfunction, chorea (extrapyramidal), hyperreflexia, mania, encephalopathy, coma, convulsion, myoclonus, tremor, dermatologic reactions, jaundice, ileus, nausea, vomiting, hyperthermia, hyponatremia, atrioventricular block, bradycardia, arrhythmia, hypotension, respiratory depression, blood dyscrasias, and oliguria. Following ingestion of extended-release form of carbamazepine, the first signs and symptoms appear after 1–3 hours. Cardiovascular disorders are generally milder, with severe cardiac complications occurring only when very high doses (>60 g) have been ingested.

Treatment: Decontamination, supportive therapy, charcoal hemoperfusion, and dialysis in case of renal failure.

Cenobamate

Therapeutic Target Range (mg/L): Not established.

Monitoring Parameters

- Liver function tests (if symptomatic)
- Serum potassium (if symptomatic)

Manifestations and Treatment of Overdose

Manifestations: There is limited clinical experience with cenobamate overdose in humans.

Treatment: Supportive measures. Dialysis may not be effective.

Eslicarbazepine Acetate

Therapeutic Target Range (mg/L): 3–26.

Toxic Concentrations (mg/L): Not well established.

Monitoring Parameters

- CBC (if symptomatic)
- Serum sodium and chloride
- Liver function tests
- Thyroid function tests (if symptomatic)

Manifestations and Treatment of Overdose

Manifestations: Hyponatremia, dizziness, nausea, vomiting, somnolence, oral paraesthesia, ataxia, walking difficulties, and diplopia.

Treatment: Decontamination (gastric lavage and/or inactivation by administering activated charcoal), supportive therapy, and hemodialysis.

Ethosuximide

Therapeutic Target Range (mg/L): 39–99.

Toxic Concentrations (mg/L): >160.

Monitoring Parameters

- CBC (if symptomatic)
- Liver function tests (if symptomatic)

Manifestations and Treatment of Overdose

Manifestations: CNS depression, excessive sedation, coma, ataxia, nausea, vomiting, hypotension, or respiratory depression (slow and shallow).

Treatment: Decontamination, supportive therapy, benzodiazepine for seizure, and hemodialysis.

Ezogabine

Therapeutic Target Range: Not well established.

Toxic Concentrations: Not well established.

Monitoring Parameters: Electrocardiogram (ECG): QT interval should be monitored in patients taking concomitant medications known to increase the QT interval or with certain heart conditions (e.g., known prolonged QT interval, congestive heart failure, ventricular hypertrophy, hypokalemia, or hypomagnesemia)

Manifestations and Treatment of Overdose

Manifestations: Cardiac arrhythmia, agitation, aggressive behavior, and irritability.

Treatment: Decontamination and supportive therapy.

Felbamate

Therapeutic Target Range (mg/L): 30–60.

Toxic Concentrations (mg/L): Not well established; probably >120.

Monitoring Parameters

- CBC
- Liver function tests

Note: Full hematologic evaluations should be performed before starting therapy and frequently during therapy. Although it might appear prudent to perform frequent CBCs in patients continuing on felbamate, there is no evidence that such monitoring will allow early detection of marrow suppression before aplastic anemia occurs. Likewise, at present, there is no way to predict who is likely to develop hepatic failure.

Manifestations and Treatment of Overdose

Manifestations: Sedation, reversible downbeat nystagmus, generalized mild motor weakness, ataxia, gastrointestinal upset, and tachycardia.

Treatment: Decontamination and supportive care.

Gabapentin

Therapeutic Target Range (mg/L): 3–21.

Toxic Concentrations: Not well established.

Monitoring Parameters: White blood count (WBC) (routine monitoring of laboratory parameters rarely necessary)

Manifestations and Treatment of Overdose

Manifestations: Somnolence, fatigue, ataxia, double vision, slurred speech, lethargy, respiratory difficulty, and diarrhea.

Treatment: Decontamination and hemodialysis.

Lacosamide

Therapeutic Target Range (mg/L): 3–10.

Toxic Concentrations: Not established.

Monitoring Parameters: ECG: In patients with cardiac disease, obtaining an ECG before beginning lacosamide and after lacosamide is titrated to steady-state is recommended.

Manifestations and Treatment of Overdose

Manifestations: Usual adverse effects.

Treatment: Decontamination, supportive measures, and possibly hemodialysis.

Lamotrigine

Therapeutic Target Range (mg/L): 3–13.

Toxic Concentrations: Not well established.

Monitoring Parameters: None

Manifestations and Treatment of Overdose

Manifestations: Ataxia, nystagmus, increased seizures, coma, and intraventricular conduction delay.

Treatment: Decontamination, supportive measures, IV sodium bicarbonate (1–2 mEq/kg) in case of wide-complex tachycardia, and possibly hemodialysis.

Levetiracetam

Therapeutic Target Range (mg/L): 5–41.

Toxic Concentrations: Not well established.

Monitoring Parameters: None

Manifestations and Treatment of Overdose

Manifestations: Somnolence, agitation, aggression, respiratory depression, and coma.

Treatment: Decontamination, supportive measures, and hemodialysis.

Oxcarbazepine

Therapeutic Target Range (mg/L): 3–36.

Toxic Concentrations: Not well established; probably >40 mg/L.

Monitoring Parameters: Serum sodium (mild hyponatremia is common, although symptomatic hyponatremia is uncommon; see Chapter 14).

Manifestations and Treatment of Overdose

Manifestations: Somnolence, ataxia, bradycardia, hypotension, vertigo, tinnitus, and CNS depression.

Treatment: Decontamination and supportive measures.

Perampanel

Therapeutic Target Range (mg/L): 0.1–1.

Toxic Concentrations: Not well established.

Monitoring Parameters: None.

Manifestations and Treatment of Overdose

Manifestations: Altered mental status, agitation, and aggressive behavior.

Treatment: Decontamination and supportive measures.

Phenobarbital

Serum phenobarbital concentrations should be used to guide therapy in all patients. Serum concentrations above 10–15 μg/mL are required for control of seizures while serious adverse effects appear when concentrations exceed 35 μg/mL. Minor sedation occurs initially at concentrations of around 5 μg/mL, which is transient. Plasma levels >50 μg/mL may produce coma or respiratory depression, and levels >80 μg/mL are potentially fatal.

Due to the long half-life of phenobarbital, several weeks of therapy may be required before the appropriate maintenance dose and therapeutic serum concentrations are achieved in the absence of the use of a loading dose.

Therapeutic Target Range (mg/L): 12–30.

Toxic Concentrations (mg/L): >50.

Monitoring Parameters

- CBC (if symptomatic)
- Liver function tests (if symptomatic)
- Serum phenobarbital concentrations

Manifestations and Treatment of Overdose

Manifestations: Unsteady gait, ataxia, hyporeflexia, asterixis, dysarthria, confusion, change in mental status, myocardial depression, hypothermia, hypotension, pulmonary edema, ptosis, miosis, and extrapyramidal reaction.

Treatment: Decontamination, supportive therapy (hypotension and other cardiopulmonary complications), repeated PO doses of activated charcoal, adequate hydration and urinary alkalinization (with IV sodium bicarbonate), and hemodialysis.

Phenytoin

Serum phenytoin concentrations should be used to monitor therapy in all patients receiving phenytoin. Therapeutic serum concentrations are generally considered to be 10–20 μg/mL (equivalent to 1–2 μg/mL unbound or free phenytoin). Free phenytoin levels may be helpful in assessing patients with hypoalbuminemia or with elevated blood urea nitrogen levels. In uremic patients, the free fraction of phenytoin may be more than doubled, leading to serious adverse reactions. It is recommended to quantitate free phenytoin in uremic patients and adjust the dose to maintain the concentration at approximately 2 mg/L (μg/mL). Achieving total serum phenytoin concentrations as high as 30–40 μg/mL may be beneficial in status epilepticus.

Due to variable metabolism and half-life, it may take several days to weeks to reach steady-state serum concentrations at a given maintenance dosage. Determining when to draw serum phenytoin concentrations is patient-specific. In emergent or noncompliant situations, serum concentrations may be drawn immediately. When evaluating maintenance doses, trough serum concentrations may be drawn 5–7 days after initiating or changing dosage. When evaluating phenytoin serum concentrations, certain patient characteristics such as fever, trauma, or hepatic disease should be considered, as well as the potential for drug or food interactions. There are marked variations among individuals with respect to plasma phenytoin concentrations and when toxicity occurs.

Therapeutic Target Range (mg/L): 10–20.

Toxic Concentrations (mg/L): >20.

Monitoring Parameters

- CBC (if symptomatic)
- Liver function tests (if symptomatic)
- Serum phenytoin concentrations

Manifestations and Treatment of Overdose

Manifestations: Manifestations of toxicity are dose dependent (Table 4.1).

Treatment: Decontamination and supportive therapy (diuresis and hemodialysis are of little value).

Table 4.1 Manifestations of phenytoin toxicity based on serum levels

Level	Manifestation
20 μg/mL	Far-lateral nystagmus
30 μg/mL	Ataxia
40 μg/mL	Change in mental status
50 μg/mL	Coma
95 μg/mL	Death (respiratory and circulatory depression)

Pregabalin

Therapeutic Target Range (mg/L): 2–6.

Toxic Concentrations: Not well established.

Monitoring Parameters

- Serum creatinine (rarely needed)
- Creatine kinase in patients with muscle pain, weakness, or tenderness

Manifestations and Treatment of Overdose

Manifestations: Somnolence, confusion, agitation, and restlessness.

Treatment: General supportive measures and hemodialysis if necessary.

Note: In overdoses up to 15 g, no unexpected adverse reactions were reported.

Primidone

Serum concentrations of both primidone and phenobarbital should be monitored in patients receiving primidone. Serum levels correlate well with clinical response. Recommended serum concentration of primidone is 8–12 μg/mL, and for phenobarbital, 15–40 μg/mL. Several weeks of therapy may be required before the appropriate maintenance dose and therapeutic serum concentrations are achieved. Symptoms and treatment of overdose are similar to those for phenobarbital.

Therapeutic Target Range (mg/L): 8–12.

Toxic Concentrations (mg/L): >15.

Monitoring Parameters

- CBC (if symptomatic)
- Liver function tests (if symptomatic)

Rufinamide

Therapeutic Target Range (mg/L): 4–31.

Toxic Concentrations: Not well established.

Monitoring Parameters: ECG: Rufinamide is contraindicated in patients with familial short QT syndrome. Caution should be used when administering rufinamide with other drugs that shorten the QT interval.

Manifestations and Treatment of Overdose

Manifestations: Usual adverse effects.

Treatment: Decontamination, supportive measures, and possibly hemodialysis.

Tiagabine

Therapeutic Target Range (µg/L): Not well established; probably 10–235.

Toxic Concentrations: Not well established.

Monitoring Parameters: Liver function tests (rarely needed)

Manifestations and Treatment of Overdose

Manifestations: Dizziness, CNS depression, agitation, ataxia, tremor, weakness, and myoclonus.

Treatment: Decontamination, multiple doses of activated charcoal, and supportive measures.

Topiramate

Therapeutic Target Range (mg/L): 2–10.

Toxic Concentrations: Not well established.

Monitoring Parameters

- Serum bicarbonate (baseline and periodic; in children; see Chapter 14)
- Serum creatinine/blood urea nitrogen (if symptomatic)

Manifestations and Management of Overdose

Manifestations: Acute neurological symptoms, abdominal pain, blurred vision, hypotension, metabolic acidosis, and stupor.

Treatment: Decontamination and hemodialysis.

Valproic Acid, Valproate, Divalproex Sodium

As with all ASMs, dosage should be individualized and adjusted to patient response and adverse effects. Therapeutic valproic acid serum concentrations for epilepsy are generally recommended to be between 50 and 100 µg/mL, although some patients may require higher serum concentrations for proper seizure control. Toxicity may be seen with concentrations exceeding 100–125 µg/mL; however, toxicity is usually seen with concentrations above 200 µg/mL.

Therapeutic Target Range (mg/L): 50–100.

Toxic Concentrations (mg/L): >200.

Monitoring Parameters

- CBC (if symptomatic)
- Liver function tests (if symptomatic)
- Serum ammonia (if symptomatic encephalopathy is present)
- Serum valproic acid concentrations

Manifestations and Treatment of Overdose

Manifestations: Somnolence, jaundice, acidosis, heart block, and deep coma.

Treatment: Decontamination, supportive measures, hemodialysis, naloxone (caution in patients with epilepsy; could reverse anticonvulsant effects), and L-carnitine (100 mg/kg loading dose, then 250 mg every 8 hours for 4 days).

Vigabatrin

Therapeutic Target Range (mg/L): 1–36.

Toxic Concentrations: Not well established.

Monitoring Parameters: CBC (if symptomatic)

Manifestations and Treatment of Overdose

Manifestations: Mood or mental status changes and delirium.

Treatment: Decontamination, supportive care, and hemodialysis.

Zonisamide

Therapeutic Target Range (mg/L): 10–38.

Toxic Concentrations (mg/L): >80.

Monitoring Parameters

- CBC (if symptomatic)
- Liver function tests (if symptomatic)

Manifestations and Treatment of Overdose

Manifestations: Confusion, loss of consciousness, difficult or labored breathing, faintness, slow or irregular heartbeat.

Treatment: Supportive measures. Dialysis may not be effective.

References

Facts and Comparisons. *Drug Facts and Comparisons*. St. Louis: Wolters Kluwer Health/Facts & Comparisons; 2007.

Johannessen SI, Battino D, Berry DJ, Bailer M, Kramer G, Tomson T, Patsalos PN. Therapeutic drug monitoring of the newer antiepileptic drugs. *Therap Drug Monitor*. 2003;25:347–363.

Johannessen SI, Tomson T. Pharmacokinetic variability of newer antiepileptic drugs. when is monitoring needed? *Clin Pharmacokin*. 2006;45:1061–1075.

Leikin JB, Paloucek FP. *Leikin & Paloucek's Poisoning & Toxicology Handbook*, 3rd ed. Hudson, OH: Lexi-Comp Inc.; 2002.

Neels HM, Sierens AC, Naelaerts K, Scharpe SL, Hatfield GM, Lambert WE. Therapeutic drug monitoring of old and newer antiepileptic drugs. *Clin Chem Lab Med*. 2004;42:1228–1255.

Reimers A, Berg JA, Burns ML, et al. Reference ranges for antiepileptic drugs revisited: A practical approach to establish national guidelines. *Drug Des Devel Ther*. 2018;12:271–280.

Thomson PDR. Felbatol. http://www.felbatol.com/pi.pdf

Online Resources

Access Data. www.accessdata.fda.gov/drugsatfda_docs/label/2018/210365lbl.pdf/2020

Brivaracetam (Briviact). www.briviact.com/2020

Cenobamate (Xcopri). www.rxlist.com › xcopri-drug/2020

Eslicarbazine (Aptiom/Sunovion). http://www.aptiom.com/2014

Ezogabine (Potiga/GSK). http://www.potiga.com/2014

Lacosamide (Vimpat/UCB). http://www.vimpat.com/2014

Perampanel (Fycompa/Eisai). http://www.fycompa.com/2014

Runfinamide (Banzel/Eisai). http://www.banzel.com/2014

Vigabatrin (Sabril/Lundbeck). http://www.sabril.net/2014

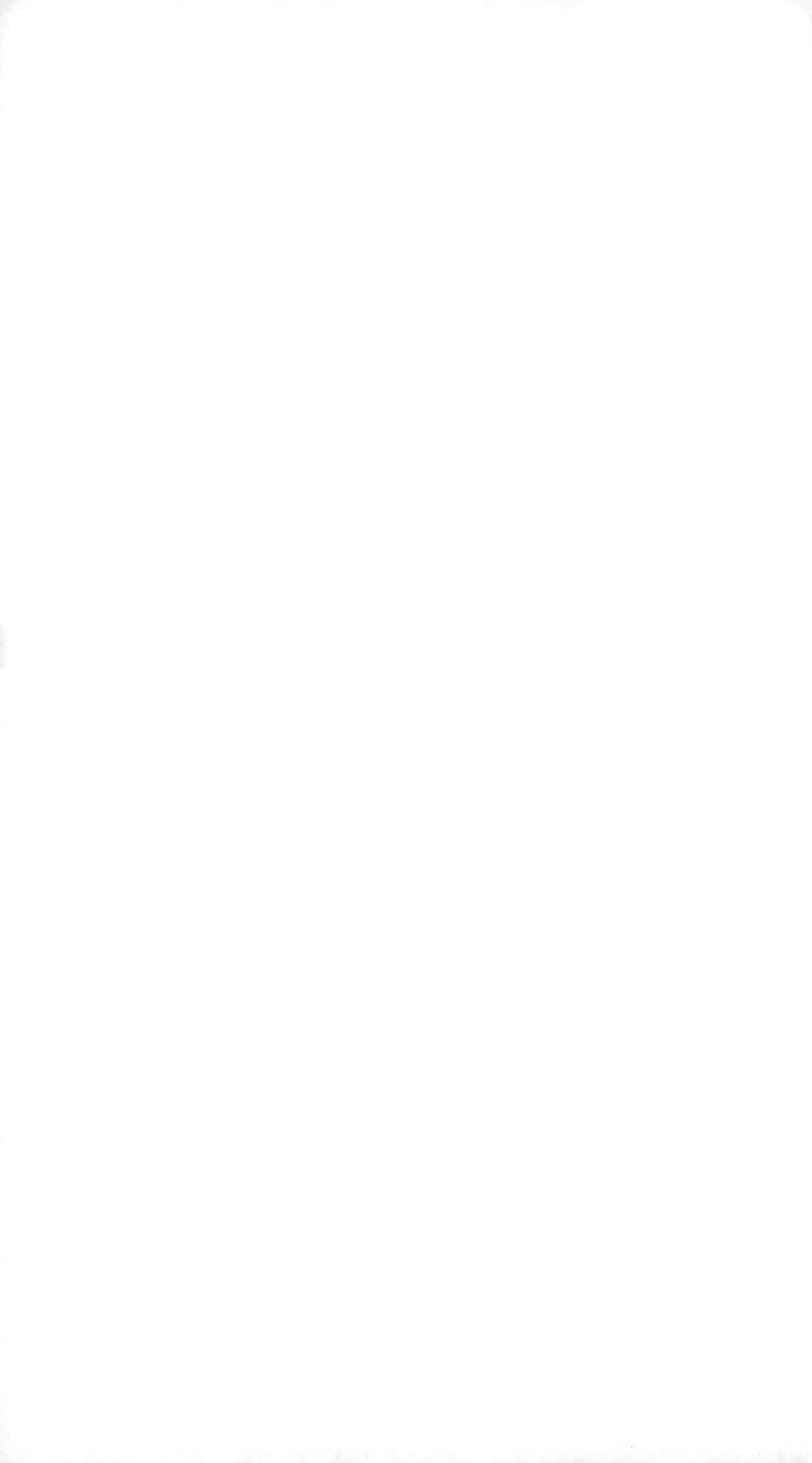

Chapter 5

Choices of Antiseizure Medications Based on Specific Epilepsy Syndromes and Seizure Types

Variables that affect the suitability of a specific antiseizure medication (ASM) for patients with epilepsy include the following (Glauser et al., 2006):

- *ASM-specific variables*: Seizure type or epilepsy syndrome, adverse effects, and drug interactions and formulations (also see Chapter 2 and Chapter 6)
- *Patient-specific variables*: Age, co-medications, and comorbidities (see other chapters)
- *Nation-specific variables*: ASM availability and cost. New ASMs are more expensive than older ASMs, and this is an important issue in some patients with limited financial resources.

Table 5.1 describes the various choices of ASMs based on specific epilepsy syndromes or seizure types according to various treatment guidelines and expert opinions.

For many patients, several agents are good choices with regard to efficacy. However, for the generalized epilepsies, valproate may have the greatest efficacy. Valproate has superior efficacy for seizure control compared with topiramate, and topiramate is better than lamotrigine. Regarding adverse effects and tolerability, lamotrigine is better than valproate, and valproate is better than topiramate. With regard to time-to-treatment failure (considering both efficacy and tolerability), valproate is the most effective drug, and lamotrigine is better than topiramate in idiopathic generalized epilepsies (IGEs) (Marson et al., 2007b). Ethosuximide is efficacious for absences but has minimal effect on generalized tonic-clonic seizures. Clonazepam is suitable mainly in pure myoclonic epilepsies with no other seizure types, although it may help absences on occasion. Lacosamide, levetiracetam, perampanel, and zonisamide are also effective for tonic-clonic seizures seen in IGE. Second-line or adjunctive drugs for IGEs include most other ASMs for generalized tonic-clonic seizures and acetazolamide for absence seizures (Panayiotopoulos, 2002). Randomized prospective studies are necessary to establish the effectiveness of brivaracetam in patients with IGE; however, because it shares a similar mechanism of action as levetiracetam, many expect that it will be

Table 5.1 Choice of antiseizure medication based on specific epilepsy syndromes or seizure types. (First-choice drug is given in italics.)

Syndrome	Treatment
Neonatal seizures	*Phenobarbital* and phenytoin are commonly used, but more than 50% of patients do not respond to either drug used alone. There are reports of nasogastric or *PO* use of topiramate or levetiracetam in neonates.
Febrile convulsions	Long-term prophylactic therapy after simple febrile seizures is not recommended. Families can be advised to have rectal diazepam available for use as needed. Usually, there is no need for any therapy.
Infantile spasms	*ACTH* is possibly the best treatment. Corticosteroids could be used instead. Vigabatrin is a first-line treatment in patients with tuberous sclerosis, but concerns about retinal toxicity suggest need for serial ophthalmologic screening. Topiramate, lamotrigine, levetiracetam, nitrazepam, pyridoxine, valproate, and zonisamide are also used.
Lennox-Gastaut syndrome (LGS)	As initial therapy, *valproate* is often a preferred first agent, but lamotrigine and topiramate are also broad-spectrum ASMs with demonstrated efficacy. Lamotrigine may exacerbate myoclonic seizures in some patients. Therapy can begin with topiramate, and low to moderate doses of lamotrigine may then be considered for synergistic action. Clonazepam (for myoclonic seizures), clobazam, and levetiracetam are also used. Felbamate is often reasonably effective although it has much greater risk. Steroids may be helpful in idiopathic/cryptogenic cases. Rufinamide is approved for adjunctive treatment of seizures associated with LGS in children *age* ≥4 years. It might be preferred to other drugs as a second-line treatment for LGS when drop-attacks are frequent. Cannabidiol is indicated for the treatment of seizures associated with LGS in patients *age* ≥2 years.
Severe myoclonic epilepsy in infancy (Dravet syndrome)	*Valproate*, topiramate, benzodiazepines, phenobarbital, ethosuximide, and levetiracetam are used with variable benefits. Carbamazepine, phenytoin, vigabatrin, and lamotrigine are probably contraindicated. Stiripentol is an effective and well-tolerated therapy that markedly reduces frequency of prolonged seizures. *Stiripentol currently has Orphan Drug Status classification in the United States, but does not have full FDA approval.* Cannabidiol is indicated for the treatment of seizures associated with Dravet syndrome in patients *age* ≥2 years.
Epilepsy with myoclonic astatic seizures (Doose syndrome)	*Valproate* is the treatment of choice. Lamotrigine, ethosuximide, Benzodiazepines, acetazolamide, levetiracetam, and topiramate are also used. Carbamazepine, phenytoin, and vigabatrin are contraindicated. Rufinamide is a promising therapeutic option.

Table 5.1 (Continued)

Syndrome	Treatment
Progressive myoclonic epilepsies	*Valproate* is usually the treatment of choice. Topiramate is also effective. Benzodiazepines, phenobarbital, piracetam, and levetiracetam are also used. Steroids can be used as a last resort in many of the refractory myoclonic epilepsies. Lamotrigine is also effective, but may exacerbate myoclonic seizures.
Landau-Kleffner syndrome	As initial therapy, valproic acid or diazepam is often empirically chosen; ethosuximide, sulthiame, and/or other benzodiazepines are used. If this fails, steroids/ACTH *are* the treatment of choice (with valproate or benzodiazepines). Carbamazepine and possibly phenobarbital and phenytoin have been reported to occasionally exacerbate the syndrome. *Sulthiame is not licensed by the FDA.*
Benign rolandic epilepsy with centrotemporal spikes (BECTS; Rolandic epilepsy)	In most patients with typical focal idiopathic epilepsy syndromes, medication is not necessary. *Carbamazepine* or oxcarbazepine is commonly used, if necessary. Gabapentin was shown to be efficacious. Valproate, lamotrigine, and levetiracetam are also used. Levetiracetam is probably a better option in children with BECTS and learning disability.
Benign occipital epilepsies	Valproate, levetiracetam, or carbamazepine are often used. Clobazam can be used in seizure clusters.
Childhood absence epilepsies (CAE) and juvenile absence epilepsies (JAE)	*Ethosuximide* (in CAE), *valproate* (in JAE), and lamotrigine are commonly used. Initial choice may be based on perception of tolerability, potential cognitive effects and systemic toxicity, and urgency of need for rapid control. Levetiracetam, topiramate, zonisamide, acetazolamide, and benzodiazepines may also be used.
Juvenile myoclonic epilepsy	*Valproate* is currently the drug of choice in men and levetiracetam is the drug of choice in women. Among newer agents, there is evidence of effectiveness of lamotrigine, topiramate, and zonisamide. Benzodiazepines are also effective (but clonazepam may aggravate generalized tonic-clonic seizures).
Children with focal-onset seizures	*Carbamazepine, lamotrigine, and levetiracetam* are considered an acceptable first drug by many, as are *oxcarbazepine and lacosamide,* with choice based on tolerability and comorbidities. Zonisamide, brivaracetam, topiramate, and perampanel may also be used. Phenytoin and phenobarbital are rarely advised as first-line agents.
Adults with focal-onset seizures	*Lamotrigine, levetiracetam, lacosamide,* brivaracetam, carbamazepine, oxcarbazepine, eslicarbazepine acetate, phenytoin, topiramate, perampanel, phenobarbital, gabapentin, tiagabine, pregabalin, cenobamate, and zonisamide may all be used, with choice based on tolerability, comorbidity, coincidental beneficial effects, and cost.
Elderly with focal-onset seizures	*Lamotrigine, levetiracetam,* and lacosamide are used. Gabapentin, zonisamide, and phenytoin are alternative agents, with choice based on tolerability and comorbidities.

(*continued*)

Table 5.1 (Continued)

Syndrome	Treatment
Children with generalized tonic-clonic (GTC) seizures	Evidence favors *topiramate* among the newer ASMs. Lamotrigine, brivaracetam, lacosamide, oxcarbazepine, levetiracetam, zonisamide, valproate, carbamazepine, phenytoin, and phenobarbital are also used. Lamotrigine and felbamate offer benefit for GTC seizures in *LGS*, and many of the others probably do as well in selected patients. Selection may be based on tolerability and comorbidities in the individual patient.
Adults with GTC seizures	Valproate, lamotrigine, levetiracetam, lacosamide, brivaracetam, topiramate, zonisamide oxcarbazepine, carbamazepine, perampanel, phenytoin, and phenobarbital are all used, with choice based on tolerability and comorbidities.
Elderly with GTC seizures	Levetiracetam and lamotrigine are effective, as are nearly all other agents, with choice based on tolerability and comorbidities.
Atonic seizures	Valproate, topiramate, rufinamide, lamotrigine, levetiracetam, cannabidiol, felbamate, phenobarbital, and zonisamide are all used, with choice based on tolerability and comorbidities.
Tonic seizures	Valproate, topiramate, rufinamide, lamotrigine, clobazam, levetiracetam, cannabidiol, felbamate, phenobarbital, and zonisamide are all used, with choice based on tolerability and comorbidities.

From Shorvon (2000), Panayiotopoulos (2002), French et al. (2004), Sankar (2004), Wheless et al. (2005), Glauser et al. (2006), von Stülpnagel et al. (2012), Wirrell et al. (2013), Conry et al. (2014), Coppola et al. (2014).

proved efficacious. In a syndromic approach, there is strong evidence-based data to support the use of valproate and ethosuximide for the treatment of childhood absence seizures; valproate, lamotrigine, and levetiracetam are appropriate agents in patients with juvenile myoclonic epilepsy; valproate, topiramate, lacosamide, lamotrigine, levetiracetam, and perampanel are appropriate drugs for patients with IGE and generalized tonic-clonic seizures only (Asadi-Pooya and Homayoun, 2020; Beydoun and D'Souza, 2012; Machado et al., 2013). Perampanel improves seizure outcomes for generalized tonic-clonic seizures, myoclonic seizures, and absence seizures in patients with IGE, with few discontinuations due to adverse events (Villanueva et al., 2018). While prospective randomized trials do not exist, carbamazepine, brivaracetam, and phenytoin can be used as an alternative treatment options for drug-resistant IGE, especially in patients in whom the main seizure type is generalized tonic-clonic seizures (Kenyon et al., 2014).

Importantly, some ASMs are generally ill-advised in IGEs. These ASMs include phenytoin, carbamazepine, oxcarbazepine, gabapentin, tiagabine, and vigabatrin, and their use is one possible cause of pseudo-intractability (Asadi-Pooya et al., 2013). These drugs may aggravate myoclonus (Sazgar and Bourgeois, 2005). Rarely, carbamazepine may exacerbate absence seizures.

In focal epilepsies, many drugs are potentially good choices with regard to efficacy, and there is probably little difference in this regard. Adverse-effect profiles, pharmacokinetic properties, and coincidental effects differ among various drugs, and these often dictate choice of therapy. We favor the use of ASMs that are neither enzyme inducers nor inhibitors and prefer those that have limited interactions with other drugs (e.g., lacosamide, lamotrigine, and levetiracetam). No studies exist that compare all drugs, and few have been conducted that compare several agents. These studies can serve to guide therapeutic choices, but clinicians must use their experience and judgment when prescribing ASMs because patient populations in the published studies may differ from theirs, and other circumstances may render study conclusions inapplicable. In a comparison study, lamotrigine had the same efficacy as carbamazepine in regard to seizure control for focal seizures, and both drugs were superior to oxcarbazepine, which had efficacy similar to topiramate. Gabapentin had the least efficacy.

With respect to adverse effects and tolerability, lamotrigine was better than gabapentin, gabapentin was better than oxcarbazepine, and oxcarbazepine was better than carbamazepine and topiramate. With regard to time-to-treatment failure (considering both efficacy and tolerability), lamotrigine was the best, oxcarbazepine and carbamazepine were next, and they were better than either topiramate or gabapentin (Marson et al., 2007a).

Table 5.2 shows various indications for ASMs in the treatment of patients with epilepsy according to US Food and Drug Administration (FDA)

Table 5.2 Government-authorized indications for marketing of drugs for epilepsy

Acetazolamide	*Absence seizures, unlocalized seizures*
Brivaracetam	*Brivaracetam is indicated for the treatment of focal-onset seizures in patients ≥4 years of age. As the safety of brivaracetam injection in pediatric patients has not been established, brivaracetam injection is indicated for the treatment of focal-onset seizures only in adult patients (≥16 years).*
Cannabidiol	*Cannabidiol is indicated for the treatment of seizures associated with Lennox-Gastaut syndrome or Dravet syndrome in patients ≥2 years of age.*
Carbamazepine	*Focal-onset seizures with complex symptomatology (psychomotor, temporal lobe). Generalized tonic-clonic seizures. Mixed seizure patterns, which include the above, or other focal-onset or generalized seizures. Absence seizures do not appear to be controlled by carbamazepine.*
Cenobamate	*Cenobamate is indicated for the treatment of focal-onset seizures in adult patients.*
Clonazepam	*Alone or as an adjunct in the treatment of Lennox-Gastaut syndrome (petit mal variant), akinetic seizures, and myoclonic seizures. In patients with absence seizures who have failed to respond to succinimides, clonazepam may be useful.*

(continued)

Table 5.2 (Continued)	
Clobazam	*Adjunctive therapy for the treatment of seizures associated with Lennox-Gastaut syndrome.*
Eslicarbazepine	*Adjunctive treatment of focal-onset seizures.*
Ethosuximide	*Absence epilepsy.*
Ezogabine	*Adjunctive treatment of focal-onset seizures in patients ≥18 years who have responded inadequately to several alternative treatments and for whom the benefits outweigh the risk of retinal abnormalities and potential decline in visual acuity. (This drug is no longer available in the United States.)*
Felbamate	*Felbamate is not indicated as a first-line antiepileptic treatment (has serious warnings). Monotherapy or adjunctive therapy in the treatment of focal-onset seizures, with and without generalization in adults with epilepsy and as adjunctive therapy in the treatment of focal-onset and generalized seizures associated with Lennox-Gastaut syndrome in children.*
Gabapentin	*Adjunctive therapy in the treatment of focal-onset seizures with and without secondary generalization in patients >12 years of age with epilepsy. Adjunctive therapy in the treatment of focal-onset seizures in pediatric patients age 3–12 years.*
Lacosamide	*Adjunctive therapy in the treatment of focal-onset seizures in patients with epilepsy aged ≥17 years. Idiopathic generalized epilepsy for generalized tonic-clonic seizures for patients aged ≥4 years.*
Lamotrigine	*Adjunctive therapy for focal-onset seizures, the generalized seizures of Lennox-Gastaut syndrome, and primary generalized tonic-clonic seizures in adults and pediatric patients (≥2 years). Conversion to monotherapy in adults with focal-onset seizures who are receiving treatment with carbamazepine, phenytoin, phenobarbital, primidone, or valproate as the single ASM.*
Levetiracetam	*Adjunctive therapy in the treatment of focal-onset seizures in adults and children ≥1 month of age. Adjunctive therapy in the treatment of myoclonic seizures in adults and adolescents ≥12 years of age with juvenile myoclonic epilepsy. Adjunctive therapy in the treatment of primary generalized tonic-clonic seizures in adults and children ≥6 years with idiopathic generalized epilepsy.*
Oxcarbazepine	*Monotherapy or adjunctive therapy in the treatment of focal-onset seizures in adults and as monotherapy in the treatment of focal-onset seizures in children aged ≥4 years, and as adjunctive therapy in children aged ≥2 years.*
Perampanel	*Adjunctive therapy for the treatment of focal-onset seizures in patients with epilepsy aged ≥4 years and primary generalized tonic-clonic seizures for patients aged ≥12 years.*
Phenobarbital	*Treatment of generalized tonic-clonic and cortical local seizures. Emergency control of certain acute convulsive episodes, such as those associated with status epilepticus, cholera, eclampsia, meningitis, tetanus, and toxic reactions to strychnine or local anesthetics.*
Phenytoin	*Control of generalized tonic-clonic and focal-onset seizures and prevention and treatment of seizures occurring during or following neurosurgery.*

Table 5.2 (Continued)	
Pregabalin	*Adjunctive therapy in the treatment of focal-onset seizures in adults.*
Rufinamide	*Adjunctive treatment of seizures associated with Lennox-Gastaut syndrome in children ≥4 years and adults.*
Tiagabine	*Adjunctive therapy in adults and children ≥12 years in the treatment of focal-onset seizures.*
Topiramate	*Topiramate is indicated for initial monotherapy in patients ≥10 years with focal-onset or generalized tonic-clonic (GTC) seizures; adjunctive therapy for adults and pediatric patients age 2–16 years with focal-onset seizures or generalized tonic-clonic seizures; adjunctive therapy for patients ≥2 years and older with seizures associated with Lennox-Gastaut syndrome.*
Valproate	*Monotherapy and adjunctive therapy in the treatment of patients with focal-onset seizures that occur either in isolation or in association with other types of seizures; sole or adjunctive therapy in the treatment of simple and complex absence seizures; adjunct for the treatment of patients with multiple seizure types that include absence seizures.*
Vigabatrin	*For focal seizures, as an adjunctive therapy, in patients ≥2 years who have responded inadequately to several alternative treatments. Also, in epileptic spasms in infants 1 month to 2 years of age.*
Zonisamide	*Adjunctive therapy in the treatment of focal-onset seizures in adults with epilepsy.*
From Beghi (2004), French et al. (2004); see also individual drug websites listed in the Online Resources at the end of this chapter and Drug Reference (http://www.neurotransmitter.net/epilepsy_drug_reference.html), and RxList (http://www.rxlist.com).	

guidelines. These "indications" are based on the studies done by pharmaceutical companies for marketing purposes and do not reflect treatment guidelines developed using expert opinion. Hence, these marketing indications are rather limited and generally do not reflect the full spectrum of efficacy or use. These indications are based on conclusions drawn from trial data submitted to government regulatory agencies. These agencies typically take a strict view and approve an ASM only for the specific circumstance tested. For example, the FDA will only approve a drug for adjunctive therapy if the investigational trial submitted for review has been conducted using that drug only as adjunctive therapy (i.e., added on to other drugs). This approach is contrary to medical experience and sensible science. Testing in experimental models does not support the concept that any drug is only effective as an adjunctive agent; every approved agent is efficacious in experimental models when given alone. In addition, human trials may have demonstrated efficacy for indications and conditions not included in official labeling; however, if a pharmaceutical company has not submitted these data to the FDA and requested approval to market the drug for that purpose, then this indication will never be noted in official regulations. Therefore, government-approved indications are often incompatible with clinical practice.

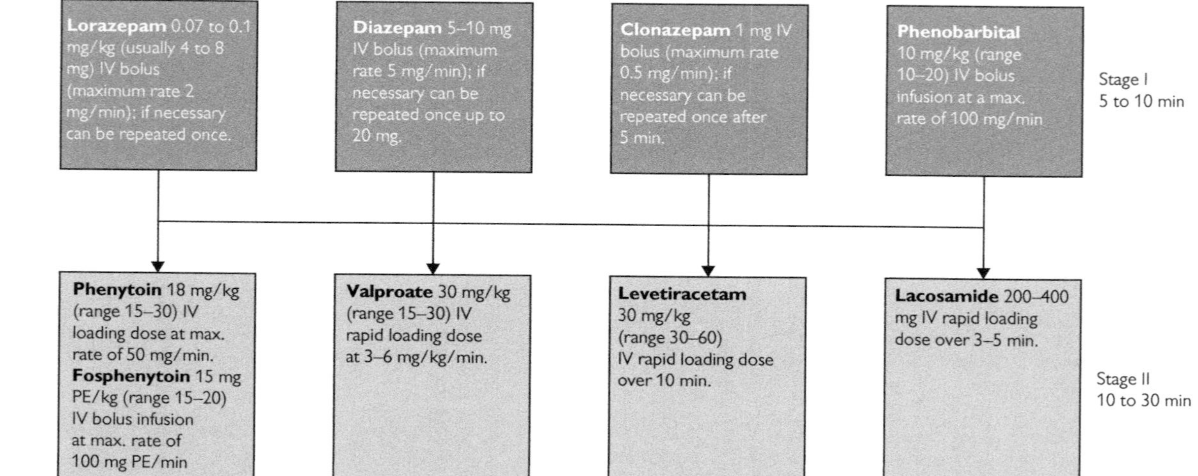

Figure 5.1 Staged treatment protocol for early (stage I) and established (stage II) convulsive status epilepticus. Timelines for stages I and II are general approximations and may vary depending on clinical circumstances, cause, and age of the patient.

Reprinted with permission from: Trinka E, Kälviäinen R. 25 years of advances in the definition, classification and treatment of status epilepticus. *Seizure*. 2017;44:65–73.

Table 5.3 Highly sedating anti-seizure medications for the treatment of refractory status epilepticus

Drug	**Loading dose**	**Maintenance infusion rate**	*Adverse effects*
Midazolam	0.2–0.4 mg/kg IV every 5 min until seizures controlled.	0.1–2.0 mg/kg/hr	*Respiratory depression, hypotension* *Maximum dose: 2 mg/kg*
Propofol	2 mg/kg IV every 5 min until seizures controlled.	30–200 µg/kg/min	*Hypotension, propofol infusion syndrome* *Maximum dose: 10 mg/kg* *Avoid ≥80 µg/kg/min for ≥48 hr*
Pentobarbital	*5 mg/kg IV up to 50 mg/min every 5 min until seizures are controlled or a maximum loading dose of 15 mg/kg*	*0.5–5 mg/kg/hr*	*Hypotension, adynamic ileus, respiratory depression, hepatotoxicity, prolonged sedation*

Reprint with permission from: Rai S, Drislane FW. Treatment of refractory and super-refractory status epilepticus. *Neurotherapeutics*. 2018;15(3):697–712.

It is worth mentioning that generalized convulsive status epilepticus (SE) is a medical emergency and should be treated as soon as possible. Urgent-control ASM treatment following administration of short-acting benzodiazepines is required in all patients who present with SE unless the immediate cause is known and corrected (e.g., hypoglycemia). There are conflicting data and differences in expert opinion about which agent is best for urgent control, and the choice often varies based on individual patient features. The preferred agents that are often used for urgent control of SE after use of benzodiazepines are IV fosphenytoin/phenytoin, valproate sodium, levetiracetam, or lacosamide; in some centers, patients with convulsive SE are promptly given IV sedative or anesthetic medications including propofol, midazolam, pentobarbital, or ketamine after failure of an initial benzodiazepine dose. In patients with known epilepsy who were taking an ASM before admission, it is reasonable to provide an IV bolus of that ASM, if available, prior to initiating an additional agent (Brophy et al., 2012). Figure 5.1 shows the staged treatment protocol for early (stage I) and established (stage II) convulsive SE (Trinka and Kälviäinen, 2017). Table 5.3 shows highly sedating ASMs for the treatment of refractory SE (Rai and Drislane, 2018).

References

Asadi-Pooya AA, Emami M, Ashjazadeh N, et al. Reasons for uncontrolled seizures in adults: The impact of pseudointractability. *Seizure*. 2013;22(4):271–274.

Asadi-Pooya AA, Homayoun M. Tonic-clonic seizures in idiopathic generalized epilepsies: Prevalence, risk factors, and outcome. *Acta Neurol Scand*. 2020 Feb 6. doi:10.1111/ane.13227. [Epub ahead of print].

Beghi E. Efficacy and tolerability of the new antiepileptic drugs: Comparison of two recent guidelines. *Lancet Neurol.* 2004;3:618–621.

Beydoun A, D'Souza J. Treatment of idiopathic generalized epilepsy: A review of the evidence. *Expert Opin Pharmacother.* 2012;13(9):1283–1298.

Brophy GM, Bell R, Claassen J, et al. Guidelines for the evaluation and management of status epilepticus. *Neurocrit Care*. 2012;17(1):3–23.

Conry JA, Ng YT, Kernitsky L, et al., OV-1004 Study Investigators. Stable dosages of clobazam for Lennox-Gastaut syndrome are associated with sustained drop-seizure and total-seizure improvements over 3 years. *Epilepsia*. 2014;55(4):558–567.

Coppola G, Besag F, Cusmai R, et al. Current role of rufinamide in the treatment of childhood epilepsy: Literature review and treatment guidelines. *Eur J Paediatr Neurol*. 2014;18(6):685–690.

Drug reference for FDA approved epilepsy drugs. Epocrates, Inc. http://www.neurotransmitter.net/epilepsy_drug_reference.html/2014.

French JA, Kanner AM, Bautista J, et al. Efficacy and tolerability of the new antiepileptic drugs, II: Treatment of refractory epilepsy: Report of the Therapeutics and Technology Assessment Subcommittee and Quality Standards Subcommittee of the American Academy of Neurology and the American Epilepsy Society. *Neurology*. 2004;62;1261–1273.

Glauser T, Ben-Menachem E, Bourgeois B, et al. ILAE treatment guidelines: Evidence-based analysis of antiepileptic drug efficacy and effectiveness as initial monotherapy for epileptic seizures and syndromes. *Epilepsia*. 2006;47:1094–1120.

Kenyon K, Mintzer S, Nei M. Carbamazepine treatment of generalized tonic-clonic seizures in idiopathic generalized epilepsy. *Seizure*. 2014;23(3):234–236.

Machado RA, García VF, Astencio AG, Cuartas VB. Efficacy and tolerability of lamotrigine in juvenile myoclonic epilepsy in adults: A prospective, unblinded randomized controlled trial. *Seizure*. 2013;22(10):846–855.

Marson AG, Al-Kharusi AM, Alwaidh M. The SANAD Study of effectiveness of carbamazepine, gabapentin, lamotrigine, oxcarbazepine, or topiramate for treatment of partial epilepsy: An unblinded randomized controlled trial. *Lancet*. 2007;369:1000–1015.a

Marson AG, Al-Kharusi AM, Alwaidh M. The SANAD study of effectiveness of valproate, lamotrigine, or topiramate for generalized and unclassifiable epilepsy: An unblinded randomized controlled trial. *Lancet*, 2007;369:1016–1026.b

Panayiotopoulos CP. *A Clinical Guide to Epileptic Syndromes and Their Treatment*. Oxford: Bladon Medical Publishing; 2002.

Rai S, Drislane FW. Treatment of refractory and super-refractory status epilepticus. *Neurotherapeutics*. 2018;15(3):697–712.

RxList. The Internet drug index. RxList Inc. http://www.rxlist.com/2014.

Sankar R. Initial treatment of epilepsy with antiepileptic drugs: pediatric issues. *Neurology*. 2004;63:S30–S39.

Sazgar M, Bourgeois BFD. Aggravation of epilepsy by antiepileptic drugs. *Pediatric Neurol*. 2005;33:227–234.

Shorvon S. *Handbook of Epilepsy Treatment*. Oxford: Blackwell Science; 2000.

Trinka E, Kälviäinen R. 25 years of advances in the definition, classification and treatment of status epilepticus. *Seizure*. 2017;44:65–73.

Villanueva V, Montoya J, Castillo A, et al. Perampanel in routine clinical use in idiopathic generalized epilepsy: The 12-month GENERAL study. *Epilepsia*. 2018;59(9):1740–1752.

von Stülpnagel C, Coppola G, Striano P, Müller A, Staudt M, Kluger G. First long-term experience with the orphan drug rufinamide in children with myoclonic-astatic epilepsy (Doose syndrome). *Eur J Paediatr Neurol*. 2012;16(5):459–463.

Wheless JW, Clarke DF, Carpenter D. Treatment of pediatric epilepsy: Expert opinion, 2005. *J Child Neurol*. 2005;20(Suppl 11):S1–S56.

Wirrell EC, Laux L, Franz DN, et al. Stiripentol in Dravet syndrome: Results of a retrospective U.S. study. *Epilepsia*. 2013;54(9):1595–1604.

Online Resources

Brivaracetam (Briviact). www.briviact.com/2020

Cannabidiol (Epidiolex). www.epidiolex.com/2020

Cenobamate (Xcopri). reference.medscape.com/drug/xcopri-cenobamate-1000328/2020

Eslicarbazine acetate (Aptiom). www.aptiom.com/2014

Ezogabine (Potiga). www.potiga.com/2014

Lacosamide (Vimpat). www.vimpat.com/2014

Perampanel (Fycompa). us.eisai.com/wps/wcm/connect/Eisai/Home/Our.../FYCOMPA/2014

Runfinamide (Banzel). www.banzel.com/2014

Vigabatrin (Sabril). drugstorenews.com/fda-approves-new-indication-lundbecks-sabril/2020

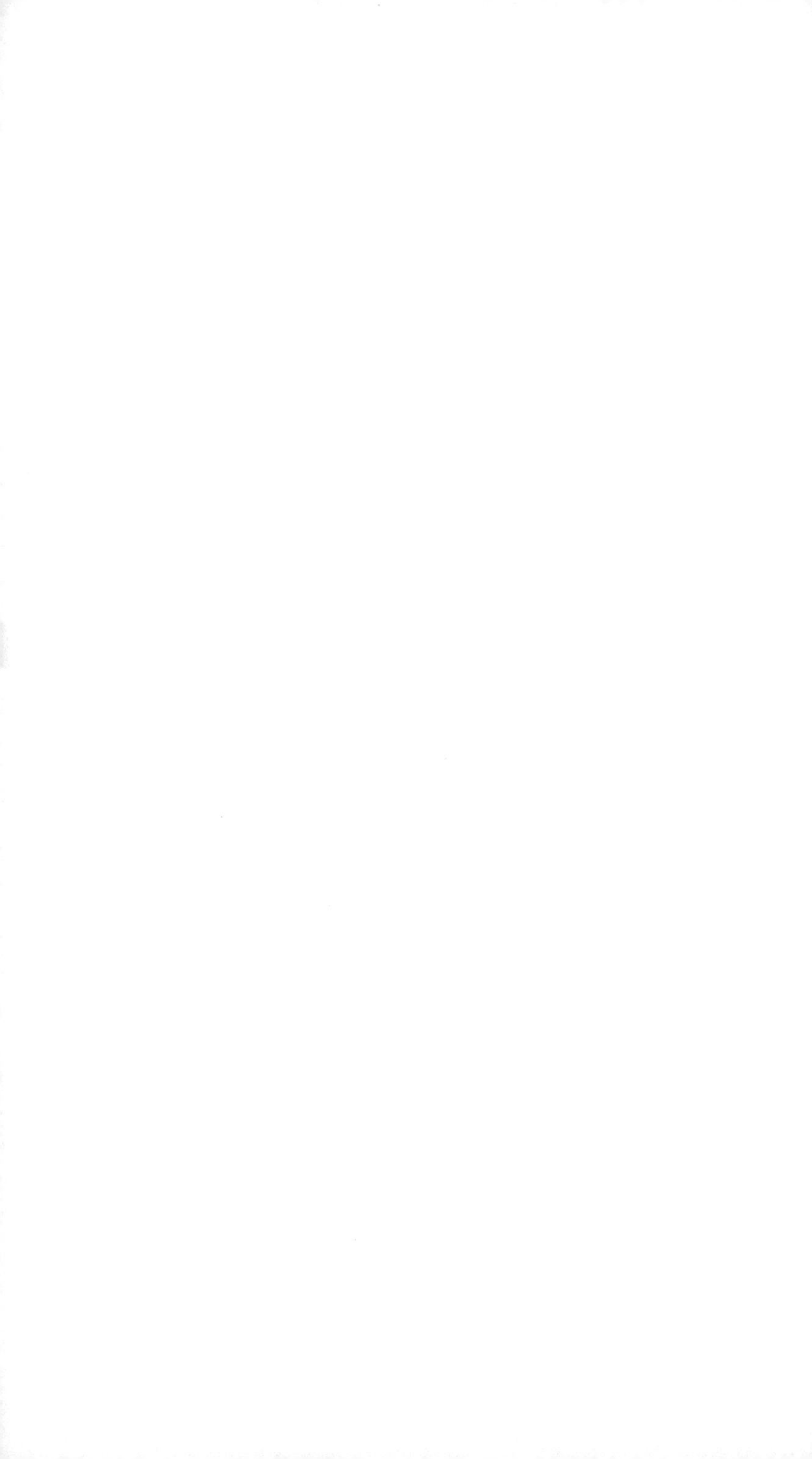

Chapter 6

Clinically Important Drug Interactions with Antiseizure Medications

Drug interactions can occur whenever two or more drugs are administered simultaneously. Most clinically important antiseizure medication (ASM) interactions with other drugs result from induction or inhibition of drug-metabolizing hepatic enzymes or significant protein binding properties. However, other mechanisms, including pharmacodynamic interactions, sometimes play a role. Unfortunately, many ASMs are substrates, inducers, or inhibitors of hepatic enzymes and have significant protein binding (Table 6.1). Therefore, drug interactions are common in patients with epilepsy (Anderson et al., 2004; Patsalos, 2013; Patsalos et al., 2002; Perucca, 2005). Drug interactions that cause a more than 50% change in drug exposure (area under the plasma drug concentration versus time curve [AUC]) or plasma levels usually require dosage adjustments (Bialer, 2005). Typically, cytochrome P-450 enzyme inducers (e.g., carbamazepine, phenytoin, phenobarbital, primidone, oxcarbazepine, topiramate) take days to weeks to upregulate the target enzymes; however, enzyme inhibitors (e.g., valproate) have a more immediate effect. Therefore, for example, initiation of as little as 500 mg of valproate per day may necessitate an immediate 50% reduction of the dose of chronically used lamotrigine (Pollard an Delanty, 2007).

Lacosamide, levetiracetam, brivaracetam, pregabalin, vigabatrin, and gabapentin rarely produce clinically significant interactions with other drugs. Lacosamide should be used with caution in patients on concomitant medications that affect cardiac conduction (sodium channel blockers, beta-blockers, calcium channel blockers, potassium channel blockers), including those that prolong PR interval (including sodium channel–blocking ASMs), because of a risk of AV block, bradycardia, or ventricular tachyarrhythmia. In such patients, obtaining an electrocardiogram (ECG) before beginning lacosamide and after lacosamide is titrated to steady-state is recommended. Patients with renal or hepatic impairment who are taking strong inhibitors of CYP3A4 and CYP2C9 (e.g., valproate) may have a significant increase in exposure to lacosamide; dose reduction may be necessary in these patients (lacosamide; www.vimpathcp.com/vimpat-prescribing-information.pdf/2020). Coadministration with rifampin decreases brivaracetam plasma concentrations, likely because of CYP2C19 induction. Because brivaracetam can increase plasma concentrations of phenytoin, phenytoin levels should be monitored in patients when

Table 6.1 Effects of antiseizure medications on hepatic enzymes and enzymes involved in antiseizure medications metabolism

Antiseizure medication	Effect		
	Induces	Inhibits	Enzymes involved in metabolism
Acetazolamide	—	CYP3A4	—
Brivaracetam	—	—	CYP2C19
Cannabidiol	CYP1A2 and CYP2B6	UGT1A9, UGT2B7, CYP2C8, CYP1A2, CYP2B6, CYP2C19 and CYP2C9	CYP3A4 and CYP2C19
Carbamazepine	CYP1A2, CYP2C, CYP3A4, UGTs	—	CYP1A2, CYP2C8, CYP3A4
Cenobamate	CYP2B6 and CYP3A4	CYP2C19	UGT2B7, UGT2B4, CYP2E1, CYP2A6, CYP2B6, CYP2C19, and CYP3A4/5
Clonazepam	—	—	CYP3A4
Eslicarbazepine acetate	CYP3A4	CYP2C19	Esterases, Uridine diphosphate-glucuronosyltransferase
Ethosuximide	—	—	CYP3A4, CYP2B, CYP2E1
Ezogabine	—	—	uridine 5'-diphosphate (UDP)-glucuronyltransferases
Phenobarbital/ primidone	CYP1A2, CYP2A6, CYP2B, CYP2C, CYP3A4, UGTs	—	CYP2C9, CYP2C19, CYP2E1
Phenytoin	CYP1A2, CYP2B, CYP2C, CYP3A4, UGTs	—	CYP2C8, CYP2C9, CYP2C19
Valproic acid	—	CYP2C9, UGTs, epoxide hydrolase	CYP2A6, CYP2C9, CYP2C19, UGTs, mitochondrial oxidases
Felbamate	CYP3 A4	CYP2C19, β-oxidation	CYP2E1, CYP3A4
Gabapentin	—	—	—
Lacosamide	—	—	CYP3A4, CYP2C9, and CYP2C19
Lamotrigine	UGTs (weak inducer)	—	UGTs
Levetiracetam	—	—	—
Oxcarbazepine	CYP3A4, UGTs	CYP2C19	UGTs

Table 6.1 (Continued)

Antiseizure medication	Effect		
	Induces	**Inhibits**	**Enzymes involved in metabolism**
Perampanel	CYP2B6 and CYP3A4/5 and UGTs (weak inducer)	CYP2C8, CYP3A4 and UGTs (weak inhibitor)	CYP3A4 and/or CYP3A5
Pregabalin	—	—	—
Rufinamide	CYP 3A4 (weakly)	CYP 2E1 (weakly)	Carboxylesterases
Tiagabine	—	—	CYP3A4
Topiramate	CYP3A4,* β-oxidation	CYP2C19	Inducible CYP isoforms
Vigabatrin	—	—	—
Zonisamide	—	—	CYP3A4

CYP, cytochrome P-450 isozyme; UGT, UDP glucuronosyltransferase.

*Dose-dependent induction.

From Patsalos et al. (2013) and Anderson (2004).

concomitant brivaracetam is added to or discontinued from ongoing phenytoin therapy. Coadministration of brivaracetam with carbamazepine may increase exposure to carbamazepine-epoxide, the active metabolite of carbamazepine, although available data did not show any safety concerns (brivaracetam; www.briviact.com/2020).

Eslicarbazepine acetate, lamotrigine, clobazam, perampanel, rufinamide, tiagabine, topiramate, and zonisamide have moderate drug interactions.

Phenobarbital, phenytoin, carbamazepine, primidone, cannabidiol, cenobamate, valproate, and felbamate have extensive and important interactions with many drugs.

Clinically Important Interactions Between Antiseizure Medications and Other Drugs

Interactions Resulting in Decreased Antiseizure Medication Plasma Levels

Coadministration of the combined contraceptive pills causes a decrease in serum lamotrigine level by about 50%, which is likely due to the stimulation of uridine glucuronosyltransferase activity by the steroids. This interaction can result in reduced seizure control in some women. Coadministration with a strong CYP3A4 or CYP2C19 inducer will decrease cannabidiol plasma concentrations (cannabidiol; www.epidiolex.com/2020). Other examples for a clinically important decrease in serum ASM concentration due to drug interactions include the marked inhibition of the gastrointestinal absorption of phenytoin, carbamazepine, and phenobarbital given concurrently with antacids; the decrease in serum valproic acid concentration after addition of some antibiotics of the carbapenem class; the decrease in serum phenytoin levels after the addition of ciprofloxacin; the decrease in serum perampanel levels after the addition of rifampin; and decreased serum carbamazepine, perampanel, and phenytoin levels due to increase in their metabolism by St. John's wort (an over-the-counter herb purported as possibly useful in mood stabilization and stress relief) (Novak et al., 2004; Patsalos, 2013; Perucca, 2005; Pollard and Delanty, 2007).

Interactions Resulting in Increased Antiseizure Medication Plasma Levels

Interactions resulting in elevated serum ASM concentrations have been reported mostly with carbamazepine, phenytoin, and phenobarbital. Clarithromycin and erythromycin can increase carbamazepine plasma levels and cause serious adverse effects by inhibiting metabolism of this agent. Similarly, fluoxetine, trazodone, fluconazole, ketoconazole, isoniazid, metronidazole, cimetidine, and verapamil can increase carbamazepine plasma levels. Omeprazole, cimetidine, allopurinol, amiodarone, ketoconazole, fluconazole, isoniazid, sertraline, fluoxetine, fluorouracil, and tamoxifen may increase phenytoin levels by inhibiting its metabolism, and sertraline and antiretroviral protease inhibitors may inhibit lamotrigine metabolism and increase its plasma concentrations (Novak et al., 2004; Perucca, 2005; Pollard and Delanty, 2007). Diltiazem, an inhibitor of CYP3A4, has been reported to increase plasma carbamazepine and phenytoin levels significantly, resulting in toxicity (Novak et al., 2004). Acetazolamide may increase plasma carbamazepine levels by a similar mechanism (Spina et al., 1996). Chloramphenicol may increase plasma phenobarbital levels, and cimetidine, isoniazid, and sertraline may increase plasma valproate levels (Pollard and Delanty, 2007). Coadministration with a moderate or strong inhibitor of CYP3A4 or CYP2C19 will increase cannabidiol plasma concentrations, which may result in a greater risk of adverse reactions (cannabidiol; www.epidiolex.com/2020).

Interactions Resulting in Decreased Plasma Levels of Other Drugs

Patients treated with enzyme-inducing ASMs are susceptible to important drug-drug interactions mediated by hepatic microsomal enzyme induction. The list of such interactions is extensive (Table 6.2). Because of practical difficulties in compensating for such interactions, effective use of some of these drugs may not be feasible in enzyme-induced patients (Novak et al., 2004). In some patients (e.g., patients with HIV/AIDS [Mullin et al., 2004; Romanelli et al., 2000] or those requiring anticancer therapy [Oberndorfer et al., 2005; Sperling and Ko, 2006]), the use of ASMs without enzyme-inducing properties is clearly preferred. ASMs that induce metabolism of at least one of the components of contraceptive pills include carbamazepine, eslicarbazepine acetate, cenobamate, felbamate, lamotrigine, oxcarbazepine, perampanel,

Table 6.2 Drugs with which hepatic enzyme inducer antiseizure medications have clinically important interactions

Drug category	Specific drugs
Anticoagulant drugs	Dicoumarol, warfarin
Antidepressant drugs	Amitriptyline, amoxapine, bupropion, clomipramine, desipramine, doxepin, imipramine, mianserin, nortriptyline, protriptyline, trimipramine
Anti-infectious agents	Albendazole, doxycycline, griseofulvin, itraconazole, ketoconazole, mebendazole, metronidazole, voriconazole
Antineoplastic agents	9-Aminocampthotecin, busulfan, ćyclophosphamide, etoposide, ifosfamide, irinotecan, methotrexate, nitrosureas, paclitaxel, procarbazine, tamoxifen, teniposide, thiotepa, topotecan, vinca alkaloids, vincristine
Antipsychotic agents	Chlorpromazine, clozapine, haloperidol, risperidone, quetiapine
Antivirals	Amprenavir, atazanavir, delavirdine, indinavir, nelfinavir, ritonavir, saquinavir, zidovudine
Benzodiazepines	Alprazolam, clonazepam, diazepam, lorazepam, midazolam
Calcium channel blockers	Amlodipine, bepridil, diltiazem, felodipine, isradipine, nisoldipine, nicardipine, nifedipine, nimodipine, nivaldipine, nisoldipine, nitrendipine, verapamil
Cardiovascular drugs	Amiodarone, atrovastatin, digoxin, disopyramide, lovastatin, procainamide, propranolol, metoprolol, timolol, quinidine, simvastatin
Corticosteroids	Cortisone, betamethasone, dexamethasone, hydrocortisone, methylprednisolone, prednisolone, prednisone, triamcinolone
Immunosuppressants	Cyclosporine, sirolimus, tacrolimus
Oral contraceptives	Conjugated estrogens, ethinyl estradiol, levonorgestrel, norethindrone
Miscellaneous	Methadone, theophylline

From Spina et al. (1996), Romanelli et al. (2000), Patsalos et al.(2002), Anderson (2004), Mullin et al. (2004), Novak et al. (2004), Bialer (2005), Oberndorfer et al. (2005), Perucca (2005), Sperling and Ko (2006), and Pollard and Delanty (2007).

phenobarbital, phenytoin, primidone, rufinamide, and topiramate (doses >200 mg/day). In patients taking both oral contraceptive pills and one of these ASMs, a double-barrier method or an interuterine device (IUD) may be necessary for effective birth control (Pollard and Delanty, 2007).

Interactions Resulting in Increased Plasma Levels of Other Drugs

Valproic acid, due to its enzyme-inhibiting properties, may increase the plasma levels of a variety of drugs, including lorazepam, nimodipine, paroxetine, amitriptyline, nortriptyline, nitrosoureas, and etoposide. For some, such as amitriptyline and nortriptyline, and for some antineoplastic drugs, these interactions may cause toxicity (Facts and Comparisons, 2007; Perucca, 2005). In addition, valproate is a highly protein-bound agent and may displace some drugs (e.g., warfarin) from their binding sites leading to an increased effect (Facts and Comparisons, 2007). The N-acetyl metabolite of ezogabine inhibited P-glycoprotein-mediated transport of digoxin in a concentration-dependent manner, indicating that this metabolite may inhibit renal clearance of digoxin. Serum levels of digoxin should be monitored when ezogabine is prescribed simultaneously. Coadministration of cannabidiol increases plasma concentrations of drugs that are metabolized by CYP2C19 (cannabidiol; www.epidiolex.com/2020).

Note: Direct oral anticoagulants (DOACs) (apixaban, dabigatran, edoxaban, and rivaroxaban) are increasingly prescribed among the general population because they are considered to be associated with lower bleeding risk than warfarin and they do not require coagulation monitoring. In addition, DOACs are increasingly concomitantly prescribed in patients with epilepsy who are taking ASMs. As a result, potential drug-drug interactions may cause an increased risk of DOAC-related bleeding or a reduced antithrombotic efficacy. Enzyme-inducing ASMs, acting on cytochrome P450 iso-enzymes, and especially on CYP3A4, such as phenobarbital, phenytoin, and carbamazepine are more likely to significantly reduce the anticoagulant effect of DOACs (especially rivaroxaban, apixaban, and edoxaban). Other ASMs not affecting CYP or P-glycoprotein significantly, such as lamotrigine, are not likely to affect DOACs efficacy. Lacosamide, which does not affect CYP activity significantly, appears to have a safe profile, even though its effects on P-glycoprotein are not well-known yet. Levetiracetam exerts only a potential effect on P-glycoprotein activity and thus it appears safe as well (Galgani et al., 2018).

Drug Interactions Between ASMs

Most clinically important ASM interactions with other ASMs result from induction or inhibition of drug metabolizing hepatic enzymes. Because often the treatment of epilepsy is life-long and patients are commonly prescribed polytherapy with other ASMs, interactions are an important consideration in the treatment of epilepsy. For new ASMs, their propensity to interact is particularly important because they are often prescribed as adjunctive polytherapy (Table 6.3) (Patsalos, 2013). For example, coadministration of cannabidiol produces a three-fold or greater increase in plasma concentrations of N-desmethylclobazam, the active metabolite of clobazam (a substrate of CYP2C19) (cannabidiol; www.epidiolex.com/2020). Cenobamate also has potential to increase drug levels of other agents, particularly phenytoin.

Table 6.3 Metabolic characteristics of new antiseizure medications (ASMs) and their propensity to interact with other ASMs

ASM	Metabolism (hepatic)	Propensity to interact metabolically with other ASMs	
		Affects other ASMs	Affected by other ASMs
Brivaracetam	Substantial (90%)	Minimal	Non-interacting
Cannabidiol	Substantial	Substantial	Substantial
Cenobamate	Substantial (>90%)	Substantial	Substantial
Eslicarbazepine acetate.	Substantial (>99%)	Minimal	Minimal
Felbamate	Moderate (50%)	Minimal	Minimal
Gabapentin	Not metabolized	Non-interacting	Non-interacting
Lacosamide	Moderate (60%; demethylation)	Non-interacting	Minimal
Lamotrigine	Substantial (90%)	Minimal	Substantial
Levetiracetam	Minimal (30%; nonhepatic)	Non-interacting	Non-interacting
Oxcarbazepine	Substantial (90%)	Minimal	Minimal
Perampanel	Substantial (>98%)	Minimal	Moderate
Pregabalin	Not metabolized	Non-interacting	Non-interacting
Retigabine (ezogabine)	Moderate (70–80%)	Minimal	Minimal
Rufinamide	Substantial (98%)	Minimal	Minimal
Stiripentol	Moderate (75%)	Substantial	Substantial
Tiagabine	Substantial (98%)	Minimal	Minimal
Topiramate	Moderate (50%)	Minimal	Minimal
Vigabatrin	Not metabolized	Non-interacting	Non-interacting
Zonisamide	Moderate (65%)	Minimal	Minimal

Adapted from: Patsalos PN. *Clin Pharmacokinet.* 2013;52(11):927–966.

References

Anderson GD. Pharmacogenetics and enzyme induction/inhibition properties of antiepileptic drugs. *Neurology*. 2004;63:S3–S8.

Bialer M. The pharmacokinetics and interactions of new antiepileptic drugs. *Therapeutic Drug Monitoring*. 2005;27:722–726.

Facts and Comparisons. *Drug Facts and Comparisons*. St. Louis: Wolters Kluwer Health/Facts and Comparisons; 2007.

Galgani A, Palleria C, Iannone LF, et al. Pharmacokinetic interactions of clinical interest between direct oral anticoagulants and antiepileptic drugs. *Front Neurol.* 2018;9:1067.

Mullin P, Green G, Bakshi R. Special populations: The management of seizures in HIV-positive patients. *Curr Neurol Neurosci Rep*. 2004;4:308–314.

Novak PH, Ekin-Daukes S, Simpson CR, Milne RM, Helms P, McLay JS. Acute drug prescribing to children on chronic antiepilepsy therapy and the potential for adverse drug interactions in primary care. *Br J Clin Pharmacol.* 2004;59:712–717.

Oberndorfer S, Piribauer M, Marosi C, Lahrmann H, Hitzenberger P, Grisold W. P-450 enzyme inducing and non-enzyme inducing antiepileptics in glioblastoma patients treated with standard chemotherapy. *J Neurooncol.* 2005;72:255–260.

Patsalos PN. Drug interactions with the newer antiepileptic drugs (AEDs). Part 1: Pharmacokinetic and pharmacodynamic interactions between AEDs. *Clin Pharmacokinet.* 2013;52(11):927–966.

Patsalos PN, Froscher W, Pisani F, van Rijn CM. The importance of drug interactions in epilepsy therapy. *Epilepsia.* 2002;43:365–385.

Perucca E. Clinically relevant drug interactions with antiepileptic drugs. *Br J Clin Pharmacol.* 2005;61:246–255.

Pollard JR, Delanty N. Antiepileptic drug interactions. *Continuum Lifelong Learning Neurol.* 2007;13:91–105.

Romanelli F, Jennings HR, Nath A, Ryan M, Berger J. Therapeutic dilemma: The use of anticonvulsants in HIV-positive individuals. *Neurology.* 2000;54:1404–1407.

Sperling MR, Ko J. Seizures and brain tumors. *Semin Oncol.* 2006;33:333–341.

Spina E, Pisani F, Perucca E. Clinically significant pharmacokinetic drug interactions with carbamazepine. *Clin Pharmacokinet.* 1996;31:198–214.

Online Resources

Brivaracetam (Briviact). www.briviact.com/2020

Cannabidiol (Epidiolex). www.epidiolex.com/2020

Cenobamate (Xcopri). https://reference.medscape.com/drug/xcopri-cenobamate-1000328/2020

Lacosamide (Vimpat). www.vimpathcp.com/vimpat-prescribing-information.pdf/2020

Chapter 7

Aggravation of Seizures by Antiseizure Medications

Drugs may sometimes aggravate seizures, defined as an increase in either the frequency or severity of existing seizures, the emergence of new types of seizures, or the occurrence of status epilepticus. Pharmacodynamic aggravation of epilepsy usually translates into both increased seizure frequency and increased interictal electroencephalographic changes. A doubling or greater increase in seizure frequency may be considered as evidence for seizure aggravation. Seizure aggravation can occur with virtually all antiseizure medications (ASMs) (Gayatri and Livingston, 2006; Somerville, 2002). Because the underlying mechanisms for antiseizure effects of ASMs are not fully understood, neither can the mechanisms involved in seizure aggravation be explained with certainty. However, mechanisms underlying ASM-induced seizure aggravation may include:

- Specific drug effects
  - Increased γ-aminobutyric acid (GABA)-mediated transmission (vigabatrin, tiagabine, and gabapentin)
  - Blockade of voltage-gated sodium channels (carbamazepine, phenobarbital, phenytoin, and lamotrigine)
- Secondary loss of efficacy due to tolerance (benzodiazepines)
- Drug-induced encephalopathy
- Drug interactions leading to diminished levels of other ASMs

In any patient with possible seizure aggravation, other potential causes should be considered (e.g., poor drug adherence, overdosage, acute idiosyncratic adverse effects, chronic dose-related adverse effects, intercurrent illness, development or progression of underlying neurological illness) (Gayatri and Livingston, 2006; Genton, 2002; Sazgar and Bourgeois, 2005). Poor adherence or compliance with the medication regimen and intercurrent illness are probably the most common causes of seizure aggravation, and aggravation by ASMs is often a diagnosis of exclusion.

ASM-induced seizure exacerbation may be observed more frequently in certain epilepsy syndromes of infancy and childhood, especially if there are multiple seizure types, even if appropriate ASMs are prescribed. These syndromes include Lennox-Gastaut, Landau-Kleffner, myoclonic-astatic epilepsy, severe myoclonic epilepsy of infancy, and electrical status epilepticus of sleep (Sazgar and Bourgeois, 2005). For example, rufinamide (a drug developed and approved for treatment of seizures in Lennox-Gastaut syndrome) has a

Table 7.1 Evidence for antiseizure medication–induced aggravation of seizures or epilepsy syndromes

	Antiseizure medication														
Seizure or Syndrome	**CBZ**	**OXC**	**PHT**	**LTG**	**VPA**	**LCS**	**GBP**	**VGB**	**TGB**	**TPM**	**BDZ**	**PB**	**ETX**	**LEV**	**RUF**
Absence	3+	1+	3+		1+	1+	1+	2+	1+			1+		1+	
Myoclonus	3+	1+	3+	1+		1+	2+	1+						1+	
GTCS											2+		2+		
JME	2+	1+	2+	1+		1+									
Infantile spasms												1+			
LGS	2+	1+	2+	1+		1+	1+	2+			2+				1+
LKS	1+		1+												
Rolandic	2+			1+	1+										
ESES	2+		2+												
Focal epilepsies	1+			1+			1+	2+	1+	1+				1+	

ASM, antiepileptic drug; BDZ, benzodiazepine; CBZ, carbamazepine; ETX, ethosuximide; GBP, gabapentin; LTG, lamotrigine; LCS, lacosamide; LEV, levetiracetam; OXC, oxcarbazepine; PB, phenobarbital; PHT, phenytoin; RUF, rufinamide; TGB, tiagabine; TPM, topiramate; VGB, vigabatrin; VPA, valproic acid; GTCS, generalized tonic-clonic seizure; ESES, electrical status epilepticus during sleep; JME, juvenile myoclonic epilepsy; LGS, Lennox-Gastaut syndrome; LKS, Landau-Kleffner syndrome.

Evidence for aggravation: 1+, limited; 2+, moderate; 3+, significant.

From Snead and Hosey (1985), Asconape et al. (2000), Genton (2002), Sazgar and Bourgeois (2005), Gayatri and Livingston (2006), Thomas et al. (2006), Kothare and Kaleyias (2007), Liu et al. (2012), Coppola et al. (2014), Birnbaum and Koubeissi (2016), Ortiz de la Rosa, et al. (2018).

low risk of aggravating seizures in patients with Lennox-Gastaut syndrome (Coppola et al., 2014). Some other patients, including patients with intellectual disability and/or behavioral disorders, may also be more exposed to the risk of pharmacodynamic aggravation of seizures. Therefore, the clinician should choose an ASM according to seizure type or, better, to epilepsy syndrome (Genton, 2002). When a definitive diagnosis is not reached in a patient, the use of ASMs with a broad spectrum of activity (e.g., valproate or levetiracetam) may be less likely to cause seizure exacerbation (Table 7.1).

References

Asconape J, Diedrich A, DellaBadia J. Myoclonus associated with the use of gabapentin. *Epilepsia*. 2000;41:479–481.

Birnbaum D, Koubeissi M. Unmasking of myoclonus by lacosamide in generalized epilepsy. *Epilepsy Behav Case Rep*. 2016;7:28–30.

Coppola G, Besag F, Cusmai R, et al. Current role of rufinamide in the treatment of childhood epilepsy: Literature review and treatment guidelines. *Eur J Paediatr Neurol*. 2014;pii S1090-3798(14)00087-7.

Gayatri NA, Livingston JH. Aggravation of epilepsy by anti-epileptic drugs. *Develop Med Child Neurol*. 2006;48:394–398.

Genton P. When antiepileptic drugs aggravate epilepsy. *Brain Develop*. 2002;22:75–80.

Kothare SV, Kaleyias J. The adverse effects of antiepileptic drugs in children. *Exp Opin Drug Safe*. 2007;6:251–265.

Liu YH, Wang XL, Deng YC, Zhao G. Levetiracetam-associated aggravation of myoclonic seizure in children. *Seizure*. 2012;21(10):807–809.

Ortiz de la Rosa JS, Ladino LD, Rodríguez PJ, et al. Efficacy of lacosamide in children and adolescents with drug-resistant epilepsy and refractory status epilepticus: A systematic review. *Seizure*. 2018;56:34–40.

Sazgar M, Bourgeois BFD. Aggravation of epilepsy by antiepileptic drugs. *Pediatr Neurol*. 2005;33:227–234.

Snead OC III, Hosey LC. Exacerbation of seizures in children by carbamazepine. *N Engl J Med*. 1985;313:916–921.

Somerville ER. Aggravation of partial seizures by antiepileptic drugs: Is there evidence from clinical trials? *Neurology*. 2002;59;79–83.

Thomas P, Valton L, Genton P. Absence and myoclonic status epilepticus precipitated by antiepileptic drugs in idiopathic generalized epilepsy. *Brain*. 2006;129:1281–1292.

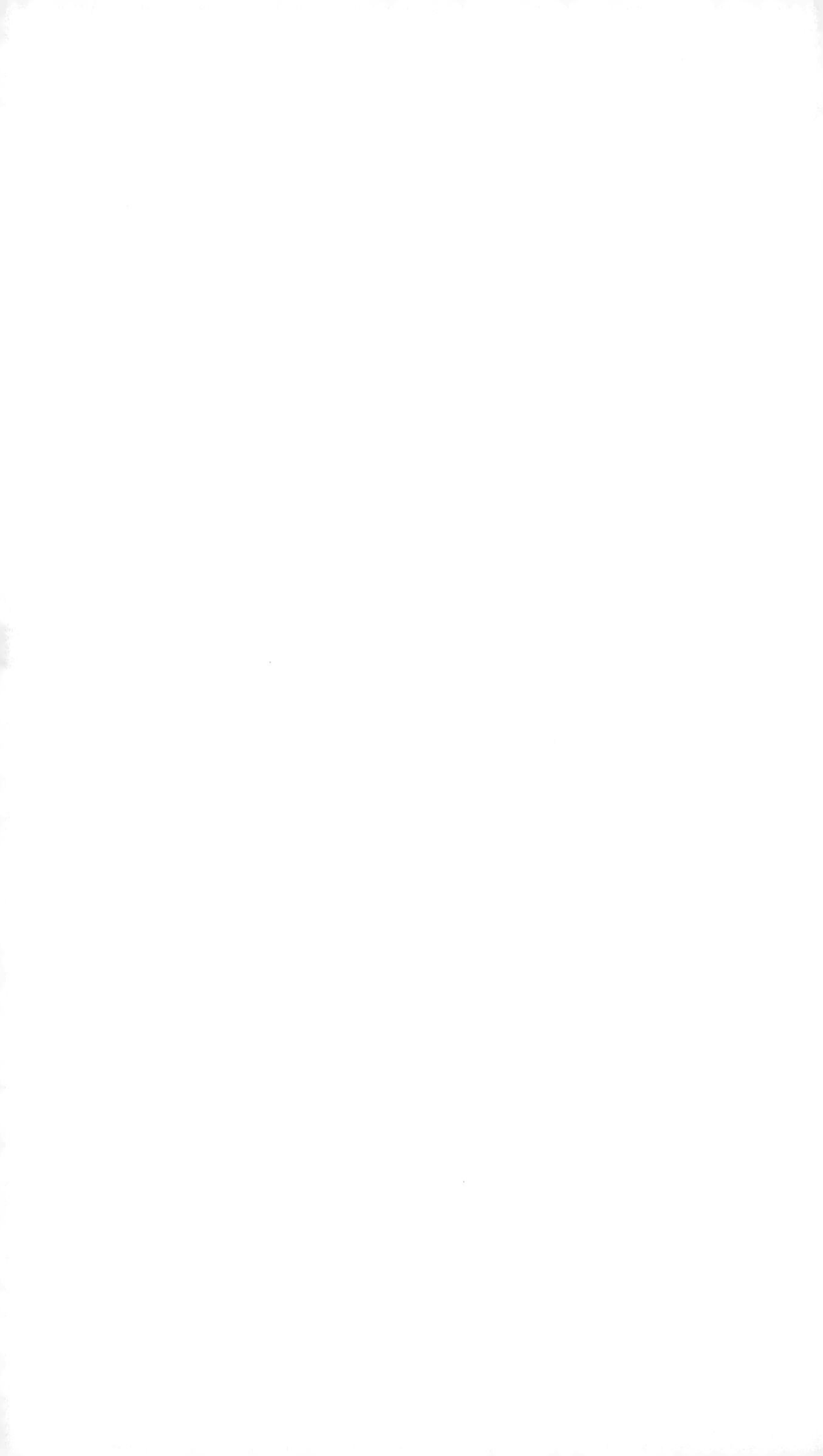

Chapter 8

Polytherapy with Antiseizure Medications

Most patients with epilepsy require prophylactic antiseizure medicine (ASM) therapy. In these patients, a single ASM should be started; treatment with a single agent is referred to as *monotherapy*. Choice of the first ASM needs to be tailored to the patient and should be based on seizure type or epilepsy syndrome, drug adverse-effect profile, age and gender of the patient, comorbidities and comedications in the patient, and, finally, cost. Most ASMs should be introduced at low doses with gradual increases in dosage, depending on the urgency of the situation, to establish an effective and tolerable regimen. Drug titration helps minimize concentration-dependent adverse effects, fosters the development of tolerance to sedation or cognitive impairment, and may aid early detection of the emergence of potentially serious adverse reactions (Brodie, 2005; Brodie and Kwan, 2002).

If the first ASM produces a significant and intolerable adverse effect or fails to improve seizure control, an alternative ASM should be substituted. The choice of an alternative ASM for patients who have not responded to the first ASM depends primarily on the seizure type and epilepsy syndrome. Therefore, as a first step, a serious effort should be made to diagnose the seizure type and syndrome (Ben-Menachem, 2014). If the first or second drug is well-tolerated, the dose can be increased by increments toward the limit of tolerability, aiming for optimal control (Brodie, 2005). However, once two drugs have failed, the chance of seizure freedom with further monotherapy options is very low (Stephen and Brodie, 2002).

Perhaps 60% of newly diagnosed patient with epilepsy will have a good response to the above-mentioned strategy and become seizure-free on a modest or moderate dose of the first or second choice of ASM without developing intolerable adverse effects. However, about 40% of patients will have "difficult-to-control" epilepsy. Focal epilepsies and symptomatic (structural-metabolic) generalized epilepsies are less likely to be controlled easily than the idiopathic (genetic) generalized epilepsies.

If control is greatly improved but seizure freedom is not achieved by monotherapy, another ASM may be added to the first agent. When *polytherapy* (use of more than one ASM) should first be tried has not been evaluated by controlled trials, but many physicians advocate combination therapy once two have failed in monotherapy. The second drug may have a different putative mechanism of action or a similar one. There is a paucity of evidence that using two drugs with differing mechanisms of action (i.e., rational polytherapy) is superior to using two drugs with similar mechanisms of action in order to bring the seizures under control; for example, carbamazepine interacts with the sodium channel and levetiracetam at the SVA2 receptor. However, adverse effects may be worse when drugs with similar mechanisms of action are used, and use of differing drug types may offer benefit with regard to adverse effects.

How should one add a second drug? The dose of the first drug might often be reduced somewhat when adding a second agent to limit the development of adverse effects. If the first ASM combination is not effective or produces untoward adverse effects, a sequence of combinations could be tried, but seizure freedom will almost certainly not result, and palliation would be the goal of this course of therapy. Triple therapy can be attempted by adding a small dose of a third ASM; however, this is to be discouraged. The greater the drug burden, the less likely that polytherapy will be tolerated (Brodie, 2005; Brodie and Kwan, 2002; Stephen and Brodie, 2002), and worsening of seizures can easily result. If polytherapy trials fail to achieve full seizure control, one should revert to the most effective, best-tolerated monotherapy. At the same time, one should consider all possible reasons for uncontrolled seizures, including functional (non-epileptic) seizures, pseudointractability (i.e., misclassification and taking a wrong medication for the specific epilepsy syndrome, taking suboptimal doses of an appropriate ASM, or poor drug adherence), and drug-resistant epilepsy. The mainstay for making a correct diagnosis is having a standardized approach, particularly with regard to taking a detailed clinical history (Asadi-Pooya et al., 2013).

Once adequate trials of two tolerated, appropriately chosen and used ASM schedules (whether as monotherapies or in combination) have failed to achieve sustained seizure freedom, other treatment options (e.g., epilepsy surgery) should be considered (Kwan et al., 2010). This is advised because the chances of permanent remission are exceedingly low after that. Additional pharmacotherapy generally should be used after failure of two ASMs only if epilepsy surgery is not possible or desired by the patient. However, more study is required as new agents are approved; for example, cenobamate appears to induce prolonged periods of seizure remission in some patients, and only time will tell whether this is a permanent effect. Neurostimulation (e.g., vagal nerve stimulation [VNS], responsive neurostimulation [RNS], deep brain stimulation [DBS]) could be considered after failure of three ASMs. Figure 8.1 shows the pathways of epilepsy management (Park et al., 2019).

There always should be a balance between efficacy, tolerability, and safety. Polytherapy with ASMs requires several considerations:

1. Knowledge of ASMs' mechanisms of action
2. Spectrum of efficacy of ASMs
3. Knowledge of the adverse-effect profiles of ASMs
4. Knowledge of drug interactions and pharmacokinetics of ASMs (Brodie, 2005; Brodie and Kwan, 2002)

Based on these considerations, some suggestions are probably useful when making a decision for polytherapy in a patient with difficult-to-control epilepsy

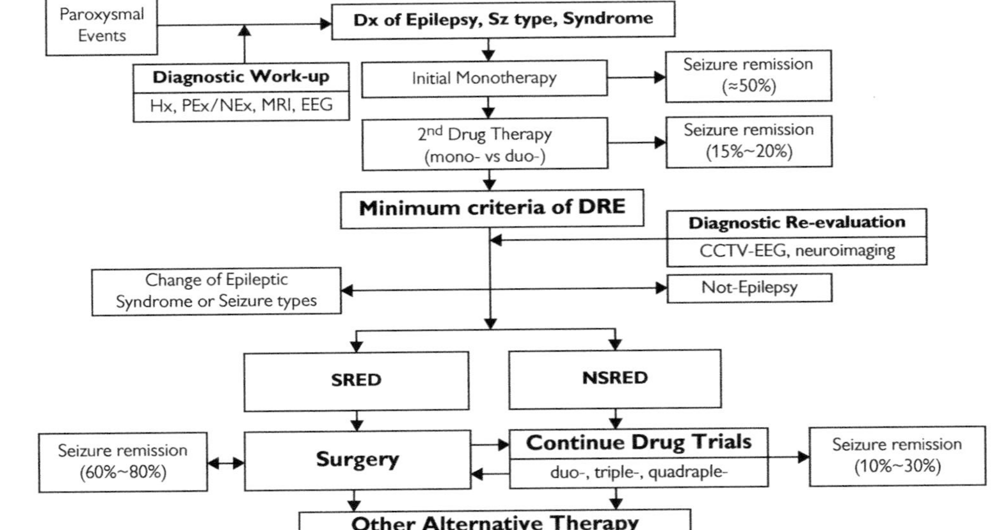

Figure 8.1 Pathways of epilepsy management. Epilepsy management starts with the accurate diagnosis of seizure type(s) and epilepsy syndrome.

Hx, history-taking; PEx/NEx, physical and neurological examination; MRI, magnetic resonance imaging of brain; EEG, electroencephalography; Dx, diagnosis; DRE, drug-resistant epilepsy; CCTV-EEG, closed circuit video-EEG recording; SRED, surgically remediable epilepsy syndrome; NSRED, not-surgically remediable epilepsy syndrome.

(Asconapé, 2002; Brodie, 2001, 2005; Kwan and Brodie, 2006; Patsalos et al., 2002; Perucca, 2001; Stephen and Brodie, 2002):

1. Treatment with two ASMs, rarely three ASMs, but not four ASMs may be a useful therapeutic option for patients who do not respond to monotherapy and are not candidates for epilepsy surgery.
2. In patients with difficult-to-control epilepsy or multiple seizure types, ASMs with different mechanisms of action could be considered for the drug regimen because this may produce fewer adverse effects.
3. Broad-spectrum drugs such as lacosamide, lamotrigine, levetiracetam, perampanel, topiramate, valproate, and zonisamide may be preferred over those with a more limited clinical efficacy profile such as eslicarbazepine acetate, oxcarbazepine, perampanel, tiagabine, gabapentin, vigabatrin, or pregabalin, particularly in patients with more than one seizure type, depending on the epilepsy syndrome.
4. Patients with a single seizure type may respond to a pairing which influences an individual ion channel or neurotransmitter system in different ways (e.g., valproate and ethosuximide for absence seizure).
5. Avoid prescribing an ASM that may worsen or aggravate the particular seizure type in the patient (e.g., carbamazepine, oxcarbazepine, phenytoin, vigabatrin, and tiagabine may worsen myoclonus and absences; refer to Chapter 7).
6. It is advisable not to prescribe enzyme-inducing ASMs (e.g., phenobarbital, phenytoin, carbamazepine) with another ASM that is a substrate for that particular enzyme system (e.g., lamotrigine, oxcarbazepine, perampanel), or at least consider the clinically important drug interactions.
7. If an enzyme-inhibiting ASM (valproate or felbamate) is included in the polytherapy regimen, clinically important drug interactions should be considered (e.g., with phenobarbital, carbamazepine, rufinamide, or lamotrigine).
8. It is usually inadvisable to prescribe together two ASMs with carbonic anhydrase-inhibiting effect (topiramate, zonisamide, and acetazolamide).
9. It is usually inadvisable to prescribe together two ASMs with significant cognitive adverse effects (benzodiazepines, topiramate, phenobarbital, and zonisamide).
10. A pharmacodynamic interaction between carbamazepine (or oxcarbazepine) and lamotrigine may result in neurotoxic reactions (e.g., headache and ataxia). If toxicity occurs, it is advisable to reduce the dose of carbamazepine or oxcarbazepine.
11. Levetiracetam does not have any significant interactions with other ASMs. Even so, pharmacodynamic interactions with carbamazepine have rarely been reported, resulting in carbamazepine toxicity.
12. Lacosamide does not have any significant interactions with other ASMs. The lack of pharmacokinetic interaction does not rule out the possibility of pharmacodynamic interactions, particularly among drugs that might affect the heart conduction system.

13. Gabapentin does not have any significant interactions with other ASMs.
14. Brivaracetam does not have any significant interactions with other ASMs other than with phenytoin and, less likely, with carbamazepine. It has no added therapeutic benefit when coadministered with levetiracetam.
15. Vigabatrin remains a drug of last resort because of its propensity to produce visual field defects.
16. Felbamate is rarely recommended because of its risk for aplastic anemia and hepatotoxicity.
17. Some combinations worth considering include
    a. For *generalized epilepsies*: Valproate and lamotrigine; valproate and levetiracetam; valproate and lacosamide; valproate and perampanel; valproate and ethosuximide; topiramate and lamotrigine; zonisamide and lamotrigine; lamotrigine and clonazepam; lamotrigine and ethosuximide; topiramate and ethosuximide; valproate and zonisamide; lamotrigine and levetiracetam depending on seizure type.
    b. For *focal epilepsies*: Brivaracetam and any agent except levetiracetam; levetiracetam and any agent except brivaracetam; perampanel and any agent; carbamazepine, lacosamide, eslicarbazepine acetate, cenobamate, perampanel, oxcarbazepine, or zonisamide with gabapentin or pregabalin.

It is worth mentioning that some combination regimens have shown synergistic interactions in clinical studies; these include valproate and lamotrigine; valproate and ethosuximide; lamotrigine and topiramate; lacosamide and levetiracetam; lamotrigine and levetiracetam; and valproate and levetiracetam (Park et al., 2019).

References

Asadi-Pooya AA, Emami M, Ashjazadeh N, et al. Reasons for uncontrolled seizures in adults: The impact of pseudointractability. *Seizure*. 2013;22(4):271–274.

Asconapé JJ. Some common issues in the use of antiepileptic drugs. *Semin Neurol*. 2002;22:27–39.

Ben-Menachem E. Medical management of refractory epilepsy: Practical treatment with novel antiepileptic drugs. *Epilepsia*. 2014;55(Suppl 1):3–8.

Brodie MJ. Management strategies for refractory localization-related epilepsies. *Epilepsia*. 2001;42(Suppl 3):27–30.

Brodie MJ. Medical therapy of epilepsy: When to initiate treatment and when to combine? *J Neurol*. 2005;252:125–130.

Brodie MJ, Kwan P. Staged approach to epilepsy management. *Neurology*. 2002;58:S2–S8.

Kwan P, Brodie MJ. Combination therapy in epilepsy: When and what to use? *Drugs*. 2006;66:1817–1829.

Kwan P, Arzimanoglou A, Berg AT, et al. Definition of drug resistant epilepsy: Consensus proposal by the ad hoc Task Force of the ILAE Commission on Therapeutic Strategies. *Epilepsia*. 2010;51(6):1069–1077.

Park KM, Kim SE, Lee BI. Antiepileptic drug therapy in patients with drug-resistant epilepsy. *J Epilepsy Res*. 2019;9(1):14–26.

Patsalos PN, Froscher W, Pisani F, van Rijn CM. The importance of drug interactions in epilepsy therapy. *Epilepsia*. 2002;43:365–385.

Perucca E. The management of refractory idiopathic epilepsies. *Epilepsia*. 2001;42(Supp1.3):31–35.

Stephen LJ, Brodie MJ. Seizure freedom with more than one antiepileptic drug. *Seizure*. 2002;11:349–351.

Chapter 9

Antiseizure Medications in Pregnancy

Due to the potential for teratogenesis and other impairments and problems (e.g., pregnancy loss), the risks and benefits of antiseizure medication (ASM) therapy should be weighed carefully in pregnant women or in women of childbearing potential. Pregnancy should be planned in a patient receiving ASMs so that appropriate measures can be taken in advance. The question should be raised whether an ASM is still required, which drug is needed, and what dose should be prescribed. Consideration must be given both to maintaining seizure control and minimizing fetal risk.

Regrettably, there is still a lack of adequate data regarding fetal risk for most ASMs, so comparisons of risk often cannot be drawn. What knowledge exists is fragmentary and limited. Many studies report only the results of the examination of newborns, so malformations and problems that first become apparent after the neonatal period are underreported. The long-term effects of most ASMs on child development are largely unknown. Therefore, the true incidence of major congenital malformations (MCMs) and other developmental problems remains uncertain.

Some general statements can be made, however. The risk of major malformation in the offspring of women in the general population is approximately 1–2%. The risk of major malformation in the offspring of women with epilepsy who take ASMs is approximately doubled or tripled, to 4–6% on average. Women who take multiple ASMs may have a 10–12% risk of having a baby with a major malformation, so polypharmacy poses a significantly greater risk. Likewise, in women with drug-resistant epilepsy and with high serum levels of ASMs, the risk is high (Penovich et al., 2004). Strong evidence now exists that ASM total daily dose is an important factor in determining the magnitude of risk for MCMs; the lowest effective dose should thus be established before pregnancy starts, regardless of which ASM the woman is taking (Campbell et al., 2014; Tomson & Xue et al., 2015). Various series report different risks for individual ASMs, but some common themes are apparent (Figure 9.1). For those drugs for which information is available, the risk of valproate appears to be the highest. Of babies born to women taking valproate, 9.3–9.7% display major malformations, and as many as one-third of children born to women taking valproate during pregnancy have measurable cognitive and learning difficulties (Campbell et al., 2014; Meador and Zupanc, 2004; Thomas, 2006). The propensity for fetal malformation with valproate may be subject to a dose effect, with problems occurring mainly in women taking doses greater

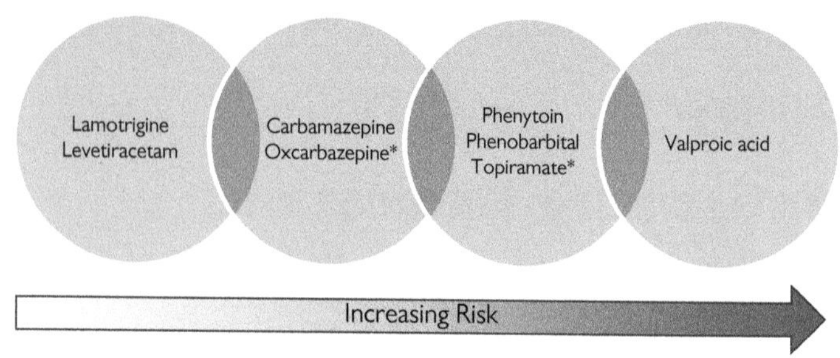

Figure 9.1. Summary of relative teratogenic risk profiles of antiseizure medications.
* Neurodevelopmental outcomes are not yet known.

Reprinted with permission: Pennell PB. Use of antiepileptic drugs during pregnancy: Evolving concepts. *Neurotherapeutics*. 2016;13(4):811–820.

than 650 mg/day. Levetiracetam appears to have a relatively low risk of producing major malformations. Lamotrigine also appears to have a relatively low risk of producing major malformations (approximately 2–2.9%); however, there may be a dose effect (≥300 mg/day may have a higher risk). Early data with regard to oxcarbazepine and gabapentin appear promising, but more studies are needed (Mølgaard-Nielsen and Hviid, 2011). Oxcarbazepine and lamotrigine were associated with greater odds of developing autism compared with controls in a single study (Veroniki et al., 2017). The other newer ASMs still lack sufficient data to draw any conclusions. The older ASMs, such as phenytoin, carbamazepine, phenobarbital, and primidone, all carry an intermediate risk—perhaps 3–6%—of producing major malformations, and some may be associated with lower IQ in children born to women taking these agents (Meador et al., 2006; Meador and Zupanc, 2004; Ornoy, 2006; Pennel, 2005; Thomas, 2006; Weiner and Buhimschi, 2004).

What is one to do? Several principles can be formulated to treat women who plan to become pregnant. First, implement appropriate treatment before pregnancy occurs (i.e., the pregnancy must be planned). Aim for therapy with a single agent, ideally one with a favorable teratogenic profile, and use the lowest possible dose of that drug. Aim for seizure freedom with that treatment because seizures may cause injury to the woman and lead to fetal abnormalities. Avoid polypharmacy, *if possible*. Place women who may become pregnant on a multivitamin and folic acid regimen before pregnancy occurs in hopes of minimizing birth defects. The optimal dose of folate is not known; most practitioners prescribe between 1 and 5 mg daily. We recommend 5 mg folate supplementation when the patient takes valproate and 1 mg while taking other ASMs as high-dose folate might have important drug interactions with some ASMs. Administration of large doses of folic acid can decrease blood levels of phenytoin, phenobarbital, and carbamazepine, potentially interfering with seizure control (Asadi-Pooya, 2015; Asadi-Pooya et al. 2008). Vitamins and folate should be continued throughout the pregnancy. Have women avoid other products known to cause birth defects or problems, such as alcohol, caffeine, tobacco, and other teratogenic drugs (if possible) (Meador et al., 2006; Meador and Zupanc, 2004; Ornoy, 2006; Pennel, 2005; Penovich et al., 2004; Thomas, 2006; Weiner and Buhimschi, 2004).

Because valproate seems at present to be the least desirable ASM, switch to another less teratogenic ASM prior to pregnancy, *if possible*. However, when the epilepsy is well controlled only with valproate and other ASMs have been proved ineffective, then valproate should be continued after discussing relevant issues with the prospective parents. Valproate is the most effective ASM to bring generalized tonic-clonic seizures under control in patients with idiopathic generalized epilepsy (IGE). Current recommendations on treatment of young women with IGE advise against the use of valproate as the first-line ASM (Tomson & Marson et al., 2015). However, we should bear in mind that these guidelines only recommend caution regarding teratogenic risks of valproate in women of child-bearing potential but do not advocate absolute avoidance. Failure to prescribe valproate for patients with IGE, particularly when other ASMs (e.g., lamotrigine or levetiracetam) have failed to bring the seizures under control, may not be in a young woman's best interests (Asadi-Pooya and Homayoun 2020). One should avoid changing to a new medication during pregnancy if possible, especially early in the pregnancy, because the consequences of using multiple drugs may be deleterious. The ASM should be given in divided doses because the effects on the fetus may depend on the concentration peaks. In addition, 10 mg of vitamin K should be administered to the mother daily starting at the 36th week of pregnancy, and the newborn should receive 1 mg of vitamin K intramuscularly at birth. This is certainly appropriate for women taking enzyme-inducing drugs; it is not known whether women taking other drugs require this regimen, but it seems sensible to follow it until more is known. The pregnancy of an ASM-treated patient has to be considered "high-risk" because there is an approximate doubling of the risk of pregnancy complications. This includes monitoring first-trimester ultrasonography and α-fetoprotein levels in maternal blood for the diagnosis of neural tube defects, ultrasound during weeks 19–23 of pregnancy to detect major anomalies, and fetal echocardiography to detect congenital cardiac defects (Ornoy, 2006; Penovich et al., 2004; Thomas, 2006).

In most women, ASM dosages must be adjusted during pregnancy. Increases in blood volume, renal clearance, hormonal interactions, and changes in hepatic metabolic activity usually lead to reductions in serum levels of ASMs. Therefore, increases in dosage may be necessary to maintain seizure control. During pregnancy, an increase in clearance and a decrease in the concentrations of lamotrigine, levetiracetam, oxcarbazepine's active metabolite licarbazepine, topiramate, and zonisamide are observed. Carbamazepine clearance remains unchanged during pregnancy. There is inadequate or no evidence for changes in the clearance or concentrations of clobazam and its active metabolite N-desmethylclobazam, gabapentin, lacosamide, perampanel, and valproate (Arfman et al., 2020). Some of the changes in drug levels may occur very early in the pregnancy. Measurement of serum levels prior to pregnancy and during pregnancy may help guide dosage. *Seizure control may be independent of serum level during pregnancy in some women.* Despite the ambiguities, we advise measuring serum levels every 2 months or so, and this may be done more often if seizures occur. For example, lamotrigine doses may need to be tripled in some women to maintain pre-pregnancy levels if that is desired. Once the pregnancy has ended, doses can usually begin to be reduced rapidly, using clinical assessment of adverse effects and therapeutic monitoring to guide adjustment in dosage. For most ASMs, maternal pharmacokinetics will return to pre-pregnancy levels within 10–14 days after delivery. Lamotrigine has been observed to return to pre-pregnancy kinetics within the first 3 postpartum days (Penovich et al., 2004; Thomas, 2006).

Food and Drug Administration (FDA) Rating for Antiseizure Medication Use in Pregnancy

1. *FDA pregnancy risk category D ASMs*: Benzodiazepines, carbamazepine, phenobarbital, phenytoin, primidone, topiramate, and valproic acid
2. *FDA pregnancy risk category C ASMs*: Acetazolamide, brivaracetam, cannabidiol, cenobamate, eslicarbazepine acetate, ethosuximide, ezogabine, felbamate, gabapentin, lacosamide, lamotrigine, levetiracetam, oxcarbazepine, perampanel, pregabalin, rufinamide, tiagabine, vigabatrin, and zonisamide

Category C means either (1) animal studies have shown an adverse effect and there are no adequate and well-controlled studies in humans or (2) no animal studies have been conducted and there are no adequate and well-controlled studies in pregnant women. Category D means that either adequate well-controlled or observational studies in pregnant women have demonstrated a risk to the fetus; however, the benefits of therapy may outweigh the potential risk. For example, a drug may be acceptable if needed in a life-threatening situation or in the presence of serious disease for which safer drugs cannot be used or are ineffective (FDA use-in-pregnancy ratings, n.d.; Weiner and Buhimschi, 2004).

Many ASMs appear to cause a similar group of minor anomalies known as the *fetal anticonvulsant syndrome*. These include craniofacial and digital anomalies, which become less apparent as the child grows. There is also a 1–6% incidence of major anomalies, including cardiac defects, cleft lip and palate, microcephaly, and developmental delay (FDA use-in-pregnancy ratings, n.d.).

Fetal Risk Summary of Antiseizure Medications Based on Human Data

- *Acetazolamide:* Data are not available.
- *Benzodiazepines:* Cardiovascular defects.
- *Carbamazepine*
  - Neural tube defects
  - Craniofacial defects
  - Cleft palate

- Cardiovascular malformations
- Urogenital anomalies
- Developmental delay
- Anomalies involving various body systems
- *Ethosuximide*
  - Cardiovascular malformations
  - Cleft lip/palate
  - Hydrocephalus
  - Mongoloid facies
- *Felbamate:* Data are not available.
- *Gabapentin:* Not enough data are available. Ventricular septal defect has been reported (Morrow et al., 2006).
- *Lamotrigine*
  - Neural tube defects
  - Esophageal malformation
  - Cleft palate
  - Club foot
  - Cardiovascular malformations
- *Levetiracetam:* Insufficient data; no significant problems found thus far.
- *Oxcarbazepine:* Data are not available.
- *Phenobarbital*
  - Cardiovascular malformations
  - Cleft lip/palate
  - Neural tube defects
  - Limb anomalies
  - Urogenital anomalies
  - Neurobehavioral developmental problems
- *Phenytoin*
  - Central nervous system anomalies
  - Craniofacial defects
  - Limb anomalies
  - Cardiovascular malformations
  - Cleft lip/palate
  - Physical and mental growth impairment
  - Many other anomalies
- *Pregabalin:* Data are not available.
- *Tiagabine:* Data are not available.
- *Topiramate:* Limited data. Cleft lip and palate and hypospadias have been reported.
- *Valproate*
  - Neural tube defects
  - Cardiovascular malformations
  - Facial defects
  - Cleft lip/palate
  - Urogenital defects
  - Developmental delay
  - Many other anomalies

- Cognitive impairment, low IQ: in a recent study, it was observed that fetal valproate exposure has dose-dependent associations with reduced cognitive abilities across a range of domains at 6 years of age. Mean IQs were higher in children exposed to periconceptional folate than they were in unexposed children (Meador et al., 2013).

- *Vigabatrin:* Congenital cardiac defects, congenital external ear anomaly, congenital hemangioma, congenital hydronephrosis, congenital male genital malformation, congenital oral malformation, congenital vesico-ureteric reflux, dentofacial anomaly, dysmorphism, fetal anticonvulsant syndrome, hamartomas, hip dysplasia, limb malformation, limb reduction defect, low-set ears, renal aplasia, retinitis pigmentosa, and supernumerary nipple have been reported.
- *Zonisamide:* A variety of fetal abnormalities, including cardiovascular defects, and embryo-fetal deaths occurred with zonisamide.
- New ASMs (i.e., brivaracetam, cannabidiol, cenobamate, eslicarbazepine acetate, ezogabine, lacosamide, perampanel, and rufinamide): not enough information is available (Meador et al., 2006; Ornoy, 2006; Pennel, 2005; Weiner and Buhimschi, 2004; see also individual drug websites listed in the Online Resources at the end of this chapter).

References

Arfman IJ, Wammes-van der Heijden EA, Ter Horst PGJ, et al. Therapeutic drug monitoring of antiepileptic drugs in women with epilepsy before, during, and after pregnancy. *Clin Pharmacokinet.* 2020. doi: 10.1007/s40262-019-00845-2. [Epub ahead of print]

Asadi-Pooya AA. High dose folic acid supplementation in women with epilepsy: Are we sure it is safe? *Seizure.* 2015;27:51–53.

Asadi-Pooya AA, Homayoun M. Tonic-clonic seizures in idiopathic generalized epilepsies: Prevalence, risk factors, and outcome. *Acta Neurol Scand.* 2020. doi:10.1111/ane.13227.

Asadi-Pooya AA, Mintzer S, Sperling, MR. Nutritional supplements, foods, and epilepsy: Is there a relationship? *Epilepsia.* 2008;49(11):1819–1827.

Campbell E, Kennedy F, Russell A, et al. Malformation risks of antiepileptic drug monotherapies in pregnancy: Updated results from the UK and Ireland Epilepsy and Pregnancy Registers. *J Neurol Neurosurg Psychiatry.* 2014;85(9):1029–1034.

FDA use-in-pregnancy ratings. Focus Information Technology, Inc. http://www.perinatology.com/exposures/Drugs/FDACategories.htm./2014

French J. Treatment with antiepileptic drugs, new and old. *Continuum Lifelong Learning Neurol.* 2007;13:71–90.

Meador KJ, Baker GA, Browning N, et al. Fetal antiepileptic drug exposure and cognitive outcomes at age 6 years (NEAD study): A prospective observational study. *Lancet Neurol.* 2013;12(3):244–252.

Meador KJ, Baker GA, Finnel RH, et al. In utero antiepileptic drug exposure: Fetal death and malformations. *Neurology.* 2006;67:407–412.

Meador LJ, Zupanc ML. Neurodevelopmental outcomes of children born to mothers with epilepsy. *Cleve Clin J Med.* 2004;71(Suppl 2):S38–S41.

Mølgaard-Nielsen D, Hviid A. Newer-generation antiepileptic drugs and the risk of major birth defects. *JAMA*. 2011;305(19):1996–2002.

Morrow J, Russell A, Guthrie E, et al. Malformations risks of antiepileptic drugs in pregnancy: A prospective study from the UK Epilepsy and Pregnancy Register. *J Neurol Neurosurg Psychiatry*. 2006;77:193–198.

Ornoy A. Neuroteratogens in man: An overview with special emphasis on the teratogenicity of antiepileptic drugs in pregnancy. *Reprod Toxicol*. 2006;22:214–226.

Pennel PB. Using current evidence in selecting antiepileptic drugs for use during pregnancy. *Epilepsy Curr*. 2005;5:45–51.

Pennell PB. Use of antiepileptic drugs during pregnancy: Evolving concepts. *Neurotherapeutics*. 2016;13(4):811–820.

Penovich PE, Eck K, Economou VV. Recommendations for the care of women with epilepsy. *Cleve Clin J Med*. 2004;71(Suppl 2):S49–S57.

Thomas SV. Management of epilepsy and pregnancy. *J Postgrad Med*. 2006;52:57–64.

Tomson T, Xue H, Battino D. Major congenital malformations in children of women with epilepsy. *Seizure*. 2015;28:46–50.

Tomson T, Marson A, Boon P, et al. Valproate in the treatment of epilepsy in girls and women of childbearing potential. *Epilepsia*. 2015;56:1006–1019.

Veroniki AA, Rios P, Cogo E, et al. Comparative safety of antiepileptic drugs for neurological development in children exposed during pregnancy and breast feeding: A systematic review and network meta-analysis. *BMJ Open*. 2017;7(7):e017248.

Weiner CP, Buhimschi C. *Drugs for Pregnant and Lactating Women*. Philadelphia: Churchill Livingstone; 2004.

Online Resources

Brivaracetam (Briviact). www.briviact.com/2020

Cannabidiol (Epidiolex). www.epidiolex.com/2020

Cenobamate (Xcopri). https://reference.medscape.com/drug/xcopri-cenobamate-1000328/2020

Vigabatrin (Sabril/Lundbeck). http://www.sabril.net/2014

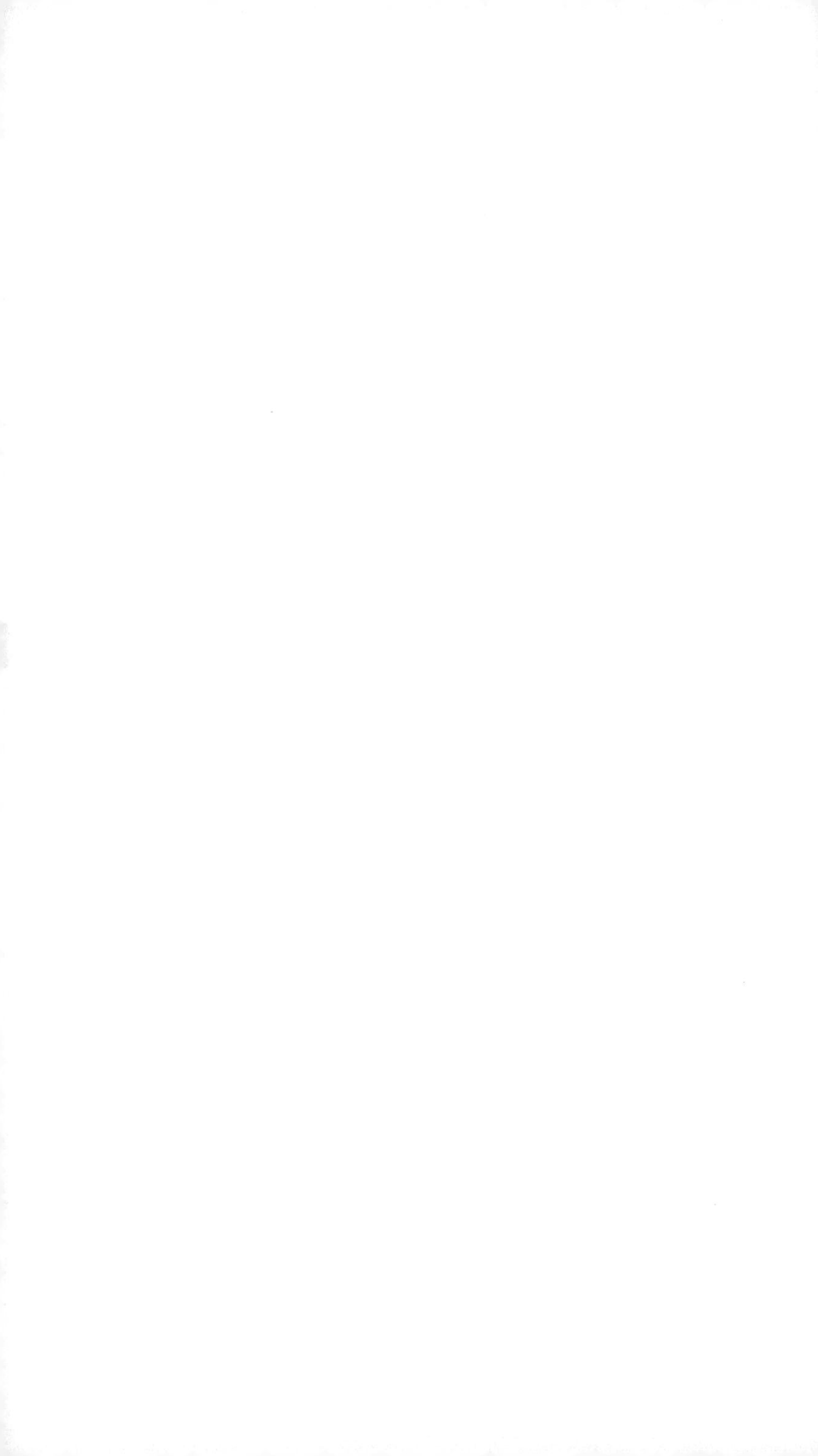

Chapter 10

Antiseizure Medications in Lactating Women

Breastfeeding is generally encouraged for a variety of health and psychological reasons. However, the breast milk of women who take antiseizure medications (ASMs) contains these drugs, which are delivered to the baby with each feeding. The obvious consequences of ASM ingestion in infants include drowsiness and other adverse effects of ASMs. However, some effects may not be readily apparent. There is evidence in animals that brain development is adversely affected in newborn animals subjected to ASM treatment after birth. Phenytoin and valproate may cause reduced brain weight and reduced incorporation of amino acids in myelin and nuclear proteins (Patsalos and Wiggins, 1982). Phenytoin may affect the posttranslational phosphorylation of actin and other cytoskeletal proteins, thereby altering dendritic patterns (Ruiz et al., 1987). Other agents, including phenobarbital, may hinder normal dendritic arborization and alter axonal development (Bergman et al., 1982; Hall et al., 2002). Moreover, some agents, particularly barbiturates, are not easily cleared by neonatal hepatic enzymes and may accumulate in the newborn. Little information is available about other newer agents; the lack of information should *not* be construed as indicating lack of risk.

Therefore, breastfeeding raises significant issues when the mother must take an ASM. Ideally, the potential benefits of breastfeeding would be weighed against the risks of the drug so a sensible decision can be made. Regrettably, scientific evidence is insufficiently robust to intelligently compare the risks and benefits of breastfeeding when the mother is taking an ASM. While the benefits of breast feeding are established, the magnitude of these benefits is difficult to measure. Similarly, data regarding risks are established only in animals. As a matter of fact, in one human study, no adverse effects of ASM (i.e., carbamazepine, lamotrigine, phenytoin, or valproate) exposure via breast milk were observed at age 6 years. In this study, breastfed children exhibited higher IQ and enhanced verbal abilities. However, the authors recommended that additional studies are needed to fully delineate the effects of all ASMs (Meador et al., 2014). Nonetheless, the animal studies raise serious concerns. Therefore, valid arguments can be made to pursue any course of action desired. It is the authors' preference to inform patients about both potential benefits of breastfeeding and risks of ASMs and let the patient help guide the decision. If a woman strongly prefers breast feeding, then certain measures, discussed next, can be taken to reduce infant exposure. If the woman is risk

Table 10.1 Antiseizure medications in breastfeeding

Antiseizure medication	Precautions
Acetazolamide	Limited data are available.
Brivaracetam	No data are available.
Cannabidiol	No data are available.
Carbamazepine	Monitor infant for jaundice, drowsiness, poor suckling, vomiting, and poor weight gain.
Cenobamate	No data are available.
Clonazepam	Monitor infant for drowsiness.
Diazepam	Avoid repeated doses, if possible. Monitor infant for drowsiness.
Eslicarbazepine acetate	No data are available. Consider discontinuation of either breastfeeding or eslicarbazepine acetate.
Ethosuximide	Monitor infant for drowsiness, poor suckling, and poor weight gain.
Ezogabine	No data are available. Consider discontinuation of either breastfeeding or ezogabine.
Felbamate	No data are available.
Phenobarbital	Monitor infant for drowsiness, poor suckling, and poor weight gain. Consider discontinuation of either breastfeeding or phenobarbital.
Phenytoin	Monitor infant for drowsiness and methemoglobinemia.
Primidone	Monitor infant for drowsiness.
Valproic acid	Monitor infant for jaundice and drowsiness.
Gabapentin	Monitor infant for drowsiness.
Lacosamide	No data are available. Consider discontinuation of either breastfeeding or lacosamide.
Lamotrigine	Monitor infant for drowsiness.
Levetiracetam	Monitor for drowsiness.
Oxcarbazepine	Monitor infant for drowsiness and lethargy.
Perampanel	No data are available.
Rufinamide	No data are available. Consider discontinuation of either breastfeeding or rufinamide.
Tiagabine	No data are available.
Topiramate	Monitor for drowsiness. No data are available.
Vigabatrin	Consider discontinuation of either breastfeeding or vigabatrin.
Zonisamide	Monitor for drowsiness. No data are available.

averse and prefers not to deliver a drug that may impair brain development, this becomes obvious during the course of a counseling session.

Should a woman choose to breastfeed, certain advice can be offered. One does not and should not choose an ASM for a prospective mother based on breast milk concentration. Therefore, the woman will likely be taking whatever medication was prescribed during pregnancy, and that drug should be continued.

Certain medications have more favorable profiles with regard to breast milk concentrations of ASMs. Medications with a short half-life and high degree of protein binding have lower concentrations in breast milk than do drugs with low or intermediate protein binding and longer half-lives (Spencer et al., 2001; Tomson, 2005; Weiner and Buhimschi, 2004). ASM concentration in breast milk is roughly inversely proportional to the extent of protein binding of the drug, although significant interindividual variability may exist. Whether lower levels of ASM concentration in breast milk convey less risk is not known, however. Nonetheless, the medication dose should be kept as low as feasible, and breast feeding should be avoided at times of peak drug levels to minimize dose to the infant. Administer single daily-dose medications just before the longest sleep interval for the infant, usually after the bedtime feeding. Feed infants immediately before medication dose when multiple daily doses are needed. In addition, one can consider using infant formula for some feedings and breast milk for others to reduce ASM delivery. Finally, closely monitor the baby for drowsiness, reduced suckling activity, and poor weight gain, particularly, those infants who are premature or in poor health. If adverse effects are suspected in the baby, consider analysis of drug serum levels in the infant. Evaluate if developmental milestones are not reached as expected (Veiby et al., 2015) (Table 10.1).

References

Bergman A, Feigenbaum JJ, Yanai J. Neuronal losses in mice following both prenatal and neonatal exposure to phenobarbital. *Acta Anatomica (Basel)*. 1982;114:185–192.

Hall AC, Brennan A, Goold RG, Cleverley K, Lucas FR, Gordon-Weeks PR, Salinas PC. Valproate regulates GSK-3-mediated axonal remodeling and synapsin I clustering in developing neurons. *Mol Cell Neuroscience*. 2002;20:257–270.

Meador KJ, Baker GA, Browning N, et al. Breastfeeding in children of women taking antiepileptic drugs: cognitive outcomes at age 6 years. *JAMA Pediatr*. 2014;168(8):729–736.

Patsalos PN, Wiggins RC. Brain maturation following administration of phenobarbital, phenytoin, and sodium valproate to developing rats or to their dams: Effects on synthesis of brain myelin and other subcellular membrane proteins. *J Neurochem*. 1982;39:915–923.

Ruiz G, Flores OG, González-Plaza R, Inestrosa NC. Effect of phenytoin on cytoskeletal protein phosphorylation and neuronal structure in the rat sensory cortex. *J Neurosci Res*. 1987;18:466–472.

Spencer JP, Gonzalez LS, Barnhart DJ. Medications in the breast-feeding mother. *Am Fam Phys*. 2001;64:119–126.

Tomson T. Gender aspects of pharmacokinetics of new and old AEDs: Pregnancy and breast-feeding. *Therap Drug Monitor*. 2005;27:718–721.

Veiby G, Bjørk M, Engelsen BA, Gilhus NE. Epilepsy and recommendations for breastfeeding. *Seizure*. 2015; 28:57–65.

Weiner CP, Buhimschi C. *Drugs for Pregnant and Lactating Women*. Philadelphia: Churchill Livingstone; 2004.

Online Resource

Vigabatrin (Sabril/Lundbeck). http://www.sabril.net/2014

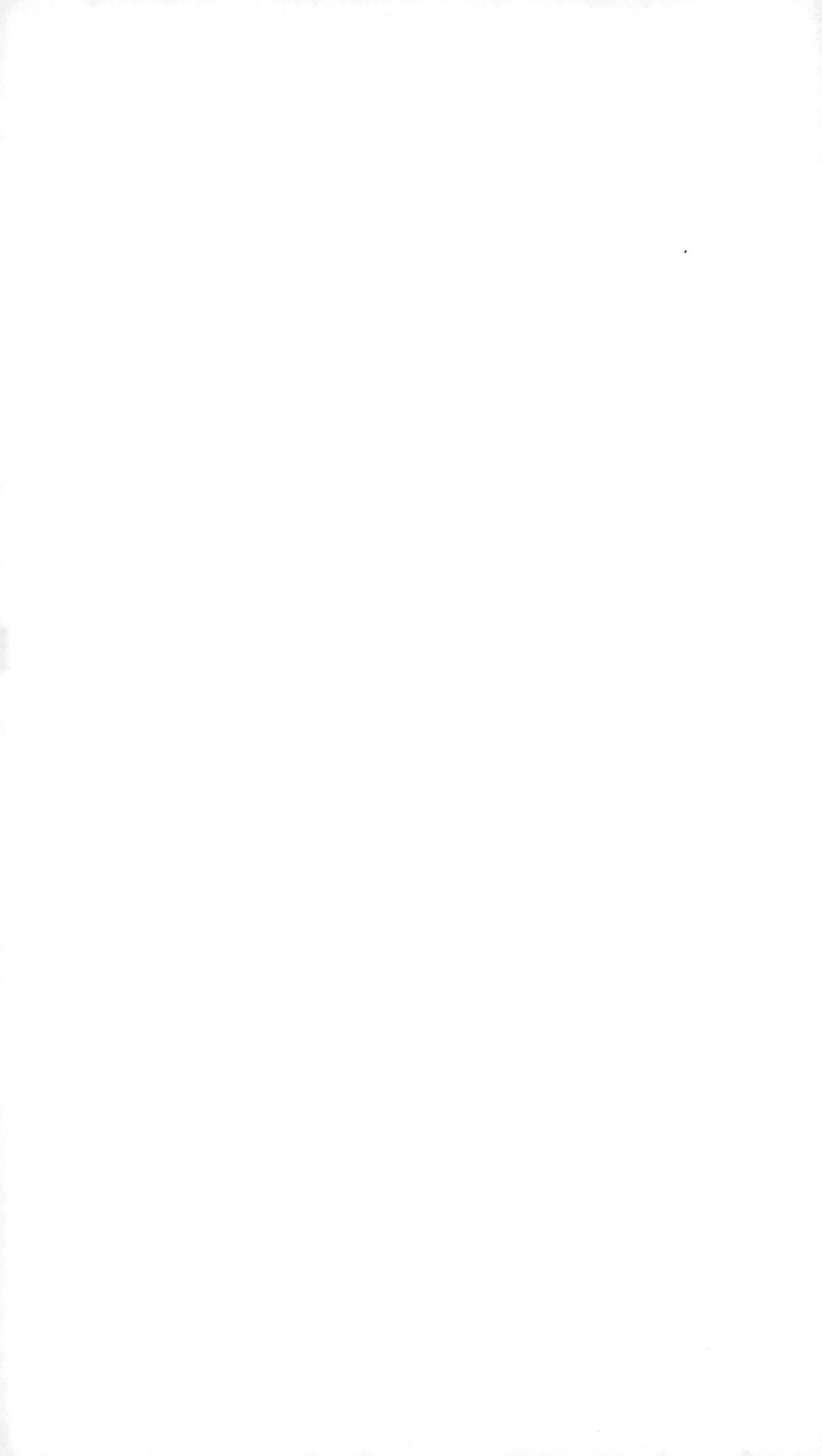

Chapter 11

Antiseizure Medications in the Elderly

Epilepsy is a common neurological problem in the elderly. The incidence of epileptic seizures rises steadily after age 60, so the need for antiseizure medications (ASMs) increases with age. Etiologies of epileptic seizures are diverse in the elderly. A study of 151 patients with new-onset seizures after age 60 reported that 32% of the seizures were caused by strokes, and 14% were caused by brain tumors. Most tumors were metastatic (71%), and 25% of patients had no identifiable cause (Luhdorf et al., 1986). Other studies have found trauma, infectious causes, toxic and metabolic causes, and degenerative diseases, among others to be causes of epilepsy in the elderly.

While similar principles of drug selection apply to elderly individuals and to younger patients, certain factors carry greater weight in the elderly. Selection of the appropriate therapy should be guided by the recognition that older patients often have comorbidity including other neurological diseases, receive multiple medications that can affect and be affected by ASMs, and have age-related changes in physiology (e.g., decreased gastrointestinal absorption and renal function). Moreover, elderly individuals may be more sensitive to the adverse effects of ASMs (Perucca, 2007; Perucca et al., 2006). In this age group, monotherapy with an ASM is desirable, and life-long therapy may be required.

Features of ASMs that are especially desirable for use in the elderly include the following:

1. Lack of significant interactions with other medications
2. Lack of induction or inhibition of hepatic microsomal enzymes
3. Minimal protein binding
4. Once- or twice-daily dosing
5. No need for laboratory monitoring
6. Adverse-effect profile with minimal effects on cognitive function and bone metabolism
7. Low cost

These considerations have practical importance. For example, ASMs with enzyme-inducing or inhibiting properties, such as phenobarbital, phenytoin, carbamazepine, primidone, and valproate, alter concentrations of other medications and may render them either less effective or toxic. They also are associated with osteoporosis, which is a significant cause of morbidity in the elderly. The elderly are particularly susceptible to sedating or cognitive adverse effects, so drugs with prominent sedation or cognitive impairment properties, such as phenobarbital, benzodiazepines, primidone, and topiramate, may cause greater problems. Because elderly patients are apt to take multiple medications, significant drug-drug interactions that occur with some drugs, such as phenytoin, carbamazepine, phenobarbital, primidone, and valproate, pose a problem.

Prolonged exposure to ASMs and potentially interacting drugs may be associated with adverse outcomes such as stroke, myocardial infarction, and mortality. Integrating neurology and clinical pharmacy consultation, combined with electronic medical records systems that alert clinicians to significant drug-drug interactions, may improve care quality and outcomes in this vulnerable population (Pugh et al., 2010).

Creatinine clearance (CrCl) is reduced in the elderly, so drugs that are primarily cleared by the kidney, such as levetiracetam, may accumulate in higher serum concentrations than expected in young patients. These considerations do not mean that drugs that might be more complicated in elderly individuals should not be used but rather that careful attention must be paid to potential interactions, toxic levels, and adverse effects and that the use of some drugs must be limited, if possible.

Some studies have been performed in older adults comparing different ASMs (Del Bianco et al., 2019; Rowan et al., 2005; Saetre et al., 2007). A systematic review and network meta-analysis was performed to estimate the comparative efficacy and safety of ASMs in the elderly with new-onset epilepsy (Lattanzi et al., 2019). This study showed no significant difference in efficacy across treatment with either carbamazepine immediate-release and extended-release, lacosamide, lamotrigine, valproate, or levetiracetam. Carbamazepine had higher risk for withdrawal due to adverse effects in elderly patients. In general, the prescribed dose of drug should be lower in the elderly than in young individuals due to progressively decreasing renal and hepatic clearance with age.

This chapter summarizes features relevant to the prescription of ASMs in older patients. Further information regarding relevant pharmacological factors can be found in some of the references (Facts and Comparisons, 2007; Perucca et al., 2006; see also individual drug websites listed in the Online Resources section at the end of this chapter). In general, when prescribing ASMs to the elderly, start with a lower dose than is used in younger patients, titrate upward more slowly, target a lower final dose, and monitor carefully for adverse effects because these may appear earlier than usual. Therapeutic monitoring of drug levels may be important for these patients to aid in drug management.

Antiseizure Medications in the Elderly

Acetazolamide

Maximum dose in the elderly is similar to that in young adults (Facts and Comparisons, 2007). However, dose reductions should be considered in this age group to compensate for age-related reductions in renal drug clearance. There is potential for renal stone formation and drug interaction.

Benzodiazepines

Because elderly patients are more likely to have decreased hepatic and/or renal function, care should be taken in using these drugs, and lower doses are used. Observe for sedating effects and avoid use if possible.

Brivaracetam

The steady-state plasma clearance of brivaracetam is slightly lower in elderly than in young healthy controls. Dose selection for an elderly patient should be judicious, usually starting at the low end of the dosing range.

Cannabidiol

In general, dose selection for an elderly patient should be cautious, usually starting at the lower end of the dosing range.

Carbamazepine

Hepatic clearance is decreased by 25–40% in elderly patients compared with younger adults so lower doses are used (Kirmani et al., 2014; Perucca et al., 2006). Due to drug interactions, use with caution.

Cenobamate

No clinically significant differences in the pharmacokinetics of cenobamate were observed based on age in subjects age 18–77 years. However, dose selection for an elderly patient should be cautious, usually targeting the lower end of the therapeutic range as an initial maintenance dose (100 mg/day).

Eslicarbazepine

Although the pharmacokinetics of eslicarbazepine are not affected by age independently, dose selection should take into consideration the greater frequency of renal impairment, medical comorbidities, and drug therapies in elderly patients.

Ethosuximide

This drug is rarely appropriate for elderly patients because they rarely have true absence seizures. Drug interactions are sometimes important.

Ezogabine

Dosage adjustment is recommended in patients age 65 years and older. Ezogabine may cause urinary retention. Elderly men with symptomatic benign prostatic hyperplasia (BPH) may be at increased risk for urinary retention.

Gabapentin

This is well-tolerated and treats concomitant neuropathy and pain. It is often a good choice if these are present. Average decrease in clearance of gabapentin in elderly patients compared with younger adults is about 30–50%, so lower doses can be used (Perucca et al., 2006). This drug is often a good choice for the elderly, particularly with appropriate comorbidity.

Lacosamide

No dose adjustment based on age is necessary. In elderly patients, dose titration should be performed with caution. This drug is a good choice.

Lamotrigine

The elderly exhibit a reduced hepatic clearance, higher peak concentrations, and longer elimination half-life compared with young adults. Average decrease in apparent clearance of lamotrigine in elderly patients compared with younger adults is about 35% (Perucca et al., 2006). It is recommended that elderly patients receive lower dosages than would be prescribed for young adults, targeting 100 mg/day as an initial maintenance dose. This drug is a good choice.

Levetiracetam

This drug has ideal pharmacological properties and is a good choice for elderly patients who require ASM therapy. Average decrease in renal clearance of levetiracetam in elderly patients compared with younger adults is about 20–40% (Perucca et al., 2006), so doses of 500–750 mg/day may be sufficient. This drug is often an excellent choice for the treatment of seizures in the elderly.

Oxcarbazepine

Average decrease in hepatic clearance of oxcarbazepine in elderly patients compared with younger adults is about 25–35% (Perucca et al., 2006). Adverse effects and drug interactions are relatively favorable; however, hyponatremia is relatively common in our experience. Use with caution because of the potential for hyponatremia.

Perampanel

In elderly patients, dose titration should be performed with caution. An increased risk of falls occurred in patients being treated with perampanel (with and without concurrent seizures). Elderly patients had an increased risk of falls compared to younger adults.

Phenobarbital

Average decrease in hepatic clearance of phenobarbital in elderly patients compared to younger adults is about 20% (Perucca et al., 2006). Sedation, hepatic enzyme induction, and drug interactions limit its use. However, this drug is quite inexpensive and may be a reasonable choice when cost poses difficulties (Kirmani et al., 2014). Lower doses, perhaps 45–90 mg/day, are effective in elderly patients.

Phenytoin

Average decrease in hepatic clearance of phenytoin in elderly patients compared with younger adults is about 25% (Perucca et al., 2006). Due to drug interactions and complicated kinetics, this drug is less than ideal. As a cytochrome P-450 enzyme inducer, it increases clearance of other hepatically metabolized drugs and is therefore suboptimal for that reason as well. This is considered a second-line drug, and better choices are available. Cost and ability to give IV doses are its major advantages (Kirmani et al., 2014).

Pregabalin

This drug is a reasonable choice for elderly patients due to minimal drug interactions and treatment of concomitant neuropathy and pain. Reduction of pregabalin dose is required in elderly patients based on CrCl so that a total dose of 150–200 mg/day may achieve levels similar to higher doses in younger patients.

Primidone

Decreased hepatic clearance mandates lower doses than in young patients. Due to sedative effects, potential for depression, and drug interactions, it should rarely be used. However, if the patient has essential tremor requiring treatment, this drug may treat both conditions.

Rufinamide

In elderly patients, dose titration should be performed with caution. Pharmacokinetics of rufinamide in the elderly is similar to that in young adults.

Tiagabine

Average decrease in clearance of tiagabine in elderly patients compared with younger adults is about 30% (Perucca et al., 2006). Elderly patients may be at increased risk for falls while on this drug (Kirmani et al., 2014). This drug is infrequently used.

Topiramate

The possibility of age-associated renal functional abnormalities should be considered. Average decrease in apparent clearance of topiramate in elderly patients compared to younger adults is about 20% (Perucca et al., 2006). Due to cognitive adverse effects and potential for renal stones, use with caution (Kirmani et al., 2014). Comorbidity of migraine and obesity may make this a good choice for some patients. Lower doses, perhaps as low as 50–75 mg/day, may be used.

Valproic Acid, Valproate, Divalproex Sodium

Average decrease in apparent clearance of valproate in elderly patients compared with younger adults is about 40% (Perucca et al., 2006). In addition, a decrease in valproic acid protein binding occurs consequent to hypoalbuminemia, and the half-life of the drug can be prolonged in geriatric patients. In general, use reduced initial dosage and slower dose titration in this age group. Target doses may be as low as 500 mg/day in some patients. Dose reductions or discontinuation should be considered in patients with decreased food or fluid intake and in patients with excessive somnolence. This drug is less than ideal in elderly patients.

Zonisamide

Dosage needs to be reduced in elderly patients because of age-related diminished renal clearance. Adverse effects are sometimes important, and the potential for renal stones should be considered.

Recommended Antiseizure Medications in Elderly Persons with Epilepsy

- *Focal epilepsies*: Lacosamide, lamotrigine, levetiracetam, gabapentin.
- *Generalized epilepsies*: These do not occur de novo in the elderly but when present consider using lower doses of existing medications if well-controlled, and valproate, lamotrigine, or levetiracetam if starting a new agent.

References

Del Bianco C, Placidi F, Liguori C, et al. Long-term efficacy and safety of lacosamide and levetiracetam monotherapy in elderly patients with focal epilepsy: A retrospective study. *Epilepsy Behav.* 2019;94:178–182.

Facts and Comparisons. *Drug Facts and Comparisons*. St. Louis: Wolters Kluwer Health/Facts & Comparisons; 2007.

Kirmani BF, Robinson DM, Kikam A, Fonkem E, Cruz D. Selection of antiepileptic drugs in older people. *Curr Treat Options Neurol*. 2014;16(6):295.

Lattanzi S, Trinka E, Del Giovane C, et al. Antiepileptic drug monotherapy for epilepsy in the elderly: A systematic review and network meta-analysis. *Epilepsia.* 2019;60(11):2245–2254.

Luhdorf K, Jensen LK, Plesner AM. Etiology of seizures in the elderly. *Epilepsia.* 1986;27:458–463.

Perucca E. Age-related changes in pharmacokinetics: predictability and assessment methods. *Int Rev Neurobiol.* 2007;81:183–199.

Perucca E, Berlowitz D, Birnbaum, et al. Pharmacological and clinical aspects of anti-epileptic drug use in the elderly. *Epilepsy Res.* 2006;68S:S49–S63.

Pugh MJ, Vancott AC, Steinman MA, et al. Choice of initial antiepileptic drug for older veterans: possible pharmacokinetic drug interactions with existing medications. *J Am Geriatr Soc.* 2010;58(3):465–471.

Rowan AJ, Ramsay RE, Collins JF, et al. New onset geriatric epilepsy: A randomized study of gabapentin, lamotrigine, and carbamazepine. *Neurology.* 2005;64:1868–1873.

Saetre E, Perucca E, Isojärvi J, Gjerstad L, LAM 40089 Study Group. An international multicenter randomized double-blind controlled trial of lamotrigine and sustained-release carbamazepine in the treatment of newly diagnosed epilepsy in the elderly. *Epilepsia.* 2007;48:1292–1302.

Online Resources

Brivaracetam (Briviact). www.briviact.com/2020

Cannabidiol (Epidiolex). www.epidiolex.com/2020

Cenobamate (Xcopri). https://reference.medscape.com/drug/xcopri-cenobamate-1000328/2020

Eslicarbazine acetate (Aptiom). www.aptiom.com/2014

Ezogabine (Potiga). www.potiga.com/2014

Lacosamide (Vimpat). www.vimpat.com/2014

Perampanel (Fycompa). us.eisai.com/wps/wcm/connect/Eisai/Home/Our.../FYCOMPA/2014

Rufinamide (Banzel). www.banzel.com/2014

Chapter 12

Antiseizure Medications in Patients with Renal Disease

The use of antiseizure medications (ASMs) in the presence of renal insufficiency is associated with an increased risk of adverse effects. Knowledge of the mechanisms of elimination of these drugs is crucial when selecting an ASM in patient with epilepsy with renal impairment (Facts and Comparisons, 2007; Kuo et al., 2002; Lacerda et al., 2006; RxList, n.d.). Drugs that are cleared by the kidneys have different pharmacokinetic properties in the presence of renal failure, and intermittent dialysis may cause significant variability in serum levels.

Moreover, renal failure is often accompanied by other medical problems, which can influence drug levels (Kuo et al., 2002). Renal failure is associated with gastroparesis, which slows absorption, and bowel edema, which may reduce absorption. There is often a decrease in gut cytochrome P-450 metabolism and P-glycoprotein active transport, which can affect how much of the drug enters the portal circulation. Renal failure is also associated with hypoalbuminemia, which may influence free plasma concentrations of ASMs that are highly protein bound. Acidosis may affect albumen-binding affinity as well.

Reduced renal function and hypoalbuminemia lead to the accumulation of renally excreted ASMs, such as eslicarbazepine acetate, gabapentin, pregabalin, vigabatrin, and levetiracetam. If there is coexisting impairment of liver function, drugs metabolized by the liver may have altered kinetics as well. ASMs that have low protein binding are largely removed through hemodialysis. Last, seizures may be caused by uremia and its associated conditions, such as intracranial hemorrhage, glucose and electrolyte imbalances, dialysis encephalopathy, primary cerebral lymphoma, opportunistic infections, and immunosuppressant toxicity in renal transplant recipients (Kuo et al., 2002).

In patients who require dialysis or in whom dialysis is anticipated, it may be wisest to use drugs that are cleared by hepatic mechanisms rather than eliminated by the kidneys. In addition, ASMs with relatively high levels of protein binding are easier to manage, although they might be less desirable for other properties; a balance must then be struck. Carbamazepine, lamotrigine, benzodiazepines (e.g., clobazam, clonazepam), and rufinamide are preferred when renal failure is present, particularly when dialysis is needed. Therapeutic monitoring of drug levels is important for these patients, and ascertainment of free levels is preferred.

Antiseizure Medications in Patients with Renal Disease

Acetazolamide

Dosage adjustment in patients with renal impairment depends on renal function and creatinine clearance of the patient (Table 12.1).

Intermittent Hemodialysis: Acetazolamide is contraindicated in patients with severe renal disease. It may potentiate acidosis and may cause central nervous system adverse effects in dialysis patients.

Peritoneal Dialysis: Acetazolamide should be avoided in patients on continuous ambulatory peritoneal dialysis (CAPD) to prevent drug-induced hyperkalemia or metabolic acidosis.

Benzodiazepines

No quantitative recommendations are available for patients with renal impairment. Due to the lack of renal excretion of unchanged drug, benzo doses do not need to be adjusted in renal dysfunction. Because active drug is not excreted by the kidneys, clonazepam doses will not need to be reduced in patients with renal dysfunction. The minimal renal excretion of lorazepam, midazolam, and diazepam or any of the active metabolites suggests that dosage adjustment is not needed in patients with renal disease (Anderson and Hakimian, 2014).

Brivaracetam

Dose adjustments are not required for patients with impaired renal function. Since there are no data available in patients with end-stage renal disease undergoing dialysis, use of brivaracetam is not recommended in this patient population (brivaracetam; www.briviact.com/2020).

Cannabidiol

Dose adjustments are not required for patients with impaired renal function. As there is minimal excretion of cannabidiol by the kidneys, doses should not need to be reduced in renal dysfunction (cannabidiol; www.epidiolex.com/2020).

Carbamazepine

No quantitative recommendations are available for patients with renal impairment. As there is minimal excretion of carbamazepine by the kidneys,

Table 12.1 Acetazolamide Dosage Adjustment Based on Renal Function

Creatinine clearance (mL/min)	Dose regimen
50 to 80	3 or 4 times/day
10 to 50	1 or 2 times/day
<10	Contraindicated

carbamazepine doses should not need to be reduced in renal dysfunction (Anderson and Hakimian, 2014).

Cenobamate

Cenobamate is primarily cleared by the liver, though a glucuronide metabolite is excreted by the kidneys. Dose reduction should be considered in patients with renal impairment. Use in patients with end-stage renal disease undergoing dialysis is not studied. The effect of hemodialysis on cenobamate pharmacokinetics has not been studied (cenobamate; https://reference.medscape.com/drug/xcopri-cenobamate-1000328/2020).

Eslicarbazepine Acetate

Clearance of eslicarbazepine is decreased in patients with impaired renal function and is correlated with creatinine clearance. Dosage should be modified depending on clinical response and degree of renal impairment. A dose reduction is recommended in patients with renal impairment (creatinine clearance <60 mL/min). Start treatment at 200 mg once daily. After two weeks, increase dosage to 400 mg once daily, which is the recommended maintenance dosage. Eslicarbazepine is not recommended in patients with creatinine clearance of less than 30 mL/min. Eslicarbazepine is dialyzable; however, no dosage adjustments have been recommended (Anderson and Hakimian, 2014).

Ethosuximide

No dosage adjustment is needed in patients with renal dysfunction since only a small percentage of ethosuximide is renally eliminated unchanged (Anderson and Hakimian, 2014).

Hemodialysis: Ethosuximide is dialyzable, however, no dosage adjustments have been recommended.

Ezogabine

Dosage adjustment is recommended for patients with CrCl of less than 50 mL/min or in patients with end-stage renal disease receiving dialysis treatments. Dosage should be modified depending on clinical response and degree of renal impairment. In patients with renal impairment (CrCL <50 mL/min or end-stage renal disease on dialysis) the initial dose is 50 mg 3 times daily (150 mg/day) and the maximum dose is 200 mg 3 times daily (600 mg/day). The effect of hemodialysis on ezogabine clearance has not been established.

Felbamate

Felbamate should be used with caution in patients with renal impairment. The starting and maintenance doses should be reduced by one-half in patients with renal impairment.

Gabapentin

Dosage adjustment in patients with renal impairment depends on renal function and CrCl of the patient. The recommendations in Table 12.2 have been made for adults and adolescents older than 12 years.

Table 12.2 Gabapentin Dosage Adjustment Based on Renal Function

Creatinine clearance (CrCl) (mL/min)	Gabapentin dosage (mg/day)	Dose regimen
≥60	900 to 3600	3 times per day
30 to 59	400 to 1400	2 times per day
15 to 29	200 to 700	Once a day
15	100 to 300	Once a day
<15	Reduce daily dose in proportion to CrCl*	Once a day

* For example, patients with a CrCl of 7.5 mL/min should receive one-half the dose that patients with CrCl of 15 mL/min receive.

Intermittent Hemodialysis: Patients on hemodialysis should receive maintenance doses based on CrCl as indicated for patients with renal impairment. A supplemental dose equal to the daily dose plus 50 mg is recommended after a 4-hour hemodialysis session (Anderson and Hakimian, 2014).

Lacosamide

No dose adjustment is necessary in patients with mild to moderate renal impairment. A maximum dose of 300 mg/day is recommended for patients with severe renal impairment (CrCl of ≤30 mL/min) and in patients with end-stage renal disease. In all renally impaired patients, the dose titration should be performed with caution. Patients with renal impairment who are taking strong inhibitors of CYP3A4 and CYP2C9 (e.g., valproate) may have a significant increase in exposure to lacosamide. Dose reduction may be necessary in these patients.

Intermittent Hemodialysis: Lacosamide is effectively removed from plasma by hemodialysis. Following a 4-hour hemodialysis treatment, dosage supplementation of up to 50% should be considered.

Lamotrigine

In patients with renal impairment, dosage should be modified depending on clinical response and degree of renal impairment. No quantitative recommendations are available.

Intermittent Hemodialysis: Hemodialysis decreases the elimination half-life of lamotrigine. Approximately 20% of lamotrigine present in the body is removed after a standard 4-hour dialysis session (Fillastre et al., 1993). An additional dose of lamotrigine is not needed to maintain therapeutic concentrations (Anderson and Hakimian, 2014). However, adjust dosage schedules to give a normally administered dosage after the hemodialysis session. No quantitative recommendations are available for adjustments.

Levetiracetam

The dosage adjustments given in Table 12.3 pertain to adults with renal impairment using estimated CrCl. Children with renal impairment also need modified dosages but no quantitative recommendations are available.

Table 12.3 Levetiracetam Dosage Adjustment Based on Renal Function

Creatinine clearance (mL/min)	Levetiracetam dosage (mg/day)	Dose regimen
>80	No need for adjustment	—
50 to 80	1000 to 2000	2 times per day
30 to 49	500 to 1500	2 times per day
<30	500 to 1000	2 times per day
ESRD patients using dialysis	500 to 1,000	Every 24 hours (Once)

Intermittent Hemodialysis: Standard hemodialysis results in a roughly 50% clearance of levetiracetam in 4 hours. A supplemental dose (50% of a single usual dose) compensating for this loss is recommended following dialysis.

Oxcarbazepine

If CrCl is greater than 30 mL/min, no dosage adjustments have been recommended. However, renal clearance of its monohydroxy derivative (MHD), the active metabolite, declines linearly with a decrease in creatinine clearance. If CrCl is less than 30 mL/min, renal clearance of MHD is decreased. Therefore, initiate therapy with 50% of the usual starting dose and slowly titrate upward as necessary.

Perampanel

No dosage adjustment is necessary for patients with mild renal impairment. Perampanel can be used in patients with moderate renal impairment with close monitoring. A slower titration may be considered based on clinical response and tolerability. Use in patients with severe renal impairment or patients undergoing hemodialysis is not recommended.

Phenobarbital

If CrCl is greater than 10 mL/min, no dosage adjustment is needed. If CrCl is less than 10 mL/min, significantly decrease dosage by increasing the interval between the doses to 12 hours or longer. Adjust dosage based on clinical response and serum concentrations. The chronic use of phenobarbital should generally be avoided in patients with renal failure.

Intermittent Hemodialysis: Phenobarbital is efficiently removed through hemodialysis. Adjust dosage schedules to give a normally administered dosage after the hemodialysis session. It is better to administer the supplementary dose after hemodialysis.

Peritoneal Dialysis: Peritoneal dialysis (as CAPD) removes phenobarbital by almost 35–50% (not as efficient as hemodialysis) (Porto et al., 1997). It is suggested that 50% of a normal dose be given after a CAPD session.

Table 12.4 Pregabalin Dosage Adjustment Based on Renal Function

Creatinine clearance (mL/min)	Pregabalin dosage (mg/day)	Dose regimen
>60	No need for adjustment	—
30 to 60	75 to 300	2 or 3 divided doses
15 to 30	25 to 150	1 or 2 times per day
<15	25 to 75	Once per day

Phenytoin

If CrCl is greater than 10 mL/min, no dosage adjustment is needed. If CrCl is less than 10 mL/min, dosage adjustment and serum concentration monitoring are necessary. Decreased protein binding occurs in uremia, and the unbound (free) fraction of phenytoin may be increased. Dosing adjustments may be required based on serum-free phenytoin level monitoring and clinical response.

Dialysis (Hemodialysis or Peritoneal Dialysis): Phenytoin is not significantly removed during a standard hemodialysis session or continuous hemodialysis or peritoneal dialysis. However, supplemental dosing after dialysis is controversial.

Pregabalin

Dose adjustments are required in patients with renal impairment with CrCl of less than 60 mL/min (Table 12.4). Reduction of pregabalin dose may be required in elderly patients based on CrCl.

Intermittent Hemodialysis: Pregabalin is effectively removed through hemodialysis because it has little plasma protein binding. Each 4-hour hemodialysis session removes 50–60% of the amount of drug present in the circulation in patients on three times per week hemodialysis. For patients undergoing hemodialysis, pregabalin daily dose should be adjusted based on renal function. In addition to the daily dose adjustment, a supplemental (single additional) dose should be given immediately following every 4-hour hemodialysis treatment as follows:

- *Patients on the 25 mg/day regimen*: Take one supplemental dose of 25 mg or 50 mg.
- *Patients on the 25–50 mg/day regimen*: Take one supplemental dose of 50 mg or 75 mg.
- *Patients on the 50–70 mg/day regimen*: Take one supplemental dose of 75 mg or 100 mg.
- *Patients on the 75 mg/day regimen*: Take one supplemental dose of 100 mg or 150 mg.

Primidone

Dose adjustments are required in patients with renal impairment with CrCl of less than 50 mL/min (Table 12.5). Monitor clinical response and serum concentrations.

Table 12.5 Primidone Dosage Adjustment Based on Renal Function	
Creatinine clearance (mL/min)	**Dose regimen**
>50	No dosage adjustment is needed
10 to 50	Every 8 to 12 hours
<10	Every 12 to 24 hours

Intermittent Hemodialysis: Primidone is partially removed through hemodialysis. Some references recommend supplementing with one-third of a routine dose after a hemodialysis session. We generally avoid prescribing this drug irrespective of diagnosis.

Rufinamide

Renally impaired patients (CrCl <30 mL/min) do not require any special dosage change. Rufinamide pharmacokinetics in patients with severe renal impairment (CrCl <30 mL/min) was similar to that of healthy subjects.

Intermittent Hemodialysis: Patients undergoing dialysis 3 hours post-rufinamide dosing showed a reduction in area under the curve (AUC) and C_{max} of 29% and 16%, respectively. Adjusting rufinamide dose for the loss of drug upon dialysis should be considered. No quantitative recommendations are available for adjustments.

Tiagabine

No initial dosage adjustment is required in patients with renal impairment. Adjust dosage according to patient's response and tolerance.

Topiramate

In adults, if CrCl is less than 70 mL/min, reduce the topiramate dose to one-half of the usual dose. In children, adjustment may be required but should be individualized because clearance rates are higher in children than in adults. Patients with renal impairment may require a longer time than patients with normal renal function to reach steady state with each topiramate dosage adjustment.

Intermittent Hemodialysis: During the hemodialysis session, adult patients clear topiramate at a rate that is 4–6 times greater than that of an adult with normal renal function. A supplemental dose of topiramate may be required during or after hemodialysis.

Valproic Acid, Valproate, Divalproex Sodium

In patients with severe renal impairment or renal failure, uremia can cause an increase in the free fraction of the drug, resulting in possible toxicity. Also, unbound valproic acid in the blood may be cleared more rapidly than bound drug. Close monitoring of valproic acid serum concentrations may be warranted to ensure adequate dosage, ensure efficacy, and limit toxicity. A supplemental dose of valproate may be required after hemodialysis in some patients.

Vigabatrin

It is recommended that the dose of vigabatrin be reduced by 25%, 50%, or 75% for patients with mild (CrCl 50–80 mL/min), moderate (CrCl 30–50 mL/min), or severe (CrCl 10–30 mL/min) renal dysfunction, respectively.

Zonisamide

Because zonisamide is excreted by the kidneys, patients with renal impairment or renal disease should be treated with caution. Slower titration and more frequent monitoring may be required. No quantitative recommendations are available.

Intermittent Hemodialysis: Zonisamide is partially removed through hemodialysis (about 50%). Adjust dosage schedules to give a normally administered dosage after the hemodialysis session.

Recommended Antiseizure Medications in Patients with Renal Failure

1. *Generalized epilepsies*: Cannabidiol (in patients with Lennox-Gastaut syndrome or Dravet syndrome), clobazam, ethosuximide, lamotrigine, rufinamide (in patients with Lennox-Gastaut syndrome)
2. *Focal epilepsies*: Brivaracetam (not in patients with end-stage renal disease undergoing dialysis), carbamazepine, clobazam, lacosamide (not in patients undergoing dialysis), lamotrigine, phenytoin

Note: Seizures are a serious complication of hemodialysis in people with epilepsy. They may occur within the first 24 hours of beginning dialysis and are usually tonic-clonic. Preexisting hypertension and the use of dialyzable ASMs are associated with dialysis-related seizures. These may be due to the removal of these drugs at a time when metabolic stress induces seizures.

In one pediatric study, phenobarbital was given at a dosage of 5 mg/kg/day orally twice daily to prevent dialysis-associated seizures. Also, diazepam (0.5 mg/kg orally) was administered 30 minutes before each dialysis session in some patients. Patients receiving diazepam prophylaxis had significantly fewer seizures than those with no treatment or patients receiving phenobarbital alone. Therefore, administration of oral diazepam, a nondialyzable ASM, 30 minutes before each dialysis may help prevent dialysis-associated seizures (Sonmez et al., 2000).

Urinary Adverse Effects of Antiseizure Medications

Many ASMs are associated with urinary and renal adverse effects (Drug Facts and Comparisons, 2007; Lacerda et al., 2006; RxList, n.d.; see also individual drug websites listed in the Online Resources section at the end of this chapter). These include:

Acetazolamide: Carbonic anhydrase inhibitors are sulfonamide derivatives that may cause crystalluria and sulfonamide-like nephrotoxicity characterized by renal tubular obstruction, hematuria, dysuria, and oliguria. An increase in calcium excretion can cause nephrolithiasis. Patients with preexisting hypercalcemia develop renal calculi most frequently.

Benzodiazepines: No significant urinary adverse effects have been reported.

Brivaracetam: No significant urinary adverse effects have been reported.

Cannabidiol: Cannabidiol can cause elevations in serum creatinine. The mechanism has not been determined. In controlled studies, an increase in serum creatinine of approximately 10% was observed within 2 weeks of starting cannabidiol.

Carbamazepine: Urinary adverse effects include increased urinary frequency, acute urinary retention, oliguria with elevated blood pressure, azotemia, and renal failure. Albuminuria, glycosuria, and microscopic deposits in the urine have also been observed. Carbamazepine may rarely cause interstitial nephritis or other renal diseases. Occasional monitoring of renal parameters or urinalysis has been recommended.

Cenobamate: No significant urinary adverse effects have been reported.

Eslicarbazepine acetate: No significant urinary adverse effects have been reported.

Ethosuximide: No significant urinary adverse effects have been reported.

Ezogabine: Because of the increased risk of urinary retention on ezogabine (in about 2% of the patients), urologic symptoms should be carefully monitored. Urinary retention was generally reported within the first 6 months of treatment, but was also observed later. Closer monitoring is recommended for patients who have other risk factors for urinary retention (e.g., benign prostatic hyperplasia), patients who are unable to communicate clinical symptoms (e.g., cognitively impaired patients), or patients who use concomitant medications that may affect voiding (e.g., anticholinergics). In these patients, a comprehensive evaluation of urologic symptoms prior to and during treatment with ezogabine may be appropriate. Hydronephrosis is a rare adverse effect in patients taking ezogabine. Dysuria and hematuria have been reported as adverse effects of ezogabine.

Felbamate: Crystalluria and urolithiasis have been reported with felbamate. Urinary tract infection and lowered blood urea nitrogen levels have been reported as a result of felbamate therapy.

Gabapentin: No significant urinary adverse effects have been reported.

Lacosamide: No significant urinary adverse effects have been reported.

Lamotrigine: No significant urinary adverse effects have been reported.

Levetiracetam: No significant urinary adverse effects have been reported.

Oxcarbazepine: Dysuria, hematuria, increased urinary frequency, urinary tract pain, polyuria, and renal calculus have been reported as adverse effects of oxcarbazepine.

Perampanel: No significant urinary adverse effects have been reported.

Phenobarbital: No significant urinary adverse effects have been reported. Reports of interstitial nephritis are rare.

Phenytoin: Phenytoin rarely causes renal complications. Glomerulonephritis, interstitial nephritis, proteinuria, and nephrotic syndrome have been reported.

Pregabalin: There are reports of increased urinary frequency and urinary incontinence with pregabalin. However, causality between pregabalin and these adverse events has not been definitively established.

Rufinamide: Urinary incontinence, dysuria, hematuria, nephrolithiasis, polyuria, enuresis, nocturia, and incontinence have infrequently been reported as adverse effects of rufinamide.

Tiagabine: No significant urinary adverse effects have been reported.

Topiramate: Nephrolithiasis, hematuria, increased urinary frequency, dysuria, and urinary incontinence have been reported as adverse effects of topiramate.

Valproate: No significant urinary adverse effects have been reported.

Vigabatrin: No significant urinary adverse effects have been reported.

Zonisamide: Increases in serum creatinine and blood urea nitrogen have been reported. Nephrolithiasis has been reported. Other infrequent adverse reactions affecting the urinary system in zonisamide-treated patients include dysuria, hematuria, nocturia, polyuria, urinary frequency, urinary incontinence, urinary retention, and urinary urgency. Rare adverse reactions include albuminuria, bladder pain, and bladder calculus.

Renal Stones

Zonisamide, topiramate, and acetazolamide, which all have carbonic anhydrase-inhibiting properties, are associated with a modest increase in the incidence of renal stones due to reduced urinary citrate excretion and increased urinary pH. Zonisamide is associated with a 4% incidence of renal stones. Approximately 1.5% of patients treated with topiramate developed kidney stones compared with the annual 0.5% incidence of renal stones in the general population. Men are at higher risk for kidney stones, and the association has also been reported for children treated with topiramate. The analyzed stones are mainly composed of calcium phosphate (Kuo et al., 2002). The ketogenic diet may also be associated with renal stones (Kossoff et al., 2002).

In general, increasing fluid intake and urine output can help reduce the risk of stone formation in patients taking zonisamide, topiramate, or acetazolamide or those on the ketogenic diet, particularly in patients with predisposing factors (Kossoff et al., 2002). If there is marked benefit with therapy with one of these drugs, and drugs that do not cause nephrolithiasis have not proved effective, the development of renal calculi is not an absolute indication to discontinue the treatment (Richards et al., 2005).

References

Anderson GD, Hakimian S. Pharmacokinetic of antiepileptic drugs in patients with hepatic or renal impairment. *Clin Pharmacokinet.* 2014;53(1):29–49.

Drug Facts and Comparisons. St. Louis: Wolters Kluwer Health/Facts and Comparisons, 2007.

Fillastre JP, Taburet AM, Fialaire A, et al. Pharmacokinetics of lamotrigine in patients with renal impairment: influence of haemodialysis. *Drugs Under Experimental and Clinical Research*. 1993;19:25–32.

Kossoff EH, Pyzik PL, Furth SL, et al. Kidney stones, carbonic anhydrase inhibitors, and the ketogenic diet. *Epilepsia*. 2002;43:1168–1171.

Kuo RL, Moran ME, Kim DH, et al. Topiramate-Induced nephrolithiasis. *Journal of Endocrinology*. 2002;16:229–231.

Lacerda G, Krummel T, Sabourdy C, et al. Optimizing therapy of seizures in patients with renal or hepatic dysfunction. *Neurology*. 2006;67:S28–S33.

Porto I, John EG, Heilliczer J. Removal of phenobarbital during continuous cycling peritoneal dialysis in a child. *Pharmacotherap*. 1997;17:832–835.

Richards KC, Smith MC, Verma A. Continued use of zonisamide following development of renal calculi. *Neurology*. 2005;64:763–764.

RxList: *The Internet drug list*. Retrieved from RxList Inc. http://www.rxlist.com/2014.

Sonmez F, Mir S, Tutuncuoglu S. Potential prophylactic use of benzodiazepines for hemodialysis-associated seizures. *Pediatric Nephrology*. 2000;14:367–369.

Online Resources

Brivaracetam (Briviact). www.briviact.com/2020

Cannabidiol (Epidiolex). www.epidiolex.com/2020

Cenobamate (Xcopri). https://reference.medscape.com/drug/xcopri-cenobamate-1000328/2020

Eslicarbazine acetate (Aptiom). www.aptiom.com/2014

Ezogabine (Potiga). www.potiga.com/2014

Lacosamide (Vimpat). www.vimpat.com/2014

Levetiracetam (Keppra). www.ucb.com/_up/ucb_com_products/documents/Keppra_IR_Current_COL_10_2019.pdf/2020

Perampanel (Fycompa). us.eisai.com/wps/wcm/connect/Eisai/Home/Our.../FYCOMPA/2014

Runfinamide (Banzel). www.banzel.com/2014

Vigabatrin (Sabril). www.lundbeck.com/upload/us/files/.../Sabril/2014

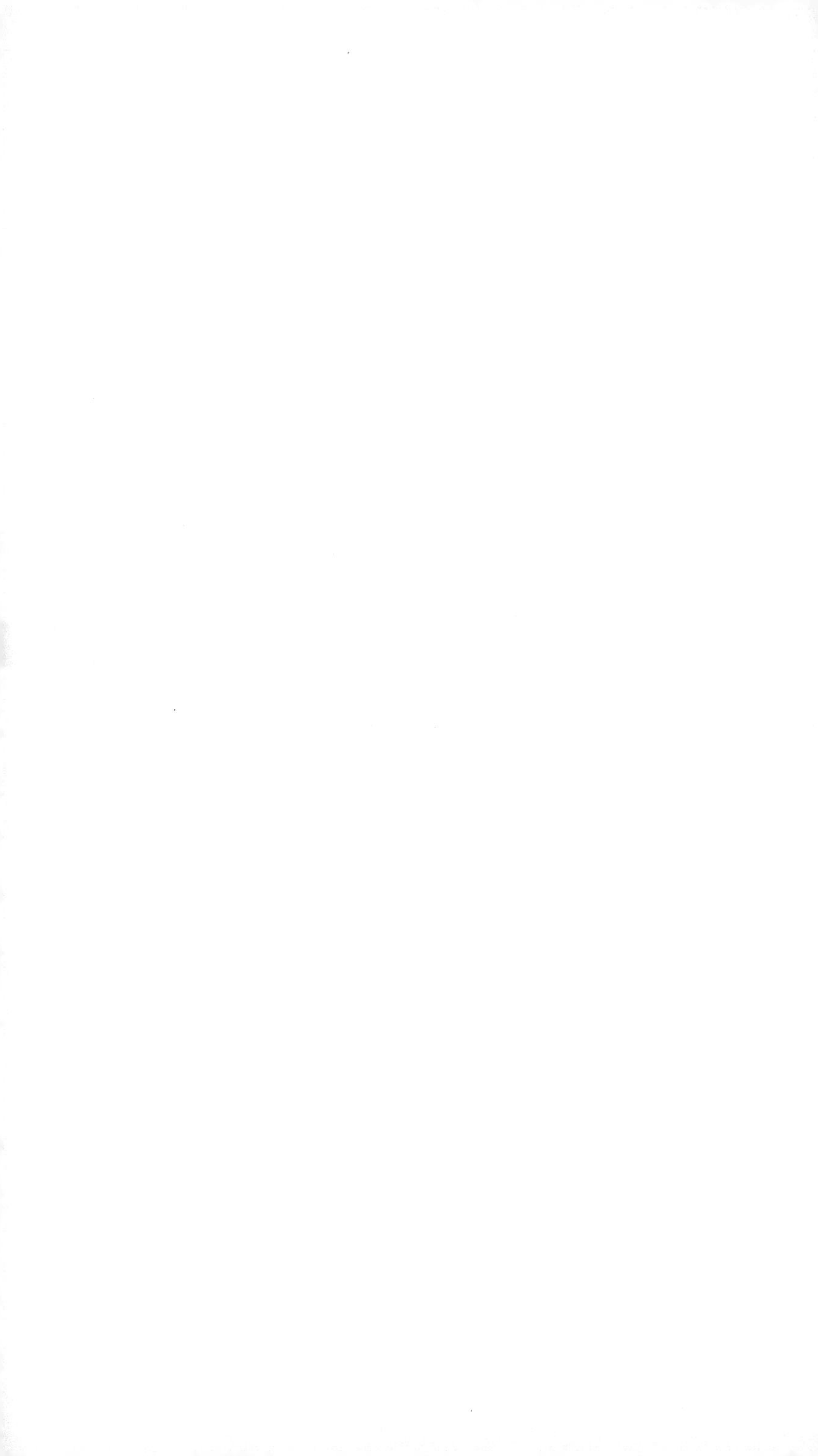

Chapter 13

Antiseizure Medications in Patients with Liver Disease

The use of antiseizure medications (ASMs) in the presence of liver diseases and hepatic dysfunction is associated with an increased risk of adverse effects. Knowledge of the mechanisms of metabolism and elimination of these drugs is crucial when selecting an ASM in patient with epilepsy with liver disease. Loss of hepatocytes and disruption of liver blood flow may alter the metabolism of some ASMs. Hypoalbuminemia and impaired metabolism by cytochrome P-450 and glucuronyl transferase enzymes may increase free ASM levels (Lacerda et al., 2006). The type of hepatic disease may also preferentially affect some enzyme systems; for example, CYP3A4 is affected more in hepatocellular dysfunction, and CYP2E1 is affected more in cholestasis. Unlike renal failure, which can be quantified, liver disease is not easily quantifiable, so adjustments in dosing are more difficult. Fortunately, even moderate liver dysfunction does not significantly impact ASM clearance, other than problems caused by the associated hypoalbuminemia, so dose adjustments are usually not needed until hepatic dysfunction is severe. In addition, some ASMs have important hepatic adverse effects (Facts and Comparisons, 2007; Lacerda et al., 2006; see also individual drug websites). Last, hepatic failure may cause renal impairment, so kidney function needs to be monitored and ASM dosing adjusted accordingly. Therapeutic monitoring of drug levels is important for these patients, and ascertainment of free levels is preferred.

In general, drugs with low protein binding that do not alter hepatic or renal clearance of other medications cleared by the kidneys, such as levetiracetam, lacosamide, and gabapentin, are preferred for ease of management, while acetazolamide, brivaracetam, cannabidiol, carbamazepine, cenobamate, felbamate, valproate, phenytoin, phenobarbital, and are less desirable. For the treatment of status epilepticus in patients with hepatic impairment, levetiracetam and lacosamide, both available in IV preparations, are reasonable second-line therapy after benzodiazepines fail to control seizures although the clinician is cautioned that randomized controlled trials do not exist for this indication (Vidaurre et al., 2017).

Antiseizure Medications in Liver Disease

Acetazolamide

Avoid acetazolamide use in patients with hepatic impairment. Patients with hepatic disease (e.g., cirrhosis) are at increased risk for hepatic encephalopathy and electrolyte imbalances (e.g., hypokalemia) (Facts and Comparisons, 2007; Lacerda et al., 2006).

Benzodiazepines

These drugs are to be avoided if possible. Dosage should be modified depending on clinical response and degree of hepatic impairment, but no quantitative recommendations are available for benzodiazepines. Hepatic dysfunction is among the adverse effects reported.

Clonazepam undergoes hepatic metabolism, and liver disease may impair clonazepam elimination. The drug should not be used in patients with significant liver dysfunction.

Lorazepam undergoes glucuronidation in the liver to inactive metabolites. However, studies in patients with cirrhosis or other significant liver diseases did not note a need for dose reduction (Facts and Comparisons, 2007; Lacerda et al., 2006). Therefore, lorazepam may be the benzodiazepine of choice (if there is no other alternative) for patients with liver disease since its half-life is minimally increased in the presence of hepatic dysfunction.

Brivaracetam

A pharmacokinetic study in adults with hepatic cirrhosis, Child-Pugh grades A, B, and C, showed 50%, 57%, and 59% increases in brivaracetam exposure, respectively, compared to matched healthy controls. Because of increases in brivaracetam exposure, dosage adjustment is recommended for all stages of hepatic impairment (brivaracetam; www.briviact.com/2020).

Cannabidiol

No effects on the exposures of cannabidiol or its metabolite were observed following administration of a single dose of cannabidiol 200 mg in patients with mild (Child-Pugh A) hepatic impairment. Patients with moderate (Child-Pugh B) or severe (Child-Pugh C) hepatic impairment had an approximately 2.5- to 5.2-fold higher area under the curve (AUC) compared with healthy volunteers with normal hepatic function. Because of an increase in exposure to cannabidiol, dosage adjustments are necessary in patients with moderate or severe hepatic impairment; its dosage does not require adjustments in patients with mild hepatic impairment (Table 13.1).

Cannabidiol causes dose-related elevations of liver transaminases (alanine aminotransferase [ALT] and/or aspartate aminotransferase [AST]). The

Table 13.1 Cannabidiol Dose Adjustment in Patients with Hepatic Impairment.

	Starting dose	Maintenance dose	Maximum dose
Moderate hepatic impairment	2.5 mg/kg/day, divided in two doses	5 mg/kg/day, divided in two doses	10 mg/kg/day, divided in two doses
Severe hepatic impairment	1 mg/kg/day, divided in two doses	2 mg/kg/day, divided in two doses	4 mg/kg/day, divided in two doses

most frequent cause of discontinuations of cannabidiol in clinical trials was transaminase elevation. In controlled studies for Lennox-Gastaut syndrome or Dravet syndrome, the incidence of ALT elevations higher than 3 times the upper limit of normal (ULN) was 13% in cannabidiol-treated patients compared with 1% in patients on placebo. Risk factors for transaminase elevations include taking concomitant valproate or clobazam, baseline transaminase levels above the ULN, and high doses of cannabidiol.

It is suggested to obtain serum transaminases (ALT and AST) and total bilirubin levels in all patients prior to starting treatment. Serum transaminases and total bilirubin levels should be checked at 1 month, 3 months, and 6 months after initiation of treatment and periodically thereafter or as clinically indicated. Serum transaminases and total bilirubin levels should also be obtained within 1 month following changes in cannabidiol dosage and addition of or changes in medications that are known to impact the liver. Consider more frequent monitoring of serum transaminases and bilirubin in patients who are taking valproate (or clobazam) or who have elevated liver enzymes at baseline. If a patient develops clinical signs or symptoms suggestive of hepatic dysfunction (e.g., unexplained nausea, vomiting, right upper quadrant abdominal pain, fatigue, anorexia, or jaundice and/or dark urine), immediately measure serum transaminases and total bilirubin and interrupt or discontinue treatment with cannabidiol as appropriate. Discontinue cannabidiol in any patient with elevations of transaminase levels greater than 3 times the ULN and bilirubin levels greater than 2 times the ULN. Patients with prolonged elevations of serum transaminases should be evaluated for other possible causes (cannabidiol; www.epidiolex.com/2020).

Carbamazepine

Carbamazepine is not recommended in patients with decompensated liver disease. Dose reductions are often necessary in patients with stable hepatic disease. Various hepatic adverse effects may occur during carbamazepine treatment, ranging from asymptomatic elevated liver enzymes to more serious derangements. Hepatitis and cholestasis have rarely been reported with carbamazepine therapy. Consider discontinuation of the drug if newly occurring or worsening clinical or laboratory evidence of liver dysfunction or hepatic damage occurs during carbamazepine treatment (Facts and Comparison, 2007; Lacerda et al., 2006).

Cenobamate

Use with caution in patients with mild to moderate hepatic impairment; a lower maintenance dosage might be required (data lacking). Use of cenobamate in patients with severe hepatic impairment is not recommended. Cenobamate may rarely cause dose-related elevations of liver transaminases (https://reference.medscape.com/drug/xcopri-cenobamate-1000328/2020).

Eslicarbazepine Acetate

Dose adjustments are not required in patients with mild to moderate hepatic impairment. Use of eslicarbazepine acetate in patients with severe hepatic impairment has not been studied and is not recommended.

Hepatic effects ranging from mild to moderate elevations in transaminases to rare cases with concomitant elevations of total bilirubin have been reported with eslicarbazepine acetate use. The combination of transaminase elevations and elevated bilirubin without evidence of obstruction is generally recognized as an important predictor of severe liver injury. Eslicarbazepine acetate should be discontinued in patients with jaundice or other evidence of significant liver injury (eslicarbazine acetate; http://www.aptiom.com/2014).

Ethosuximide

Specific guidelines for dosage adjustments of ethosuximide in hepatic impairment are not available. Dosage adjustment may be needed in moderate and severe cirrhosis, and ethosuximide plasma concentrations should be monitored (Anderson and Hakimian, 2014).

Elevated hepatic enzymes have been reported with ethosuximide treatment. Serious hepatic dysfunction may be an indication of drug hypersensitivity reaction and may require drug discontinuation (Facts and Comparisons, 2007; Knowles et al., 1999; Lacerda et al., 2006).

Ezogabine

No dosage adjustment is required for patients with mild hepatic impairment. In patients with moderate or severe hepatic impairment, the initial and maintenance dosage of ezogabine should be reduced. In patients with hepatic impairment and Child-Pugh 7–9, the initial dose is 50 mg 3 times daily (150 mg/day) and the maximum dose is 250 mg 3 times daily (750 mg/day). In patients with hepatic impairment and Child-Pugh greater than 9, the initial dose is 50 mg 3 times daily (150 mg/day) and the maximum dose is 200 mg 3 times daily (600 mg/day). Elevated hepatic enzymes have been reported with ezogabine treatment (ezobagine; http://www.potiga.com/2014).

Felbamate

Felbamate may cause idiosyncratic hepatotoxicity and massive hepatic necrosis (O'Neil et al., 1996). Felbamate may be contraindicated in patients with a history of hepatic impairment, although there are little data to support this recommendation. *It should be used only in the treatment of severe epilepsy refractory to other ASMs because of the risk of acute liver failure.* Patients or their caregivers should be advised of the symptoms of liver disease. Liver function tests are recommended before beginning treatment and regularly during treatment. Felbamate should be stopped if there is any evidence of liver abnormalities (Facts and Comparisons, 2007; Lacerda et al., 2006).

Gabapentin

No dosage adjustment is necessary in patients with hepatic impairment since gabapentin is not metabolized by the liver. Hepatic adverse effects have rarely been reported (Facts and Comparisons, 2007; Lacerda et al., 2006).

Lacosamide

The dose titration should be performed with caution in patients with hepatic impairment. A maximum dose of 300 mg/day is recommended for patients with mild or moderate hepatic impairment. Lacosamide use is not recommended in patients with severe hepatic impairment. Patients with hepatic impairment who are taking strong inhibitors of CYP3A4 and CYP2C9 (e.g., valproate) may have a significant increase in exposure to lacosamide. Dose reduction may be necessary in these patients. Elevated hepatic enzymes have been reported with lacosamide treatment (lacosamide; http://www.vimpat.com/2020).

Lamotrigine

Initial escalation and maintenance doses should be reduced by approximately 50% in patients with moderate hepatic impairment (Child-Pugh Grade B) and by 75% in patients with severe (Child-Pugh Grade C) hepatic impairment. Doses of lamotrigine should be reduced by one- third in patients with Gilbert's syndrome. Adjust doses as needed according to clinical response. Abnormal liver function tests have been reported with lamotrigine treatment (Anderson and Hakimian, 2014; Facts and Comparisons, 2007; Lacerda et al., 2006).

Levetiracetam

No dosage adjustment is necessary in patients with mild to moderate hepatic impairment. Levetiracetam is not extensively metabolized by the liver. The dose of levetiracetam should be reduced by 50% in patients with severe hepatic dysfunction (Anderson and Hakimian, 2014; Facts and Comparisons, 2007; Lacerda et al., 2006).

Oxcarbazepine

No dosage adjustments are recommended for mild to moderate hepatic impairment. The effects of severe hepatic impairment have not been evaluated. Hepatic adverse effects have rarely been reported with oxcarbazepine treatment. Abnormal liver function tests have been reported (Facts and Comparisons, 2007; Lacerda et al., 2006).

Perampanel

Because perampanel has higher exposure and longer half-life in patients with mild and moderate hepatic impairment, dosage adjustment is recommended. Starting dose should be 2 mg/day, with weekly increments of 2 mg/day every 2 weeks until target dose is achieved. The maximum recommended daily dose is 6 mg for patients with mild hepatic impairment and 4 mg for patients with moderate hepatic impairment. Dose increases in patients with mild and moderate hepatic impairment, as with all patients, should be based on clinical response and tolerability. Use in patients with severe hepatic impairment is not recommended (perampanel; http://www.fycompa.com/2014).

Phenobarbital/Primidone

These drugs should be avoided in patients with hepatic disease due to sedative effects and decreased protein binding. Modify initial dose depending on degree of hepatic impairment. A 50% reduction in dose may be needed in patients with moderate to severe hepatic cirrhosis. Initiate phenobarbital cautiously and adjust the dose based on clinical response and serum concentrations. Hepatic adverse effects have rarely been reported. Because of sedating effects, it may precipitate coma in hepatic encephalopathy and is not recommended (Anderson and Hakimian, 2014; Facts and Comparisons, 2007; Lacerda et al., 2006).

Phenytoin

Phenytoin is primarily metabolized in the liver, and patients with hepatic disease may rapidly show signs of phenytoin toxicity. In addition, serum concentrations of free phenytoin may be increased due to hypoalbuminemia that is commonly present in cirrhotic liver diseases. Dosing adjustments may be required based on serum phenytoin level monitoring and clinical response.

Phenytoin is potentially hepatotoxic. It can cause elevated hepatic enzymes or more serious manifestations of hepatitis such as focal hepatic necrosis and hepatomegaly. Cholestasis with jaundice can occur. Hepatotoxicity may also be a component of a severe hypersensitivity reaction (*antiepileptic hypersensitivity syndrome*) (Knowles et al., 1999). Careful investigation should be considered in case of any evidence suggestive of hepatic injury (Facts and Comparisons, 2007; Lacerda et al., 2006).

Pregabalin

This drug is cleared by the kidneys and has low protein binding. No dosage adjustments are required (Facts and Comparisons, 2007; Lacerda et al., 2006).

Rufinamide

Use of rufinamide in patients with hepatic impairment has not been studied. Therefore, use in patients with severe hepatic impairment is not recommended. Caution should be exercised in treating patients with mild to moderate hepatic impairment (rufinamide; http://www.banzel.com/2014).

Tiagabine

Because the half-life of tiagabine is prolonged in patients with hepatic disease, dosage reduction and longer dosing intervals may be necessary. However, specific dosing guidelines have not been established (Facts and Comparisons, 2007; Lacerda et al., 2006).

Topiramate

While mostly excreted by the kidneys, topiramate is partially metabolized by the liver. In liver failure, topiramate half-life may be lengthened, and dosage reduction may be required. Elevated hepatic enzymes, hepatic failure, and hepatitis have been rarely reported with topiramate treatment (Facts and Comparisons, 2007; Lacerda et al., 2006). Topiramate (as well as potentially other drugs with carbonic anhydrase inhibitory activity, such as zonisamide and acetazolamide) may affect the clearance of ammonia via their effects on renal carbonic anhydrase activity, leading to worsening hepatic encephalopathy (Anderson and Hakimian, 2014).

Valproic Acid, Valproate, Divalproex Sodium

Drug clearance may be decreased by 50% in cirrhosis because it is cleared by the liver. Therefore, dosage reductions may be required in hepatic failure.

In rare cases, valproate may cause liver failure, mainly in children. Hepatotoxicity due to valproate is most likely to occur within the first 6 months of treatment. Idiosyncratic hepatotoxicity is rare and not predictable on the basis of laboratory monitoring. Risk factors for hepatotoxicity include

- children, especially those younger than 2 years of age
- patients receiving multiple ASMs
- patients with other complicating factors (e.g., metabolic diseases, mental retardation, and organic brain syndromes)
- mitochondrial disease
- genetic factors

Because liver dysfunction associated with valproic acid is likely dose-related, titrate dose slowly in susceptible patients. Changes in hepatic function may be indicated by loss of seizure control, jaundice, malaise, weakness, lethargy, facial edema, anorexia, or vomiting. The most serious adverse reaction induced by valproic acid is hepatic failure. The formation of valproate reactive metabolites, inhibition of fatty acid β-oxidation, excessive oxidative stress, and genetic variants of some enzymes, such as CPS1, POLG, GSTs, SOD2, UGT, and CYP genes, have been reported to be associated with valproate-induced hepatotoxicity. L-carnitine supplementation and antioxidants administration may be beneficial treatment strategies in case of valproate-induced hepatotoxicity (Fenichel and Greene, 1985; Facts and Comparisons, 2007; Guo et al., 2019; Lacerda et al., 2006; Verrotti et al., 2002).

Vigabatrin

Vigabatrin is not significantly metabolized. With negligible protein binding and minimal to no hepatic metabolism, dose adjustment is not necessary in hepatic diseases. It should be used only in the treatment of severe epilepsy refractory to other ASMs because of the risk of visual field defect.

Vigabatrin decreases ALT and AST plasma activity in up to 90% of patients. In some patients, these enzymes become undetectable. The suppression of ALT and AST activity may preclude the use of these markers to detect early hepatic injury (vigabatrin; http://www.sabril.net/2014).

Zonisamide

Because zonisamide is hepatically metabolized, patients with hepatic disease should be treated with caution. Slower titration and more frequent monitoring may be required. However, no quantitative recommendations are available.

Elevated hepatic enzymes, hepatitis, fulminant hepatic necrosis, cholangitis, and cholecystitis have been rarely reported with zonisamide treatment (Facts and Comparisons, 2007; Lacerda et al., 2006).

Preferred Antiseizure Medications in Patients with Severe Liver Disease

- *Generalized epilepsies*: Levetiracetam, lacosamide
- *Focal epilepsies*: Lacosamide, levetiracetam, oxcarbazepine, gabapentin

Note: Other agents metabolized by the liver may be used but dose adjustments are required

References

Anderson GD, Hakimian S. Pharmacokinetic of antiepileptic drugs in patients with hepatic or renal impairment. *Clin Pharmacokinet.* 2014;53(1):29–49.

Facts and Comparison. *Drug Facts and Comparisons.* St. Louis: Wolters Kluwer Health/Facts and Comparisons; 2007.

Fenichel GM, Greene HL. Valproate hepatotoxicity: Two new cases, a summary of others, and recommendations. *Pediatr Neurol*. 1985;1:109–113.

Guo HL, Jing X, Sun JY, et al. Valproic acid and the liver injury in patients with epilepsy: An update. *Curr Pharm Des*. 2019;25(3):343–351.

Knowles SR, Shapiro LE, Shear NH. Anticonvulsant hypersensitivity syndrome: Incidence, prevention and management. *Drug Safety*. 1999;21:489–501.

Lacerda G, Krummel T, Sabourdy C, Ryvlin P, Hirsch E. Optimizing therapy of seizures in patients with renal or hepatic dysfunction. *Neurology*. 2006;67:S28–S33.

O'Neil MG, Perdun CS, Wilson MB, et al. Felbamate-associated fatal acute hepatic necrosis. *Neurology.* 1996;46:1457–1459.

Verrotti A, Trota D, Morgese G, Chiarelli F. Valproate-induced hyperammonemic encephalopathy. *Metab Brain Dis*. 2002;17 367–373.

Vidaurre J, Gedela S, Yarosz S. Antiepileptic drugs and liver disease. *Pediatr Neurol*. 2017;77:23–36.

Online Resources

Brivaracetam (Briviact). www.briviact.com/2020

Cannabidiol (Epidiolex). www.epidiolex.com/2020

Cenobamate (Xcopri). https://reference.medscape.com/drug/xcopri-cenobamate-1000328/,2020

Eslicarbazine acetate (Aptiom). www.aptiom.com/2014

Ezogabine (Potiga). www.potiga.com/2014

Lacosamide (Vimpat). www.vimpat.com/2020

Perampanel (Fycompa). us.eisai.com/wps/wcm/connect/Eisai/Home/Our.../FYCOMPA/2014

Rufinamide (Banzel). www.banzel.com/2014

Vigabatrin (Sabril). http://www.sabril.net/2014

Chapter 14

Antiseizure Medications and Metabolic Disorders

Metabolic Acidosis

Three antiseizure medications (ASMs)—acetazolamide, topiramate, and zonisamide—are typically associated with metabolic acidosis due to their property of inhibiting the enzyme carbonic anhydrase. All are associated with various degrees of renal tubular acidosis (Sheth, 2004).

Topiramate is associated with a mild hyperchloremic, non–anion gap metabolic acidosis manifest by a persistently low bicarbonate level. Bicarbonate decrements are usually mild to moderate, with an average decrease of 4 mEq/L at daily doses of 400 mg in adults and approximately 6 mg/kg/day in pediatric patients. Decreases of more than 10 mEq/L can be found in rare cases. The metabolic acidosis typically occurs soon after initiation of therapy. Conditions or therapies that predispose to acidosis such as renal diseases, severe respiratory disorders, diarrhea, surgery, ketogenic diet, or other drugs may add to the bicarbonate-lowering effects of topiramate.

Baseline and periodic measurements of serum bicarbonate levels during topiramate, zonisamide, and acetazolamide treatment are recommended, especially in children. If metabolic acidosis develops and persists, consideration should be given to reducing the dosage or discontinuing these ASMs, especially topiramate, considering the adverse effects of chronic metabolic acidosis on kidney, bone, heart, and growth (in children). If the decision is made to continue topiramate therapy despite persistent acidosis, alkali treatment should be considered (Groeper and McCann, 2005; Sheth, 2004).

It is reasonable to avoid prescribing these three ASMs (acetazolamide, topiramate, and zonisamide) in patients with preexisting disorders with metabolic acidosis (e.g., inborn errors of metabolism, renal tubular acidosis).

Hyponatremia

Hyponatremia occurs in patients treated with carbamazepine, oxcarbazepine, or eslicarbazepine acetate. In most patients, the hyponatremia is transient, mild, and asymptomatic. In our experience, the hyponatremia associated with oxcarbazepine is enduring and variable in severity. In one study, it was observed that mild hyponatremia is associated with an increased risk of death in an ambulatory setting (Gankam-Kengne et al., 2013).

Hyponatremia occurs more frequently with oxcarbazepine than with carbamazepine. This adverse effect typically occurs during the first 3 months of treatment; rare cases of symptomatic hyponatremia beginning more than 1 year after treatment initiation have been observed. The mechanism by which carbamazepine and oxcarbazepine cause hyponatremia is not completely understood. Patients typically present with findings similar to the syndrome of inappropriate secretion of antidiuretic hormone (SIADH) (Asconapé, 2002). However, a mechanism other than SIADH may be partially responsible because some cases of hyponatremia without abnormal ADH levels have been observed (Sachdeo et al., 2002). The risk of developing significant hyponatremia with the use of oxcarbazepine is age=related, more common in the elderly (Dong et al., 2005). In a study of 97 oxcarbazepine-treated and 451 carbamazepine-treated patients (Dong et al., 2005), the prevalence of hyponatremia, defined as serum sodium of less than 134 mEq/L, was 29.9% among oxcarbazepine-treated patients and 13.5% among carbamazepine-treated patients. Severe hyponatremia, defined by the authors as serum sodium less than 128 mEq/L, was found in 12.4% of oxcarbazepine-treated patients and 2.8% of carbamazepine-treated patients.

Periodic monitoring of sodium levels is recommended during the first 3 months of therapy with oxcarbazepine in elderly patients, patients with renal failure, and patients on other medications associated with hyponatremia. Patients with stable sodium levels of greater than 130 mEq/L during the first 3 months are at minimal risk for late development of hyponatremia, and no further monitoring is usually necessary. In patients with sodium levels between 125 and 130 mEq/L, repeat measurements are recommended to confirm that hyponatremia is not worsening. When the serum sodium level falls below 125 mEq/L or hyponatremic symptoms appear, intervention is necessary, consisting either of water restriction or change in medication (Asconapé, 2002).

Clinically significant hyponatremia (sodium <125 mEq/L) can develop in patients taking eslicarbazepine acetate. This effect is dose-related and generally appears within the first 8 weeks of treatment (as early as after 3 days). Serious, life-threatening complications were reported with eslicarbazepine-associated hyponatremia (as low as 112 mEq/L), including seizures and severe nausea and vomiting leading to dehydration. Concurrent hypochloremia was also present in patients with hyponatremia. Depending on the severity of hyponatremia, the dose of eslicarbazepine may need to be reduced or discontinued. Measurement of serum sodium and chloride levels should be considered during maintenance treatment with eslicarbazepine, particularly if the patient is receiving other medications known to decrease serum sodium levels, and these measurements should be performed if symptoms of hyponatremia develop (e.g., nausea/vomiting, malaise, headache, lethargy, confusion, irritability, muscle weakness/spasms, obtundation, or increase in seizure frequency or severity).

Oligohidrosis

Cases of oligohidrosis, hyperthermia, and heat stroke have been reported with topiramate and zonisamide. All patients with dehydration, hypovolemia, or other predisposing factors to heat intolerance should have their condition corrected before using topiramate or zonisamide. All patients, especially children, should be instructed to limit exposure to high temperatures. The concurrent use of drugs that predispose patients to heat intolerance, such as anticholinergic medications and carbonic anhydrase inhibitors, should be avoided when topiramate and zonisamide are taken. To help prevent oligohidrosis and hyperthermia in patients treated with either drug, proper hydration is suggested before and during strenuous activity or exposure to warm temperatures (Facts and Comparisons, 2007).

Hyperammonemia

Hyperammonemia can occur in as many as half of the patients receiving valproic acid regardless of liver function status. There is a dose-dependent association between valproic acid and blood ammonia level. In most patients, elevated ammonia levels are minimal and benign, but in some patients lethargy and/or coma have been reported. Early recognition of subtle cognitive and behavioral changes in patients taking valproate and early therapeutic interventions may prevent the development of more severe problems. L-carnitine treatment in doses ranging from 1,000 to 3,000 mg/day usually normalizes serum ammonia levels and may enhance the survival of patients with valproate-induced hyperammonemia and encephalopathy (Verrotti et al., 2002). If symptomatic hyperammonemia occurs, L-carnitine at a dosage of 330–990 mg three times daily can be given, usually with prompt resolution of symptoms.

Patients with *urea cycle disorders* (UCD) should not receive valproate. These individuals have a genetic enzyme defect leading to an impaired ability to produce urea. Hyperammonemic encephalopathy has been reported following initiation of valproate therapy in patients with UCD (Thakur et al., 2006).

Hyperammonemia and encephalopathy are reported with concomitant valproic acid and topiramate use in patients who have tolerated either drug alone. Clinical symptoms include acute alteration in level of consciousness and/or cognitive function with lethargy or vomiting. In most patients, symptoms and signs abated with discontinuation of either drug (Facts and Comparisons, 2007).

Acetazolamide can also cause hepatic difficulties. In patients with hepatic disease, especially cirrhosis, hepatic encephalopathy can occur as a result of hypokalemia and elevations in serum ammonia concentrations during acetazolamide therapy. Disorientation, possibly due to elevated ammonia concentrations, has also been observed in these patients (Facts and Comparisons, 2007).

Mitochondrial Disorders

Epilepsy is a common manifestation of mitochondrial disorders. Patients with mitochondrial disorder–related epilepsy are largely treated in the same way as any other patient with epilepsy. However, some ASMs are mitochondrial toxic and care is needed when administering these ASMs to patients with mitochondrial disorders. The ASM with the most well-known mitochondrial toxicity is valproate, which may produce deleterious effects in patients with POLG1 mutations and patients with myoclonic epilepsy with ragged red fibers syndrome. Other ASMs that may affect mitochondrial function include phenobarbital, carbamazepine, phenytoin, oxcarbazepine, ethosuximide, and topiramate (Finsterer & Zarrouk Mahjoub, 2012). Lamotrigine and levetiracetam are good ASM choices in patients with mitochondrial disorder—related epilepsy (Finsterer & Scorza, 2017).

Other Metabolic Adverse Effects of Antiseizure Medications

Acetazolamide: Metabolic adverse effects of acetazolamide may include hypokalemia, hyperglycemia, glycosuria in patients with diabetes, hyperuricemia, and hyperchloremia.

Cannabidiol: Metabolic adverse effects of cannabidiol may include elevations in serum creatinine.

Lacosamide: Lacosamide oral solution contains aspartame, a source of phenylalanine. Patients with phenylketonuria should be advised.

Oxcarbazepine: Metabolic adverse effects of oxcarbazepine may include hyperglycemia, hypocalcemia, hypoglycemia, and hypokalemia.

Phenobarbital: Phenobarbital, like other barbiturates, can exacerbate porphyria, causing a buildup of porphyrin precursors and enhancing porphyrin synthesis.

Phenytoin: Phenytoin can interfere with glucose metabolism. Phenytoin can stimulate glucagon secretion, impair insulin secretion, and cause a post-binding defect at the peripheral insulin receptor by affecting [^{14}C]3,0-methylglucose transport. Any of these effects could increase serum glucose. Blood sugar should be monitored closely when phenytoin is administered to patients with diabetes mellitus, and this drug is less than desirable for diabetic patients.

Valproate: Other metabolic adverse effects of valproate may include Fanconi syndrome, hyperglycinemia, and decreased carnitine concentrations.

Vigabatrin: Vigabatrin may increase the amount of amino acids in the urine, possibly leading to a false positive test for certain rare genetic metabolic diseases (e.g., alpha aminoadipic aciduria) (al-Rubeaan and Ryan, 1991; Drug Facts and Comparisons, 2007; see also individual drug websites listed in the Online Resources section at the end of this chapter).

Zonisamide: Rare metabolic adverse effects of zonisamide may include hypoglycemia and hyponatremia.

References

al-Rubeaan K, Ryan EA. Phenytoin-induced insulin insensitivity. *Diabetic Med.* 1991;8:968–970.

Asconapé JJ. Some common issues in the use of antiepileptic drugs. *Semin Neurol.* 2002;22:27–39.

Dong X, Leppik IE, White J, Parick J. Hyponatremia from oxcarbazepine and carbam-azepine. *Neurology.* 2005;65:1967–1978.

Facts and Comparisons. *Drug Facts and Comparisons.* St. Louis: Wolters Kluwer Health/Facts & Comparisons; 2007.

Finsterer J, Zarrouk Mahjoub S. Mitochondrial toxicity of antiepileptic drugs and their tolerability in mitochondrial disorders. *Expert Opin Drug Metab Toxicol.* 2012; 8(1):71–79.

Finsterer J, Scorza FA. Effects of antiepileptic drugs on mitochondrial functions, morphology, kinetics, biogenesis, and survival. *Epilepsy Res.* 2017;136:5–11.

Gankam-Kengne F, Ayers C, Khera A, de Lemos J, Maalouf NM. Mild hyponatremia is associated with an increased risk of death in an ambulatory setting. *Kidney Int.* 2013;83(4):700–706.

Groeper K, McCann ME. Topiramate and metabolic acidosis: a case series and review of the literature. *Pediatr Anesth.* 2005;15:167–170.

Sachdeo RC, Wasserstein A, Mesenbrink PJ, D'Souza J. Effects of oxcarbazepine on sodium concentration and water handling. *Ann Neurol.* 2002;51:613–620.

Sheth RD. Metabolic concerns associated with antiepileptic medications. *Neurology.* 2004;63:S24–S29.

Thakur V, Rupar A, Ramsay DA, Singh R, Fraser DD. Fatal cerebral edema from late-onset ornithine transcarbamylase deficiency in a juvenile male patient receiving valproic acid. *Pediatr Crit Care Med.* 2006;7:273–276.

Verrotti A, Trota D, Morgese G, Chiarelli F. Valproate-induced hyperammonemic encephalopathy. *Metab Brain Dis.* 2002;17:367–373.

Online Resources

Cannabidiol (Epidiolex). www.epidiolex.com/2020

Cenobamate (Xcopri). https://reference.medscape.com/drug/xcopri-cenobamate-1000328/2020

Eslicarbazine acetate (Aptiom). www.aptiom.com/2014

Ezogabine (Potiga). www.potiga.com/2014

Lacosamide (Vimpat). www.vimpat.com/2014

Perampanel (Fycompa). us.eisai.com/wps/wcm/connect/Eisai/Home/Our.../FYCOMPA/2014

Rufinamide (Banzel). www.banzel.com/2014

Vigabatrin (Sabril). www.lundbeck.com/upload/us/files/.../Sabril/2014

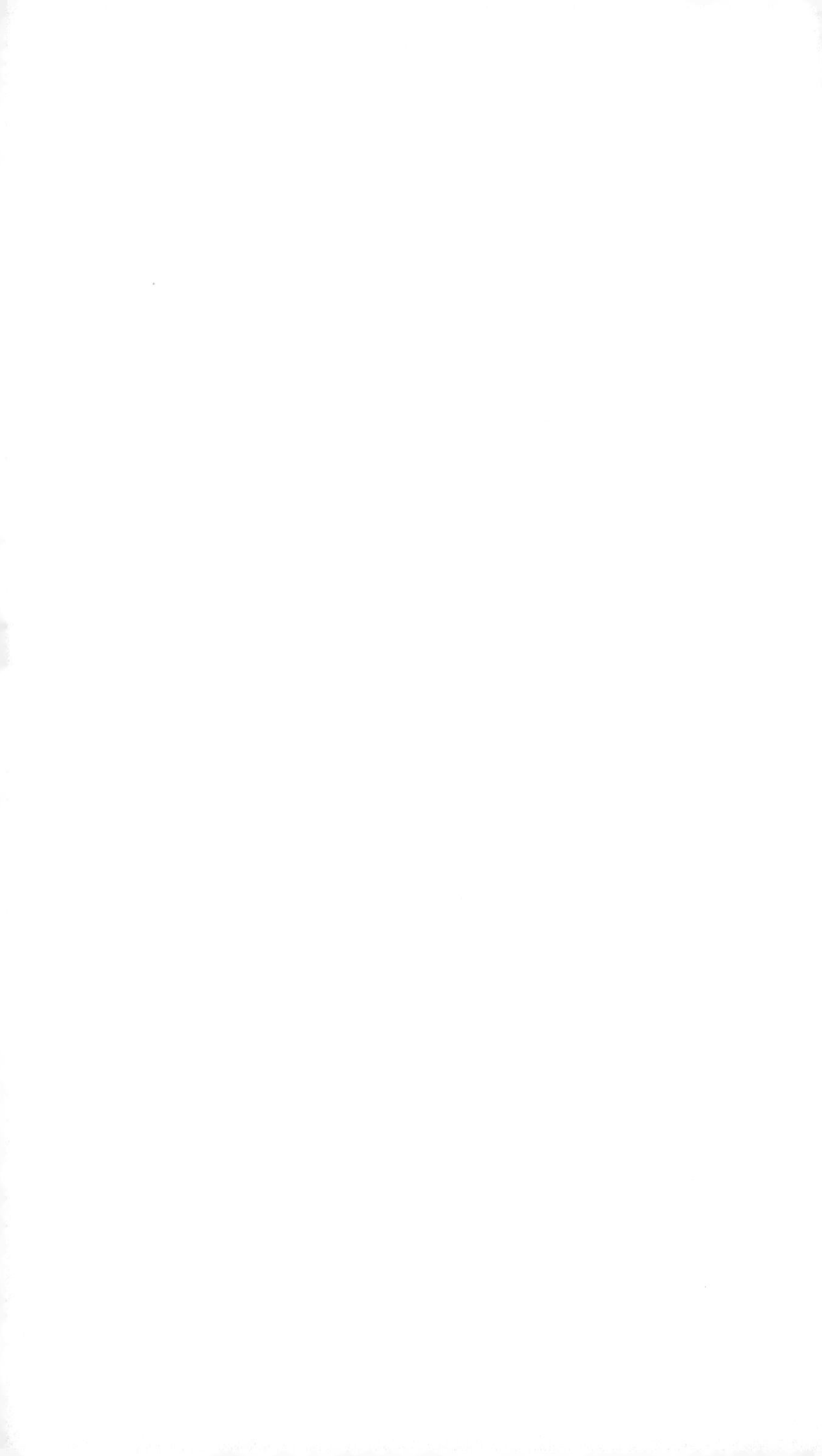

Chapter 15

Antiseizure Medications in Patients with Hyperlipidemia

Several reports have already shown that chronic treatment with some antiseizure medications (ASMs) influences serum lipid profile. There have been reports of high total cholesterol concentrations in patients receiving carbamazepine, phenytoin, phenobarbital, or primidone; high levels of HDL cholesterol in normal subjects receiving phenobarbital and in patients treated with carbamazepine or phenytoin; and high levels of LDL cholesterol in patients treated with carbamazepine and phenobarbital, as well as high triglyceride levels in patients receiving carbamazepine, phenobarbital, or phenytoin. An investigation examined lipid levels in adult patients with epilepsy taking phenytoin or carbamazepine who were subsequently switched over to the non-inducing agents lamotrigine or levetiracetam and found that the change from enzyme-inducing to non–enzyme-inducing ASM led to a decline in total cholesterol averaging 26 mg/dL after only 6 weeks (Mintzer et al., 2009). A later prospective randomized controlled trial comparing lacosamide and carbamazepine provided class II evidence that carbamazepine elevates serum lipids, whereas lacosamide had no effect on lipids (Mintzer et al., 2020). Influence of valproic acid on serum lipid profiles is controversial (Karikas et al., 2006; Nikolaos et al., 2004; Sonmez et al., 2006). Valproate may have adverse long-term metabolic consequences, including obesity, insulin resistance, and the metabolic syndrome, via mechanisms that are presumably distinct from those activated by the inducing drugs (Mintzer et al., 2009).

The effects of ASMs on the serum levels of lipids and lipoproteins may have different mechanisms. Carbamazepine, phenytoin, and phenobarbital alter hepatic P-450 microsomal enzyme activity and are metabolized by this same system. This enzyme system catalyzes cholesterol. Thus, carbamazepine, phenytoin, and phenobarbital might compete with cholesterol for utilization of these enzymes and change cholesterol metabolism by altering enzyme levels. The high level of HDL cholesterol could be attributed to the enzyme-inducing properties of carbamazepine, phenytoin, and phenobarbital, which results in an increased hepatic synthesis of apolipoprotein A_1, the major component of HDL cholesterol (Nikolaos et al., 2004). Last, the widely prescribed lipid-lowering agents, statins, are metabolized by the cytochrome P-450 complex (Prueksaritanont et al., 1997). Therefore, enzyme-inducing ASMs enhance the clearance of these cholesterol-lowering agents and reduce their effectiveness. For example, comedication with phenytoin resulted in significant (approximately 50%) reductions in the systemic exposure of atorvastatin (Miller et al., 2008). While eslicarbazepine acetate may positively affect the lipid metabolism profile in patients with epilepsy, in vivo studies suggest that eslicarbazepine acetate can induce CYP3A4, decreasing plasma concentrations of drugs that are metabolized by this isoenzyme (e.g., simvastatin). Patients receiving enzyme-inducing ASMs are significantly more likely to require multiple upward dose adjustments of their statin medication (Candrilli et al., 2010; Pulitano et al., 2017).

One should assess the serum lipid profile in patients treated with enzyme-inducing ASMs. In patients with hyperlipidemia it is reasonable to consider switching the patient to a non-inducing ASM. A low-cholesterol diet is recommended for patients receiving carbamazepine, phenytoin, phenobarbital, or primidone. Oxcarbazepine and topiramate in high doses (>1,200 mg and >200 mg, respectively) are also enzyme inducers, so lipid assessments should be performed as well when enzyme-inducing doses are reached. Treatment with a cholesterol-lowering agent may be indicated as well. Addition of an enzyme-inducing ASM may necessitate raising the dose of a cholesterol-lowering agent that has been prescribed.

Recommended Antiseizure Medications in Patients with Hyperlipidemia

- *Generalized epilepsies*: Ethosuximide, lacosamide, lamotrigine, levetiracetam, perampanel, rufinamide (in patients with Lennox-Gastaut syndrome), zonisamide
- *Focal epilepsies*: Brivaracetam, gabapentin, lacosamide, lamotrigine, levetiracetam, perampanel, zonisamide

References

Candrilli SD, Manjunath R, Davis KL, Gidal BE. The association between antiepileptic drug and HMG-CoA reductase inhibitor co-medication and cholesterol management in patients with epilepsy. *Epilepsy Res.* 2010;91(2–3):260–266.

Karikas GA, Schulpis KH, Bartzeliotou A, et al. Lipids, lipoproteins, apolipoproteins, selected elements and minerals in the serum of children on valproic acid mono-therapy. *Basic Clin Pharmacol Toxicol.* 2006;98:599–603.

Miller JM, Bullman JN, Alexander S, VanLandingham KE. A prospective assessment of the effect of phenytoin on the pharmacokinetics of atorvastatin. *Epilepsia.* 2008;49:444.

Mintzer S, Dimova S, Zhang Y, Steiniger-Brach B, Ce Backer M, Chellun D, Roebling R. Effects of lacosamide and carbamazepine on lipids in a randomized trial. *Epilepsia.* 2020;61:2696–2704.

Mintzer S, Skidmore CT, Abidin CJ, Morales MC, Chervoneva I, Capuzzi DM, Sperling MR. Effects of antiepileptic drugs on lipids, homocysteine, and C-reactive protein. *Ann Neurol.* 2009:65:448–456.

Nikolaos T, Stylianos G, Chryssoula N, et al. The effect of long-term antiepileptic treatment on serum cholesterol (TC, HDL, LDL) and triglyceride levels in adult epileptic patients on monotherapy. *Med Sci Monitor*. 2004;10:MT50–MT52.

Pulitano P, Franco V, Mecarelli O, et al. Effects of eslicarbazepine acetate on lipid profile and sodium levels in patients with epilepsy. *Seizure*. 2017;53:1–3.

Prueksaritanont T, Gorham LM, Ma B, et al. In vitro metabolism of simvastatin in humans: Identification of metabolizing enzymes and effect of the drug on hepatic P450s. *Drug Metab Disposition*. 1997;25:1191–1199.

Sonmez FM, Demir E, Orem A, et al. Effect of antiepileptic drugs on plasma lipids, lipoprotein (a), and liver enzymes. *J Child Neurol*. 2006;21:70–74.

Online Resources

Brivaracetam (Briviact). www.briviact.com/2020

Eslicarbazine acetate (Aptiom). www.aptiom.com/2014

Lacosamide (Vimpat). www.vimpat.com/2014

Perampanel (Fycompa). us.eisai.com/wps/wcm/connect/Eisai/Home/Our.../FYCOMPA/2014

Rufinamide (Banzel). www.banzel.com/2014

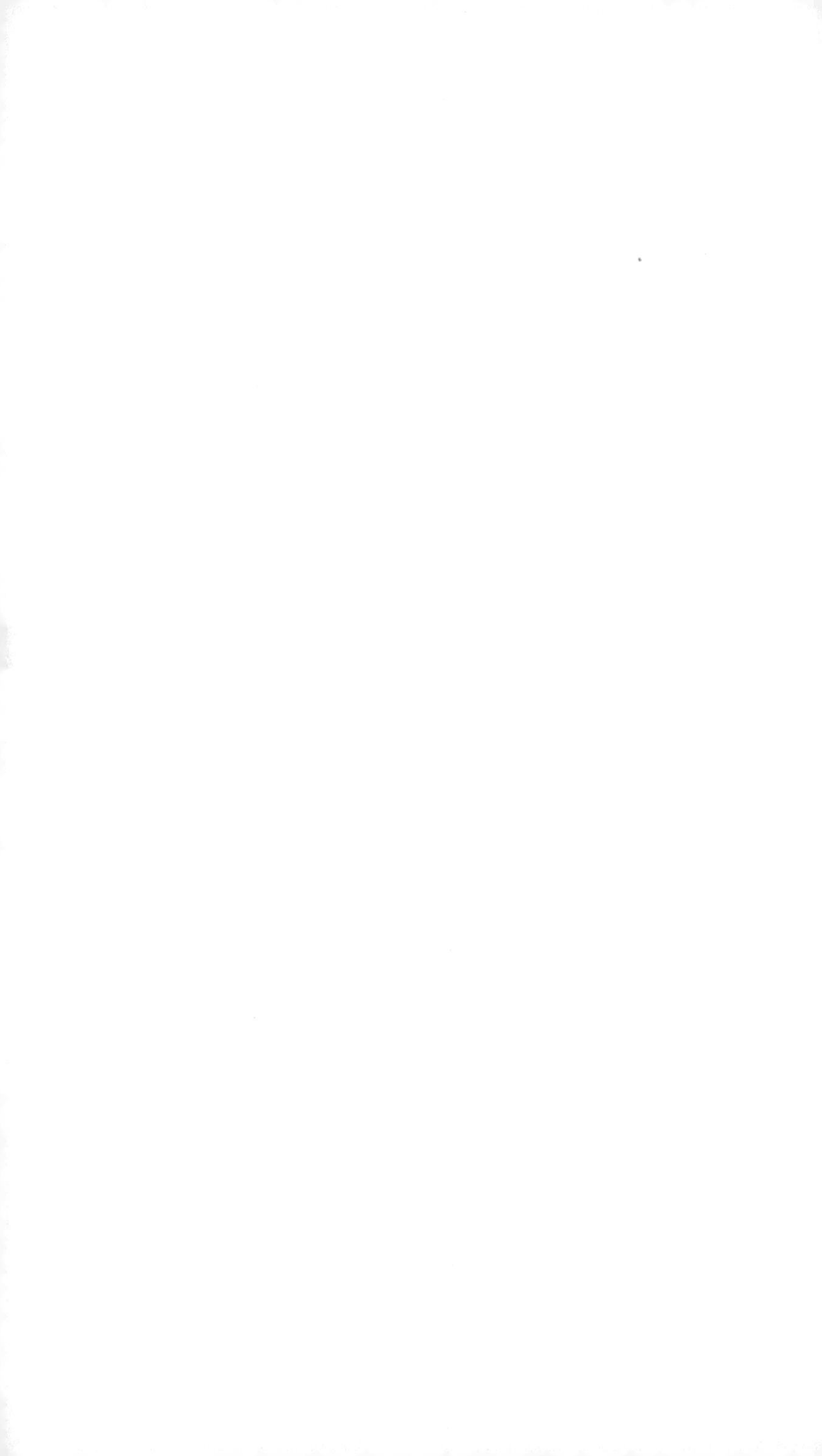

Chapter 16

Antiseizure Medications in Patients with Diabetes Mellitus

Selection of the appropriate antiseizure medication (ASM) should be guided by the recognition that some patients have multiple comorbidities and receive multiple medications. People with type 1 diabetes mellitus (DM) have a two- to six-fold higher risk of epilepsy than the general population. These two conditions share four potential pathogenic factors: (a) genetic predisposition, (b) autoimmune responses (i.e., anti-glutamic acid decarboxylase antibodies), (c) effects of hypo-/hyperglycemia, and (d) cerebrovascular damage resulting in ischemic processes (Marcovecchio et al., 2015; Mastrangelo et al., 2019). ASMs may have various adverse or beneficial effects in patients with DM. Nutritional recommendations, weight management, and physical activity may also produce significant benefits in these patients (Mastrangelo et al., 2019).

Antiseizure Medications in Diabetes

Acetazolamide

Acetazolamide has rarely caused severe metabolic acidosis in patients with DM (Zaidi and Kinnear, 2004). Diabetic patients should be monitored for a loss of blood glucose control and electrolyte disturbances.

Cannabidiol

Cannabidiol may cause weight loss (cannabidiol; www.epidiolex.com/2020). Cannabidiol has wide range of therapeutic properties, including mitigation of diabetes and neurodegeneration in animal studies (Zorzenon et al., 2019).

Carbamazepine

Carbamazepine may help painful diabetic neuropathy (Maizels and McCarberg, 2005; Vinik, 2005). Because this agent is a sodium channel blocker, this has a theoretical risk of producing arrhythmias in patients with comorbid cardiovascular disease.

Eslicarbazepine

Because this agent is a sodium channel blocker, this has a theoretical risk of producing arrhythmias in patients with comorbid cardiovascular disease.

Ezogabine

Ezogabine was associated with dose-related weight gain. It is not an optimal drug for patients with DM.

Gabapentin

Gabapentin is useful for postherpetic neuralgia and may also be appropriate for painful diabetic neuropathy (Maizels and McCarberg, 2005; Vinik, 2005). However, it causes weight gain in some patients and is therefore suboptimal as a first-line choice for epilepsy treatment. Studies have reported fluctuations in blood sugar levels, and this should be considered in diabetic patients.

Lacosamide

Because this agent is a sodium channel blocker, this has a theoretical risk of producing arrhythmias in patients with comorbid cardiovascular disease.

Lamotrigine

Lamotrigine does not pose problems with regard to diabetes and may be appropriate for painful diabetic neuropathy (Vinik, 2005). Because this agent is a sodium channel blocker, this has a theoretical risk of producing arrhythmias in patients with co-morbid cardiovascular disease.

Levetiracetam

Levetiracetam induced an antihyperalgesic effect in two models of human neuropathic pain, suggesting a therapeutic potential in neuropathic pain patients (Ardid et al., 2003). Human studies are scarce and conflicting.

Oxcarbazepine

Because this agent is a sodium channel blocker, this has a theoretical risk of producing arrhythmias in patients with comorbid cardiovascular disease.

Perampanel

Perampanel was associated with weight gain. It is not an optimal drug for patients with DM.

Phenytoin

Phenytoin may impair insulin release and cause insulin insensitivity and hyperglycemia, so this drug should be avoided in patients with diabetes. These adverse effects may cause temporary loss of glycemic control in diabetic patients. Close observation is necessary to maintain adequate glycemic control in patients with DM (al-Rubeaan and Rayan, 1991). Because this agent is a sodium channel blocker, it has a theoretical risk of producing arrhythmias in patients with comorbid cardiovascular disease.

Pregabalin

Pregabalin is efficacious for painful diabetic neuropathy (Maizels and McCarberg, 2005; Vinik, 2005). Pregabalin treatment did not appear to be associated with loss of glycemic control. However, as the thiazolidin-edione class of antidiabetic drugs can cause weight gain and fluid retention, possibly exacerbating diabetes or leading to heart failure, it should not be considered a first-line drug for primary treatment of seizures (Laustsen et al., 2006). Pregabalin has the potential to cause an increase in appetite (in 5% of patients) and might cause weight gain (in 4–12%).

Topiramate

Topiramate may occasionally be helpful in controlling the pain of diabetic neuropathy (Vinik, 2005). In addition, topiramate treatment of overweight diabetic patients can result in significant weight reduction and loss of body fat, leading to improvement in the glycemic control (Eliasson et al., 2007).

Valproic Acid, Valproate, Divalproex Sodium

Valproate is associated with weight gain, alteration of adipocytokine homeostasis, insulin resistance, and non-alcoholic fatty liver disease (Rauchenzauner et al., 2013). Therefore it is not an optimal drug for patients with DM.

Vigabatrin

Vigabatrin causes weight gain in adult and pediatric patients. Weight gain is not related to the occurrence of edema. In addition, it may cause symptoms of peripheral neuropathy. Therefore, it is not an optimal drug for patients with DM.

Zonisamide

Zonisamide may lead to weight loss in some individuals, leading to improvement in glycemic control.

Recommended Antiseizure Medications in Patients with Diabetes Mellitus

- *Generalized epilepsies*: Cannabidiol (in Lennox-Gastaut syndrome and Dravet syndrome), lamotrigine, levetiracetam, topiramate, zonisamide
- *Focal epilepsies*: Brivaracetam, levetiracetam, lacosamide, lamotrigine, topiramate, zonisamide

Note: Carbamazepine, valproate, pregabalin, and gabapentin may cause weight gain, which is not desirable in diabetic patients. In contrast, topiramate and zonisamide may cause weight loss, which may be favorable in diabetic patients if this is sustained (Biton, 2006).

References

al-Rubeaan K, Rayan EA. Phenytoin-induced insulin insensitivity. *Diabetic Med.* 1991;8:968–970.

Ardid D, Lamberty Y, Alloui A, Coudore-Civiale MA, Klitgaard H, Eschalier A. Antihyperalgesic effect of levetiracetam in neuropathic pain models in rats. *Eur J Pharmacol.* 2003;473(1):27–33.

Biton V. Weight change and antiepileptic drugs. *Neurologist.* 2006;10:163–167.

Eliasson B, Gudbjornsdottir S, Cederholm J, Liang Y, Vercruysse F, Smith U. Weight loss and metabolic effects of topiramate in overweight and obese type

2 diabetic patients: Randomized double-blind placebo-controlled trial. *Int J Obesity*. 2007;31:1140–1147.

Laustsen G, Gilbert M, Wimett L. A look back at the influential drug approvals of 2005. *Nurse Pract*. 2006;31:29–36.

Maizels M, McCarberg B. Antidepressants and antiepileptic drugs for chronic non-cancer pain. *Am Fam Phys*. 2005;71:483–490.

Marcovecchio ML, Petrosino MI, Chiarelli F. Diabetes and epilepsy in children and adolescents. *Curr Diab Rep*. 2015;15(4):21.

Mastrangelo M, Tromba V, Silvestri F, Costantino F. Epilepsy in children with type 1 diabetes mellitus: Pathophysiological basis and clinical hallmarks. *Eur J Paediatr Neurol*. 2019;23(2):240–247.

Rauchenzauner M, Laimer M, Wiedmann M, et al. The novel insulin resistance parameters RBP4 and GLP-1 in patients treated with valproic acid: Just a side-step? *Epilepsy Res*. 2013;104(3):285–288.

Vinik A. Clinical review: Use of antiepileptic drugs in the treatment of chronic painful diabetic neuropathy. *J Clin Endocrinol Metabol*. 2005;90:4936–4945.

Zaidi FH, Kinnear PE. Acetazolamide, alternate carbonic anhydrase inhibitors and hypoglycaemic agents: Comparing enzymatic with diuresis induced metabolic acidosis following intraocular surgery in diabetes. *Br J Ophthalmol*. 2004;88:714–715.

Zorzenon MRT, Santiago AN, Mori MA, et al. Cannabidiol improves metabolic dysfunction in middle-aged diabetic rats submitted to a chronic cerebral hypoperfusion. *Chem Biol Interact*. 2019;312:108819.

Online Resources

Cannabidiol (Epidiolex). www.epidiolex.com/2020

Ezogabine (Potiga). www.potiga.com/2014

Perampanel (Fycompa). us.eisai.com/wps/wcm/connect/Eisai/Home/Our.../FYCOMPA/2014

Vigabatrin (Sabril). www.lundbeck.com/upload/us/files/.../Sabril/2014

Chapter 17

Antiseizure Medications in Patients with Cardiovascular Disorders

The selection of appropriate antiseizure medications (ASMs) should be guided by the recognition that some patients have multiple comorbidities and receive multiple medications. ASMs may have adverse effects on the cardiovascular system. While there is no evidence for clinical effect, sodium channel blockers have a theoretical risk of producing arrhythmias in patients with comorbid cardiac rhythm disturbances. In addition, patients with cardiovascular disorders are usually on antihypertensive, anticoagulant, or cardiac drugs, which may have significant interactions with ASMs (Zaccara et al., 2020).

A number of serologic markers relevant to cardiovascular risk have been found to be affected by the CYP450-inducing ASMs. These include cholesterol and specific atherogenic lipid fractions, lipoprotein(a), C reactive protein (CRP), and homocysteine. These alterations suggest that enzyme-inducing ASMs might produce elevations in cardiovascular risk, a notion reinforced by the epidemiologic data. Monitoring vascular risk factors in patients receiving CYP450-inducing ASMs may be beneficial. In addition, newer non–enzyme-inducing ASMs such as lamotrigine and levetiracetam may be safer when prescribed to patients with a high risk of developing atherosclerosis as indicated by a family history of occlusive vascular disease or genetic disorders that lead to hyperhomocysteinemia, but whether the newer ASMs are clearly beneficial in this context remains to be evaluated (Jakubus et al., 2009; Mintzer 2010; Svalheim et al., 2010).

The major class of drug-drug interaction is between ASMs that induce or inhibit the cytochrome P-450 enzyme system and cardiovascular medications that are metabolized by these enzymes. Therefore, it is best to avoid enzyme-altering ASMs if possible. Some cardiovascular drugs inhibit these hepatic enzymes and so may produce ASM adverse effects and toxicity. Similarly, ASMs that are highly protein bound have interactions with cardiovascular drugs that bind to serum proteins and similar cautions apply. Specific drug-disease and drug-drug interactions of ASMs with cardiovascular system and drugs are listed here (Dhatt et al., 1979; Facts and Comparisons, 2007; Kenneback et al., 1991; Laine et al., 2000; Parrish et al., 2006; see also individual drugs websites listed in the Online Resources section at the end of this chapter).

Antiseizure Medications in Cardiovascular Disorders

Acetazolamide

Acetazolamide can cause hypokalemia. Therefore, patients receiving acetazolamide concurrently with cardiac glycosides are at an increased risk for cardiac toxicity if hypokalemia develops during treatment.

Benzodiazepines

CYP3A4 inhibitors may reduce the metabolism of clonazepam and increase the probability for benzodiazepine toxicity. Examples of CYP3A4 inhibitors include amiodarone, diltiazem, nicardipine, and verapamil. Monitor patients who receive concurrent therapy.

Carbamazepine

Cardiovascular adverse effects that can develop during carbamazepine therapy include atrioventricular block, cardiac arrhythmias or arrhythmia exacerbation, congestive heart failure, edema, aggravation of hypertension, hypotension, syncope, thrombophlebitis, and thromboembolism. Some cardiovascular complications have resulted in death. However, severe cardiac complications generally occur only when very high doses (>60 g) have been ingested. Carbamazepine should be used with caution in any patient with cardiac disease, such as cardiac arrhythmias, congestive heart failure, or coronary artery disease. The drug should not be used in patients with atrioventricular block or other conduction abnormalities (bundle-branch block) (Kenneback et al., 1991). Carbamazepine is an enzyme-inducing ASM and may affect serologic markers that are relevant to cardiovascular risk.

Carbamazepine is metabolized by the hepatic isoenzyme CYP3A4. Many drugs (e.g., diltiazem and verapamil) are known to inhibit CYP3A4 and may decrease carbamazepine metabolism thereby increasing carbamazepine plasma concentrations. Serum carbamazepine concentrations should be monitored closely if any of these agents are added during carbamazepine therapy. It may be necessary to reduce the dose of carbamazepine in this situation. Conversely, carbamazepine may induce the hepatic metabolism of calcium channel blockers, which reduces the levels of these drugs. Carbamazepine is also protein bound, and its concentration may be altered by or alter that of other protein-bound drugs.

Carbamazepine induces the metabolism of warfarin and dicumarol, thus requiring the dosage of anticoagulants to be increased over several weeks after initiating carbamazepine therapy. If carbamazepine is discontinued, dosage reductions of warfarin or dicumarol are usually necessary. Patients on oral anticoagulation should be monitored closely for changes in their international normalized ratio (INR) when carbamazepine is added to or discontinued from a patient's drug therapy regimen (Parrish et al., 2006). Enzyme-inducing ASMs, such as phenobarbital, phenytoin, and carbamazepine, are likely to significantly reduce the anticoagulant effect of direct oral anticoagulants (especially rivaroxaban, apixaban, and edoxaban) (Galgani et al., 2018).

Cenobamate

Patients who take cenobamate (31% at 200 mg and 66% at 500 mg) may have a QT shortening of greater than 20 msec. Patients with familial short QT syndrome should not be treated with cenobamate. Caution should be used when coadministering cenobamate and other drugs that shorten the QT interval. Cenobamate is extensively metabolized; its metabolism could be affected by other drugs. Cenobamate may affect the metabolism of other drugs as well (https://reference.medscape.com/drug/xcopri-cenobamate-1000328/2020).

Eslicarbazepine Acetate

Compared to placebo, eslicarbazepine acetate use was associated with slightly higher frequencies of increases in total cholesterol, triglycerides, and LDL. Patients receiving warfarin should be monitored to maintain INR. Because this agent is a sodium channel blocker, this has a theoretical risk of producing arrhythmias in patients with comorbid cardiac rhythm disturbances.

Ezogabine

Ezogabine might cause QT prolongation. The QT interval should be monitored when ezogabine is prescribed with medicines known to increase QT interval and in patients with known prolonged QT interval, congestive heart failure, ventricular hypertrophy, hypokalemia, or hypomagnesemia.

Data from an in vitro study showed that the N-acetyl metabolite of ezogabine inhibited P-glycoprotein-mediated transport of digoxin in a concentration-dependent manner. Administration of ezogabine at therapeutic doses may increase digoxin serum concentrations. Serum levels of digoxin should be monitored.

Gabapentin

Hypertension has been reported with gabapentin therapy, occurring at an incidence of greater than 1%.

The combination of propranolol and gabapentin may induce dystonia via a pharmacodynamic interaction.

Lacosamide

Dose-dependent prolongations in PR interval with lacosamide have been observed. First-degree, second-degree, and complete atrioventricular (AV) blocks have been reported. Lacosamide should be used with caution in patients with known conduction problems (e.g., marked first-degree AV block, second-degree or higher AV block, and sick sinus syndrome without pacemaker), sodium channelopathies (e.g., Brugada syndrome), on concomitant medications that prolong PR interval, or with severe cardiac disease such as myocardial ischemia or heart failure, or structural heart disease. In such patients, obtaining an ECG before beginning lacosamide and after lacosamide is titrated to steady-state is recommended. Lacosamide administration may predispose the patient to atrial arrhythmias (atrial fibrillation or flutter), especially in those with diabetic neuropathy and/or cardiovascular disease. Lacosamide may rarely cause palpitation, bradycardia, or syncope.

Lamotrigine

Because this agent is a sodium channel blocker, this has a theoretical risk of producing arrhythmias in patients with comorbid cardiac rhythm disturbances.

Oxcarbazepine

Sinus bradycardia, sinus tachycardia, heart failure, hypertension, orthostatic hypotension, palpitations, and syncope have been reported with oxcarbazepine. However, the role of oxcarbazepine in their causation cannot be reliably determined. Hepatic enzyme inhibitors may delay conversion of oxcarbazepine to its active metabolite. Because this agent is a sodium channel blocker, this has a theoretical risk of producing arrhythmias in patients with comorbid cardiac rhythm disturbances.

Phenobarbital/Primidone

Phenobarbital and primidone are enzyme-inducing ASMs and may affect serologic markers that are relevant to cardiovascular risk.

A serious drug interaction can occur between barbiturates and warfarin. All barbiturates are hepatic enzyme inducers, and the clinical effects of warfarin can be compromised if a barbiturate is added. More importantly, discontinuation of a barbiturate during warfarin therapy may lead to fatal bleeding. Warfarin doses require readjustment if a barbiturate is added or discontinued during warfarin therapy (Laine et al., 2000).

Barbiturates can enhance the hepatic metabolism of β-blockers that are significantly metabolized by the liver (betaxolol, labetalol, metoprolol, pindolol, propranolol, and timolol). Patient should be monitored for loss of β-blockade.

Barbiturates may interact with cardiac glycosides. Barbiturates can accelerate the metabolism of digoxin, thus decreasing digoxin serum concentrations.

Concurrent use of phenobarbital with some antihypertensive agents may lead to excessive hypotension. In addition, barbiturates have been shown to enhance the hepatic clearance of calcium channel blockers (e.g., diltiazem, nifedipine, and verapamil). When selecting alternative therapy to a barbiturate is not possible, patients should be monitored for the desired cardiovascular effects of these drugs.

Parenteral administration of barbiturates should be given cautiously to patients with hypertension, hypotension, cardiac disease, or other hemodynamically unstable conditions (i.e., heart failure, shock).

Phenytoin

Phenytoin should be used with caution in patients with cardiac disease (e.g., cardiac arrhythmias, congestive heart failure, or coronary artery disease). This drug should not be used in patients with cardiac conduction abnormalities (e.g., bundle-branch block) (Dhatt et al., 1979). Phenytoin is an enzyme-inducing ASM and may affect serologic markers that are relevant to cardiovascular risk.

Parenteral phenytoin should be used with caution in patients with cardiac disease, because it can cause atrial and ventricular conduction depression, hypotension, ventricular fibrillation, and reduced cardiac output. The rate of

IV administration of phenytoin is important (i.e., maximum infusion rate is 50 mg/min in adults).

The interaction between warfarin and phenytoin is complex. An immediate interaction may occur as phenytoin can displace warfarin from its protein-binding sites, causing rapid increases in the INR. After prolonged administration, phenytoin may reduce the effectiveness of warfarin by inducing the hepatic metabolism of warfarin. Warfarin dosage adjustments may be necessary if phenytoin is added. Competitive inhibition may also occur since phenytoin and warfarin are both substrates for cytochrome P-450 2C9. Warfarin may alter phenytoin serum concentrations as well. Phenytoin also may deplete vitamin K–dependent clotting factors after prolonged therapy. Similar interactions may occur between phenytoin or fosphenytoin and dicumarol. Oral anticoagulant dosage adjustments may also be necessary on discontinuation of phenytoin or fosphenytoin therapy.

Phenytoin clearance can be decreased by drugs that inhibit hepatic microsomal enzymes, particularly those drugs that significantly inhibit the cytochrome P-450 2C subset of isoenzymes (e.g., amiodarone and ticlopidine). Phenytoin or fosphenytoin dosage adjustments may be necessary in patients who receive any of these drugs concurrently. Monitor the patient for signs of phenytoin toxicity.

Hydantoin anticonvulsants induce hepatic microsomal enzymes and may increase the metabolism of cardiac glycosides, atorvastatin, simvastatin, and calcium channel blockers.

Pregabalin

Pregabalin should be used cautiously in patients with severe heart failure. Dose-related weight gain and peripheral edema have been noted with pregabalin.

Rufinamide

ECG studies demonstrated shortening of the QT interval with rufinamide treatment. However, there was no signal for drug-induced sudden death or ventricular arrhythmias. The degree of QT shortening induced by rufinamide is without any known clinical risk. Familial short QT syndrome is associated with an increased risk of sudden death and ventricular arrhythmias, particularly ventricular fibrillation. Patients with familial short QT syndrome should not be treated with rufinamide. Caution should be used when administering rufinamide with other drugs that shorten the QT interval.

Topiramate

Hypertension and bradycardia are among infrequent adverse effects of topiramate. Although the clinical relevance has not been determined, the clinician should be aware that serum digoxin concentrations may be decreased when digoxin and topiramate are used concomitantly.

Valproic Acid, Valproate, Divalproex Sodium

Cardiovascular adverse effects of valproate include hypertension, palpitation, tachycardia, and bradycardia.

Valproic acid, due to its enzyme-inhibiting properties, may increase the plasma levels of a variety of drugs. Concurrent administration of highly protein-bound agents such as valproate may displace warfarin from its binding sites, leading to increased anticoagulation. Monitor INR closely when valproate therapy is introduced or stopped.

Zonisamide

Cardiovascular adverse effects have been infrequently reported with zonisamide therapy. These adverse effects included hypertension, hypotension, palpitation, sinus bradycardia, sinus tachycardia, syncope, thrombophlebitis, and vascular insufficiency. Rare cardiovascular adverse reactions include atrial fibrillation, heart failure, pulmonary embolus, and ventricular extrasystole.

Zonisamide is metabolized by hepatic CYP3A4. Inhibitors including diltiazem, nicardipine, ranolazine, and verapamil can increase the systemic exposure of zonisamide by decreasing the metabolism of the drug.

Recommended Antiseizure Medications in Patients with Cardiovascular Disorders

- *Generalized epilepsies*: Ethosuximide, levetiracetam, perampanel
- *Focal epilepsies*: Brivaracetam, levetiracetam, perampanel

References

Dhatt MS, Gomes JA, Reddy CP, Akhtar M, Caracta AR, Lau SH, Damato AN. Effects of phenytoin on refractoriness and conduction in the human heart. *J Cardiovasc Pharmacol.* 1979;1:3–18.

Facts and Comparisons. *Drug Facts and Comparisons*. St. Louis: Wolters Kluwer Health/Facts & Comparisons, St. Louis; 2007.

Galgani A, Palleria C, Iannone LF, et al. Pharmacokinetic interactions of clinical interest between direct oral anticoagulants and antiepileptic drugs. *Front Neurol.* 2018;9:1067.

Jakubus T, Michalska-Jakubus M, Lukawski K, Janowska A, Czuczwar SJ. Atherosclerotic risk among children taking antiepileptic drugs. *Pharmacol Rep.* 2009;61(3):411–423.

Kenneback G, Bergfeldt L, Vallin H, Tomson T, Edhag O. Electrophysiologic effects and clinical hazards of carbamazepine treatment for neurologic disorders in patients with abnormalities of the cardiac conduction system. *Am Heart J.* 1991;121:1421–1429.

Laine K, Forsstrom J, Gronroos P, Irjala K, Kailajarvi M, Scheinin M. Frequency and clinical outcome of potentially harmful drug metabolic interactions in patients hospitalized on internal and pulmonary medicine wards: Focus on warfarin and cisapride. *Therap Drug Monitor.* 2000;22:503–509.

Mintzer S. Metabolic consequences of antiepileptic drugs. *Curr Opin Neurol.* 2010;23:164–169.

Parrish RH, Pazdur DE, O'Donnell PJ. Effect of carbamazepine initiation and discontinuation on antithrombotic control in a patient receiving warfarin: Case report and review of the literature. *Pharmacotherapy*. 2006;26:1650–1653.

Svalheim S, Luef G, Rauchenzauner M, Mørkrid L, Gjerstad L, Tauboll E. Cardiovascular risk factors in epilepsy patients taking levetiracetam, carbamazepine or lamotrigine. *Acta Neurol Scand*. 2010;122 (Suppl. 190):30–33.

Zaccara G, Lattanzi S, Cincotta M, Russo E. Drug treatments in patients with cardiac diseases and epilepsy. *Acta Neurol Scand*. 2020 Apr 7. doi:10.1111/ane.13249. [Epub ahead of print]

Online Resources

Brivaracetam (Briviact). www.briviact.com/2020

Cenobamate (Xcopri). https://reference.medscape.com/drug/xcopri-cenobamate-1000328/2020

Eslicarbazine acetate (Aptiom). www.aptiom.com/2014

Ezogabine (Potiga). www.potiga.com/2014

Lacosamide (Vimpat). www.vimpat.com/2014

Rufinamide (Banzel). www.banzel.com/2014

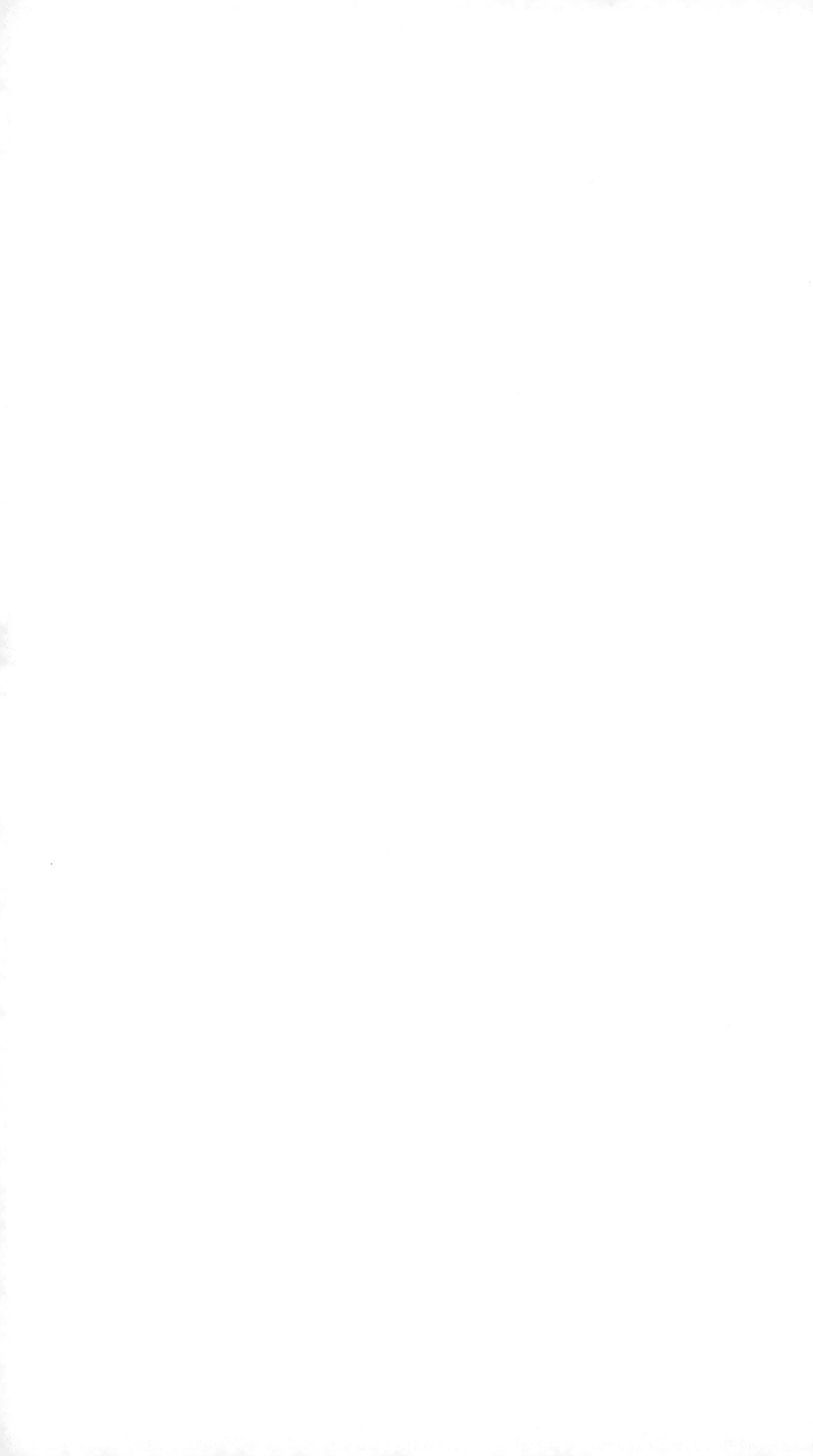

Chapter 18

Antiseizure Medications in Patients with Hematological Disorders

Many antiseizure medications (ASMs) are associated with hematological adverse effects (Facts and Comparisons, 2007; Levy et al., 2002; Verrotti et al., 2014; see also individual drug websites listed in the Online Resources section at the end of this chapter). A wide spectrum of hematological abnormalities can be seen after prescribing an ASM, ranging from mild thrombocytopenia or neutropenia to anemia, red cell aplasia, or even bone marrow failure. The magnitude of the problem is illustrated by the fact that at least one hematological abnormality was noted in 33% of patients taking valproate in one study (May and Sunder, 1993). Transient leukopenia has been reported in 12% of patients taking carbamazepine (Asadi-Pooya and Ghetmiri, 2006), while persistent leukopenia may occur in 2% of patients (Verrotti et al., 2014). Phenytoin produces similar rates of leukopenia. These abnormalities are usually inconsequential, but as noted, serious life-threatening illnesses may be provoked by ASM therapy. Fortunately, potentially fatal hematological disorders are rare; for example, aplastic anemia has an incidence of only a few cases per million per year. Nonetheless, knowledge of the hematological adverse effects of these drugs is crucial when selecting ASMs in patients with epilepsy.

Cytochrome P-450 enzymes are hemoproteins and play an important role in drug metabolism, particularly in the liver. As a result of enzyme induction, more of these hemoproteins are synthesized, which in turn induces heme synthesis. Increased heme synthesis then leads to accelerated porphyrin production and may result in an acute attack of porphyria. Many drugs that either influence hepatic metabolism or are metabolized by liver are potentially porphyrinogenic and may pose rise for with porphyria; these are best avoided though objective data regarding their risks are lacking for many of agents. ASMs of concern include carbamazepine, cenobamate, eslicarbazepine, lamotrigine, oxcarbazepine, phenobarbital, phenytoin, primidone, topiramate, valproate, and zonisamide. ASMs such as levetiracetam, perampanel, pregabalin, and gabapentin are preferred in patients with porphyria due to their negligible hepatic metabolism (Ruiz-Giménez et al., 2010).

Whether patients with underlying primary hematological disorders are at greater risk for adverse effects when prescribed ASMs is uncertain. Due to the relatively common provocation of hematological abnormalities by some drugs, however, it seems prudent to avoid their use in patients who have less functional reserve. This chapter reviews hematological adverse effects known to be associated with the use of ASMs.

Antiseizure Medications and Hematological Disorders

Acetazolamide

Acetazolamide rarely induces bone marrow suppression; cases of fatal aplastic anemia and thrombocytopenia have been reported. Patients with hematological disease should have periodic hematological evaluations, probably no more often than warranted for their clinical condition, however.

Benzodiazepines

Significant hematological adverse effects, such as thrombocytopenia, leucopenia, agranulocytosis, and pancytopenia are quite rare (Verrotti et al., 2014).

Brivaracetam

Brivaracetam may infrequently cause hematologic abnormalities; 1.8% of brivaracetam-treated patients had decreased white blood cell count ($<3.0 \times 10^9$/L).

Cannabidiol

Cannabidiol may cause decreases in hemoglobin and hematocrit (i.e., anemia) in 30% of patients.

Carbamazepine

Carbamazepine should be used with caution in patients with blood dyscrasias caused by drugs or other hematological diseases. The overall incidence of severe hematological adverse effects of carbamazepine is estimated to be 1:38,000 to 1:10,800 in various studies. These serious adverse effects include aplastic anemia, agranulocytosis, and pancytopenia. Carbamazepine has also been associated with thrombocytopenia. Mild anemia has been reported in fewer than 5% of the patients taking carbamazepine, and mild leukopenia is not uncommon as well. The risk of developing these adverse reactions is 5–8 times greater in patients treated with carbamazepine than in the general population. If pretreatment baseline complete blood counts are abnormal, periodic monitoring of blood counts is advisable. No objective data exist to advise a desirable monitoring regimen; we check the blood count 1 month or so after initiating therapy and then every few months for the first year. Then the blood count is checked yearly in those patients with abnormal pretreatment baseline complete blood counts, assuming no problems are detected. If neutropenia or thrombocytopenia develops, the patient should be closely monitored. Discontinuation of carbamazepine is advisable if the total leukocyte (white blood cell [WBC]) count falls below 2,000/mL, the neutrophil (polymorphonuclear cell [PMN]) count falls below 1,000/mL, the erythrocyte count falls below 3.5×10^6/mL, the platelet count falls below 80,000/mL, or the hemoglobin concentration falls below 11 g/dL. In most cases, leukopenia, thrombocytopenia, and other adverse effects are usually mild and transient, and cessation is rarely necessary (Joffe et al., 1985; Olcay et al., 1995; Rush and Beran, 1984; Tohen et al., 1995; Verrotti et al., 2014). These guidelines are applicable for all ASMs. Folate supplementation may prevent carbamazepine-induced leukopenia or anemia (Asadi-Pooya and Ghetmiri, 2006). Because carbamazepine may exacerbate porphyria, this drug should be avoided in that disease.

Cenobamate

Hematological adverse events are quite rare and no significant hematological concerns have arisen thus far in this relatively new agent.

Eslicarbazepine Acetate

Hematological adverse events are quite rare. Compared to placebo, eslicarbazepine acetate use was associated with a slightly higher frequency of anemia.

Ethosuximide

Ethosuximide should be used with caution in patients with bone marrow suppression or any hematological disease. Blood dyscrasias including leukopenia, eosinophilia, agranulocytosis, aplastic anemia, and pancytopenia have been reported to be associated with ethosuximide treatment. Discontinue the drug if counts fall below the parameters mentioned in the preceding paragraph (see "Carbamazepine").

Ezogabine

Hematological adverse events are quite rare. Leukopenia, neutropenia, and thrombocytopenia have been reported rarely.

Felbamate

Treatment with felbamate has been associated with an increase in the incidence of aplastic anemia. The incidence of aplastic anemia has been reported to be 27–209 per million users for those receiving felbamate (most probable value of 127 per million users) versus about 2–2.5 per million persons in the general population (Kaufman et al., 1997). The aplastic anemia population risk for felbamate treatment is 20 times greater than that for carbamazepine (Kaufman et al., 1997). Therefore, felbamate should only be used in patients with severe epilepsy posing significant risk of injury and harm that is unresponsive to other ASMs. It is not certain whether the risk of developing aplastic anemia changes with the duration of treatment or dose of felbamate, but nearly all reported cases have occurred within the first year of treatment. Routine blood testing cannot reliably predict the incidence of aplastic anemia but allows the detection of the hematological changes early in their course. Felbamate should be discontinued if any evidence of bone marrow suppression occurs.

Other infrequent hematological adverse effects of felbamate include lymphadenopathy, leukocytosis, and thrombocytopenia. Antinuclear factor test–positive, qualitative platelet disorder, and agranulocytosis have been rarely reported.

Gabapentin

Hematological adverse events are quite rare. The reported incidence of leukopenia with gabapentin treatment is about 1.1%, and it is usually mild. The hematological adverse effect more often reported is purpura or bruising from physical trauma. Reports of thrombocytopenia, anemia, and lymphadenopathy have been rare.

Lacosamide

Hematological adverse events are quite rare. Rarely, agranulocytosis, neutropenia, and anemia have been reported.

Lamotrigine

Hematological adverse effects observed during lamotrigine therapy include anemia, eosinophilia, leukopenia, thrombocytopenia, and disseminated intravascular coagulation. These adverse reactions are rare. Although lamotrigine has weak antifolate activity, no clinically significant alterations in serum or erythrocyte folate concentrations have been identified with lamotrigine therapy (Gidal et al., 2005).

Levetiracetam

Leukopenia and neutropenia have been infrequently reported in adults and children receiving levetiracetam. Most of these reactions are transient, and usually there is no need for drug discontinuation. Mild anemia has also been reported in adults. Pancytopenia has been reported in post-marketing reports; however, no causal relationship has been established. Levetiracetam seems to inhibit thromboxane-dependent platelet activation and aggregation. Caution should be exercised when levetiracetam is used concomitantly with antithrombotic drugs, especially with antiplatelet agents such as clopidogrel, because of an expected additive effect (Verrotti et al., 2014).

Oxcarbazepine

Leukopenia and thrombocytopenia have been reported with oxcarbazepine treatment, but are rare.

Perampanel

Hematological adverse events are quite rare.

Phenobarbital

Megaloblastic anemia, leukopenia, agranulocytosis, and thrombocytopenia have been reported with phenobarbital treatment. Megaloblastic anemia may respond to folate supplementation, allowing continued phenobarbital therapy. Because phenobarbital may exacerbate porphyria, this drug should be avoided in that disease.

Phenytoin

Phenytoin should be used with caution in patients with blood dyscrasias caused by drugs or other hematological diseases. Phenytoin can cause hematological adverse effects including thrombocytopenia, leukopenia, neutropenia, agranulocytosis, pancytopenia, macrocytosis, and megaloblastic anemia.

However, serious blood dyscrasias are rare in patients taking phenytoin (Blackburn et al., 1998). Monitoring guidelines are similar to those for carbamazepine. Although macrocytosis and megaloblastic anemia usually respond to therapy with folate, they are uncommon, and folate need not be administered routinely to patients receiving phenytoin. Folate has potential detrimental effects on phenytoin plasma levels and efficacy that may cause seizure exacerbation (Steinweg and Bentley, 2005).

Because phenytoin may exacerbate porphyria, this drug should be avoided in that disease. Phenytoin may rarely cause hemolysis as an adverse reaction; use with caution in patients with hemolytic anemia. Methemoglobinemia is rare with normal therapeutic doses of phenytoin; however, this adverse effect has occasionally been reported, especially in the setting of overdose or in patients with methemoglobin reductase deficiency.

There are some reports about a relationship between phenytoin and the development of lymphadenopathy (local or generalized) including benign lymph node hyperplasia, pseudolymphoma, lymphoma, and Hodgkin's disease. Although a cause-and-effect relationship has not been established, the occurrence of lymphadenopathy requires investigation, and phenytoin should be stopped.

Pregabalin

Pregabalin treatment has been associated with thrombocytopenia, although this is rare.

Rufinamide

Anemia has been reported with rufinamide use. Other hematological adverse effects are infrequent and include lymphadenopathy, leucopenia, neutropenia, and thrombocytopenia.

Topiramate

Epistaxis has been reported to occur in 1–4% of patients with topiramate treatment. Topiramate may modulate voltage-gated L-type calcium ion channels located on vascular smooth muscle and platelets. Bleeding tendency associated with topiramate may be more pronounced in patients receiving concomitant antiplatelet therapy. Hematological complications (e.g., anemia) are rare.

Valproate

Thrombocytopenia (dose-dependent), inhibition of the secondary phase of platelet aggregation, and abnormal coagulation parameters (e.g., low fibrinogen) have been reported with valproate treatment. A decrease in platelet count is the most common hematological adverse effect of valproate. While the reported incidence varies from 5% to 60%, this is usually transient, and sustained thrombocytopenia is uncommon in our experience. Clinically significant bleeding is uncommon because the thrombocytopenia is usually not severe. Thrombocytopenia usually develops after several months of high valproate levels (>100 µg/mL) but resolves within a few days after dose reduction (Gerstner et al., 2006; Suchitra and James, 2000). Platelet counts are recommended before initiating valproic acid therapy and at periodic intervals if clinical signs appear. If an increased bleeding tendency is observed before surgical procedures, it is recommended to assess platelet count, thromboelastography, PT, aPTT, TT, fibrinogen, vWF, and factor XIII. Hemorrhages, hematomas, petechiae, bruising, and prolonged bleeding time are indications for dosage reduction or withdrawal of therapy (Verrotti et al., 2014).

Mild leukopenia, neutropenia, bone marrow suppression, lymphadenopathy, and exacerbation of acute intermittent porphyria have been reported with valproic acid therapy (Suchitra and James, 2000). Any evidence of hemorrhage, bruising, hematomas, petechiae, or a disorder of hemostasis or coagulation (e.g., prolonged bleeding time) is an indication for reduction of the dosage or withdrawal of therapy.

Vigabatrin

Anemia has been reported with vigabatrin use. Other hematological adverse events are quite rare.

Zonisamide

Ecchymosis is a hematological adverse reaction occasionally associated with zonisamide therapy. Also, anemia, immunodeficiency, leukopenia, and lymphadenopathy have rarely been reported. Rare adverse reactions include microcytic anemia, petechiae, and thrombocytopenia.

Recommended Antiseizure Medications in Patients with Bone Marrow Suppression or Hematological Disorders

- *Generalized epilepsies*: Benzodiazepines, lamotrigine, levetiracetam
- *Focal epilepsies*: Brivaracetam, cenobamate, eslicarbazepine acetate, gabapentin, lacosamide, lamotrigine, levetiracetam, oxcarbazepine, perampanel

References

Asadi-Pooya AA, Ghetmiri E. Folic acid supplementation reduces the development of some blood cell abnormalities in children receiving carbamazepine. *Epilepsy Behav*. 2006;8:228–231.

Blackburn SC, Oliart AD, Garcia Rodriguez LA. Antiepileptics and blood dyscrasias: A cohort study. *Pharmacotherapy*. 1998;18:1277–1283.

Facts and Comparisons. *Drug Facts and Comparisons*. St. Louis: Wolters Kluwer Health/Facts and Comparisons; 2007.

Gerstner T, Teich M, Bell N, Longin E, Dempfle CE, Brand J, Konig S. Valproate-associated coagulopathies are frequent and variable in children. *Epilepsia*. 2006;47:1136–1143.

Gidal BE, Tamura T, Hammer A, Vuong A. Blood homocysteine, folate and vitamin B-12 concentrations in patients with epilepsy receiving lamotrigine or sodium valproate for initial monotherapy. *Epilepsy Res*. 2005;64:161–166.

Joffe RT, Post RM, Roy-Byrne PP, et al. Hematological effects of carbamazepine in patients with affective illness. *Am J Psychiatry*. 1985;142:1196–1199.

Kaufman DW, Kelly JP, Anderson T, et al. Evaluation of case reports of aplastic anemia among patients treated with felbamate. *Epilepsia*. 1997;38:1265–1269.

Levy RH, Mattson RH, Meldrum BS, Perucca E. *Antiepileptic Drugs*, 5th ed. Philadelphia: Lippincott Williams and Wilkins; 2002.

May R, Sunder TR. Hematologic manifestations of long-term valproate therapy. *Epilepsia*. 1993;34:1098–1101.

Olcay L, Pekcan S, Yalnizoglu D, et al. Fatal agranulocytosis developed in the course of carbamazepine therapy. *Turkish J Pediatr*. 1995;37:73–77.

Ruiz-Giménez J, Sánchez-Alvarez JC, Cañadillas-Hidalgo F, et al. Antiepileptic treatment in patients with epilepsy and other comorbidities. *Seizure*. 2010;19(7):375–382.

Rush JA, Beran RG. Leucopenia as an adverse reaction to carbamazepine therapy. *Med J Austral*. 1984;140:426–428.

Steinweg DL, Bentley ML. Seizures following reduction in phenytoin level after orally administered folic acid. *Neurology*. 2005;64:1982.

Suchitra A, James B. Hematologic toxicity of sodium valproate. *J Pediatr Hematol*. 2000;22:62–65.

Tohen M, Castillo PHJ, Baldessarini RJ, et al. Blood dyscrasias with carbamazepine and valproate: A pharmacoepidemiological study of 2228 patients at risk. *Am J Psychiatry*. 1995;152:413–418.

Verrotti A, Scaparrotta A, Grosso S, Chiarelli F, Coppola G. Anticonvulsant drugs and hematological disease. *Neurol Sci*. 2014;35(7):983–993.

Online Resources

Brivaracetam (Briviact). www.briviact.com/2020

Cannabidiol (Epidiolex). www.epidiolex.com/2020

Cenobamate (Sabril). www.lundbeck.com/upload/us/files/.../Sabril/2014

Cenobamate (Xcopri). https://reference.medscape.com/drug/xcopri-cenobamate-1000328/2020

Eslicarbazine acetate (Aptiom). www.aptiom.com/2014

Ezogabine (Potiga). www.potiga.com/2014

Lacosamide (Vimpat). www.vimpat.com/2014

Perampanel (Fycompa). us.eisai.com/wps/wcm/connect/Eisai/Home/Our.../FYCOMPA/2014

Runfiamide (Banzel). www.banzel.com/2014

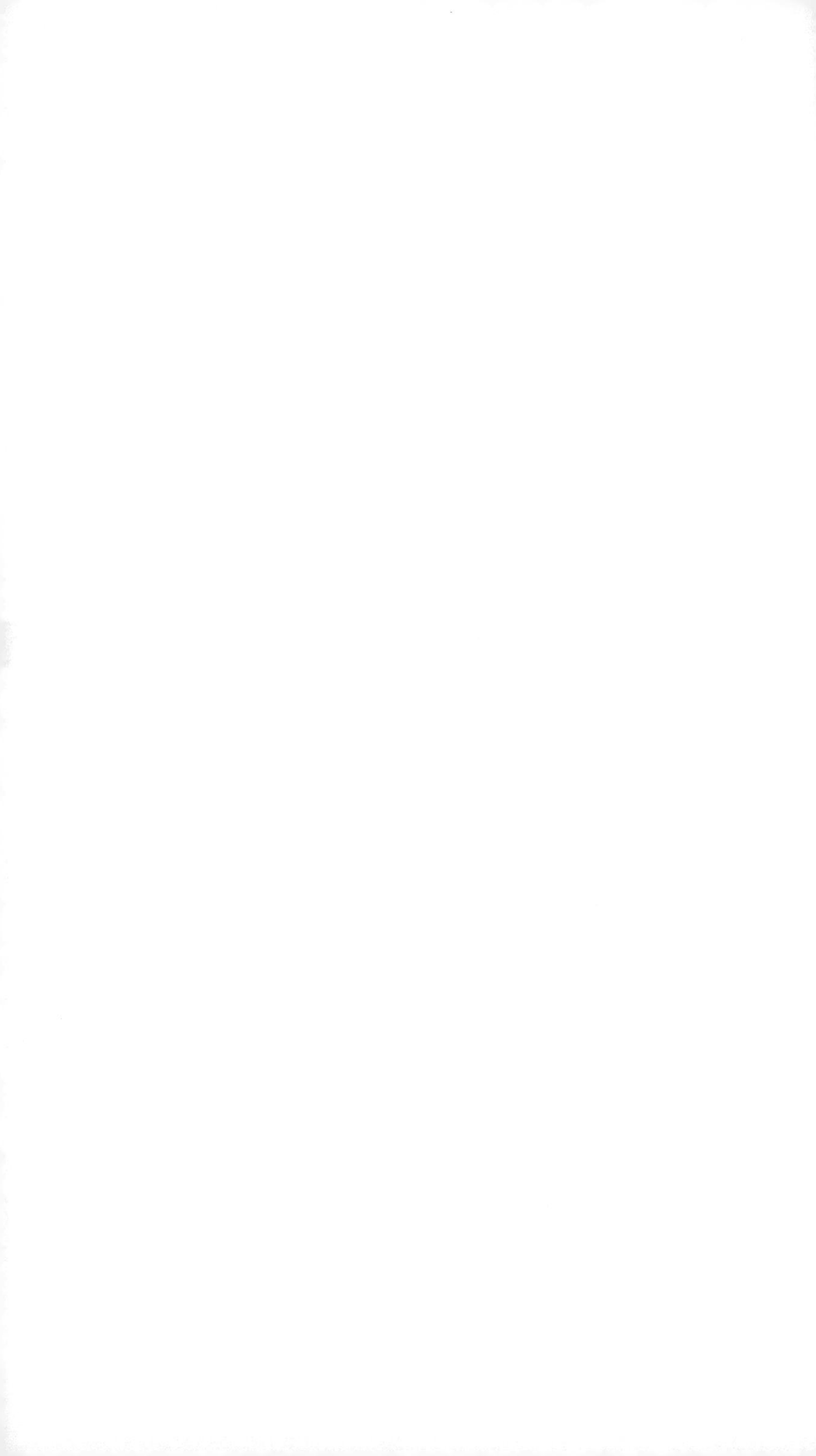

Chapter 19

Antiseizure Medications in Patients on Chemotherapy or Immunosuppressive Therapy

Seizures may occur in patients with cancer as a consequence of direct central nervous system (CNS) invasion by tumor cells, adverse effects of treatment (surgery, radiation, systemic therapies), systemic infections in immunocompromised patients, or metabolic derangements resulting from the effects of systemic cancer (e.g., hypocalcemia, hyponatremia) (Gonzalez Castro and Milligan, 2020). On the other hand, patients with cancer are at high risk for drug-drug interactions because anticancer drugs not only possess a complex pharmacologic profile but also may possess a narrow therapeutic index and a steep dose toxicity curve. While antiseizure medications (ASMs) are indicated in patients with cancer who present with epilepsy, chemotherapeutic agents may lose effectiveness when enzyme-inducing ASMs are prescribed because many chemotherapeutic agents are also metabolized by the cytochrome P-450 enzyme system (Box 19.1). These ASMs include phenobarbital, primidone, phenytoin, and carbamazepine, as well as eslicarbazepine, oxcarbazepine, and topiramate in higher doses, and cenobamate (CYP2B6 and CYP3A substrates). On the other hand, enzyme-inhibiting ASMs, such as valproic acid, stiripentol, and cannabidiol, may amplify hematologic and other toxicities of chemotherapeutic agents (e.g., nitrosoureas or etoposide). Cenobamate inhibits CYP2C19 and has interaction with its substrates. It is therefore advisable to use ASMs that do not interfere with the cytochrome P-450 enzyme complex and have low protein binding when treating patients who require chemotherapy (Oberndorfer et al., 2005; Patsalos et al., 2002; Perucca, 2013; Vecht and van Breemen, 2006; Yap et al., 2008). It is important to remember that some chemotherapeutic agents and systemic cancer therapies are associated with seizures (Table 19.1). It is even advisable to start prophylactic treatment with an appropriate ASM in patients who are going to receive busulfan or chimeric antigen receptor T cells (Gonzalez Castro and Milligan, 2020). Chimeric antigen receptor T-cell therapies are used for the treatment of refractory acute lymphocytic leukemia and lymphoma. Their neurotoxicity is characterized by aphasia, encephalopathy, and seizures (Gonzalez Castro and Milligan, 2020).

Box 19.1 Commonly Used Anticancer Drugs Negatively Affected by Comedication with Enzyme-Inducing Antiseizure Medications

Alkylating Agents

Carmustine, lomustine, nimustine, fotemustine (nitrosoureas), thiotepa, cyclophosphamide, ifosfamide

Mitotic Inhibitors

Vincristine, vinorelbine (vinca-alkaloids), paclitaxel, docetaxel

Topoisomerase Inhibitors/DNA-Damaging Agents

Irinotecan, topotecan, etoposide, doxorubicin

Antimetabolites

Methotrexate pemetrexed

Signal Transduction Inhibitors

Imatinib, erlotinib, gefinitib, sorafenib, temsirolimus, everolimus, vemurafenib

Proteasome Inhibitors

Bortezomib

Adapted from: Weller M, Stupp R, Wick W. Epilepsy meets cancer: when, why, and what to do about it? *Lancet Oncol.* 2012;13(9):e375–e382.

Table 19.1 Systemic cancer therapies commonly associated with seizures

Drug	Mechanism of action	Indications
Busulfan	Alkylating agent	CML, preconditioning for SCT
L-Asparaginase	Antimetabolite	All, AML
Cisplatin	Platinum-based agent	Ovarian cancer, testicular cancer, bladder caner
5-Fluoracil	Antimetabolite	Colorectal cancer, pancreatic cancer, breast cancer, gastric, sarcomas
Ifosfamide	Alkylating agent	Testicular cancer, sarcomas
Etoposide	Inhibitor of DNA replication	Testicular cancer, SCLC, medulloblastoma, pineoblastoma, ependymoma
Methotrexate (intrathecal)	Antimetabolite	Lymphoma
Chimeric antigen receptor T cells	Cell-based immunotherapy	B-cell ALL, B-cell lymphoma
Blinatumumab	Bispecific T-cell engager Ab, anti-CD3/CD19 Ab	Multiple myeloma

Ab, antibody; ALL, acute lymphocytic leukemia; AML, acute myelogenous leukemia; CML, chronic myelogenous leukemia; SCLC, small-cell lung cancer; SCT, stem cell transplantation.

Reprinted with permission: Gonzalez Castro LN, Milligan TA. Seizures in patients with cancer. *Cancer*. 2020;126:1379–1389.

Similar recommendations are applicable for patients on immunosuppressive therapy (e.g., transplant patients). For example, carbamazepine, oxcarbazepine, phenobarbital, and phenytoin reduce cyclosporine, tacrolimus, and corticosteroid blood levels. However, there are other considerations in transplant patients (Chabolla and Wszolek, 2006).

1. Toxicity from ASMs is more common in patients with coexisting hepatic or renal dysfunction.
2. Drugs such as phenytoin, carbamazepine, and valproate are heavily protein-bound; only unbound or free drug is pharmacologically active. Although free drug concentration can be estimated from total concentration, for strongly bound drugs the prediction of free level is not always possible. Conditions like uremia, liver disease, and hypoalbuminemia, which are commonly observed in transplant patients, can lead to significant increases in free drug levels, resulting in drug toxicity even if the serum concentration of total drug is within therapeutic range (Chabolla and Wszolek, 2006; Dasgupta, 2007).
3. Hypersensitivity can occur with agents such as carbamazepine, oxcarbazepine, phenobarbital, and lamotrigine, with fever, rash, and eosinophilia. This may contribute to the morbidity of transplantation (Asconapé, 2002; Chabolla and Wszolek, 2006).
4. Azathioprine, mycophenolate mofetil, and muromonab (OKT3) metabolism is not significantly affected by ASMs (Chabolla and Wszolek, 2006).
5. Most transplant patients who experience one or two seizures during the peritransplantation period typically do not have long-term risk for recurrent seizures. A 1- to 3-month course of ASM therapy is often sufficient to provide protection during a vulnerable period. Patients with potentially epileptogenic brain lesions or who are critically ill may need a longer course of ASM therapy (Chabolla and Wszolek, 2006).
6. Most chemotherapeutic agents and immunosuppressant drugs have potential for bone marrow suppression. This adverse effect should be considered at the time of ASM selection for patient with epilepsy.

Antiseizure Medications in Patients on Chemotherapy or Immunosuppressive Therapy

Acetazolamide

Acetazolamide is known to inhibit CYP3A4 and may decrease metabolism of other drugs and increase their plasma concentrations (Spina et al., 1996). This may amplify the toxicity of chemotherapeutic and immunosuppressive agents.

Brivaracetam

Brivaracetam rarely produces clinically significant interactions with other drugs (brivaracetam; www.briviact.com/2020).

Cannabidiol

This drug is suboptimal in patients who receive chemotherapy or immunosuppressive therapy. Because of potential inhibition of enzyme activity, consider a reduction in dosage of substrates of UGT1A9, UGT2B7, CYP2C8, CYP2C9, and CYP2C19 if adverse reactions are experienced when administered concomitantly with cannabidiol. Because of potential for both induction and inhibition of enzyme activity, consider adjusting dosage of substrates of CYP1A2 and CYP2B6, as clinically appropriate (cannabidiol; www.epidiolex.com/2020).

Carbamazepine

This drug is suboptimal in patients who receive chemotherapy or immunosuppressive therapy. Carbamazepine induces hepatic microsomal enzymes, which, in turn, accelerates the metabolism of other drugs, including many of antineoplastic drugs. This drug is 76% protein-bound in adults. Carbamazepine may interact with chemotherapeutic agents via different mechanisms. For example, myelosuppressive antineoplastic agents and radiation therapy possess hematologic toxicities similar to carbamazepine and should be used concomitantly with caution. Cisplatin and doxorubicin may increase the rate of carbamazepine metabolism because these antineoplastics induce hepatic microsomal enzymes (e.g., CYP3A). Dosage adjustments (either in carbamazepine or in antineoplastic agents) may be necessary, and closer monitoring of clinical and/or adverse effects is warranted when carbamazepine is used with any of the agents mentioned.

Cenobamate

This drug is suboptimal in patients who receive chemotherapy or immunosuppressive therapy. Increase the dosage of CYP2B6 or CYP3A4 substrates, as needed, when used concomitantly with cenobamate (it is an inducer). Consider a reduction in dosage of CYP2C19 substrates, as clinically appropriate, when used concomitantly with cenobamate (it is an inhibitor) (https://reference.medscape.com/drug/xcopri-cenobamate-1000328/2020).

Eslicarbazepine Acetate

This is a less-than-ideal choice for patients receiving chemotherapy or immunosuppressive therapy due to hepatic metabolism and potential for drug interactions. Eslicarbazepine acetate can inhibit CYP2C19, which can cause increased plasma concentrations of drugs that are metabolized by this isoenzyme. In vivo studies suggest that eslicarbazepine acetate can induce CYP3A4, thus decreasing plasma concentrations of drugs that are metabolized by this isoenzyme.

Ethosuximide

This drug is a good choice for patients who require chemotherapy or immunosuppressive therapy.

Gabapentin

This drug is a good choice for patients with normal renal function who require chemotherapy or immunosuppressive therapy.

Lacosamide

This drug is a good choice for patients who require chemotherapy or immunosuppressive therapy.

Lamotrigine

This is a less-than-ideal choice for patients receiving chemotherapy or immunosuppressive therapy due to hepatic metabolism and potential for drug interactions. Lamotrigine inhibits dihydrofolate reductase. Caution should be exercised when administering other drugs (e.g., fluorouracil or methotrexate), which may inhibit this enzyme.

Levetiracetam

This drug is a good choice for patients with normal renal function who receive chemotherapy or immunosuppressive therapy.

Oxcarbazepine

This is a suboptimal choice for patients receiving chemotherapy or immunosuppressive therapy due to hepatic metabolism and potential for drug interactions. Oxcarbazepine and its metabolite 10-monohydroxy metabolite (MHD) produce a dose-related inhibition of CYP2C19 and induction of CYP3A4. The effectiveness of immunosuppressive medications such as cyclosporine, sirolimus, and tacrolimus could be decreased by the coadministration of oxcarbazepine (Rosche et al., 2001).

Perampanel

This drug is a reasonable choice for patients who receive chemotherapy or immunosuppressive therapy, although protein binding could be an issue. Perampanel is approximately 95% bound to plasma proteins.

Phenobarbital

This drug is suboptimal in patients who receive chemotherapy or immunosuppressive therapy. Phenobarbital accelerates the clearance of other drugs metabolized via hepatic microsomal enzymes (e.g., uridine 5'-diphospho-glucuronosyltransferase [UGT] enzymes, CYP2C-family enzymes, CYP3A-family enzymes, and CYP1A2). This drug is about 20–45% bound to plasma proteins.

Phenytoin

This drug is suboptimal in patients who receive chemotherapy or immunosuppressive therapy. Mechanisms of drug interactions with phenytoin may be complex. In general, phenytoin is an inducer of the hepatic cytochrome P-450 microsomal enzymes including CYP3A4, CYP2C9, and CYP2C19 isoenzymes. This drug is about 90–95% bound to plasma proteins.

Pregabalin

This drug is a reasonable choice in patients who receive chemotherapy or immunosuppressive therapy.

Rufinamide

This drug is an acceptable choice for patients who require chemotherapy or immunosuppressive therapy. Rufinamide is a weak inducer of the CYP3A4 enzyme and can decrease exposure of drugs that are substrates of CYP3A4. Only a small fraction of rufinamide (34%) is bound to serum proteins.

Tiagabine

Tiagabine does not inhibit or induce the hepatic CYP-450 microsomal enzymes or UGT. Tiagabine is extensively bound to plasma proteins (96%), mainly to serum albumin and α_1-acid glycoprotein.

Topiramate

Topiramate is not metabolized to a great extent. Its protein binding range is 13–41% to plasma proteins. Topiramate may induce hepatic enzymes with dosages of greater than 200 mg/day. Because of potential for interactions, high doses of this drug are less than ideal in patients who receive chemotherapy or immunosuppressive therapy.

Valproic Acid, Valproate, Divalproex Sodium

This drug is suboptimal in patients who receive chemotherapy or immunosuppressive therapy because of interactions and enzyme inhibition. Valproic acid inhibits the activity of CYP2C9 and UGT at clinically relevant concentrations in human liver microsomes. Inhibition of CYP2C9 can explain some of the effects of valproic acid on the pharmacokinetics of other drugs. Valproic acid is about 90% protein bound.

Vigabatrin

This drug is an acceptable choice for patients who require chemotherapy or immunosuppressive therapy with regard to drug interactions. However, it should be used only in the treatment of severe epilepsy refractory to other ASMs because of the risk of visual field defect.

Zonisamide

This drug is a reasonable choice for patients who receive chemotherapy or immunosuppressive therapy although protein binding could be an issue. In vitro data suggest that zonisamide does not inhibit or induce cytochrome P-450 enzymes or UGT. Zonisamide is not likely to interfere with the hepatic metabolic clearance of drugs metabolized by these enzyme systems. Zonisamide is approximately 40–60% bound to human plasma proteins. (Facts and Comparisons, 2007; Perucca, 2005; van Breemen et al., 2007; see also individual drug websites listed in the Online Resources at the end of this chapter).

Recommended Antiseizure Medications in Patients on Chemotherapy or Immunosuppressive Therapy

- *Generalized epilepsies*: Ethosuximide, levetiracetam, rufinamide (in Lennox-Gastaut syndrome), topiramate (low doses)
- *Focal epilepsies*: Brivaracetam, gabapentin, lacosamide, levetiracetam, perampanel, zonisamide

References

Asconapé JJ. Some common issues in the use of antiepileptic drugs. *Semin Neurol.* 2002;22:27–39.

Chabolla DR, Wszolek ZK. Pharmacologic management of seizures in organ transplant. *Neurology.* 2006;67:S34–S38.

Dasgupta A. Usefulness of monitoring free (unbound) concentrations of therapeutic drugs in patient management. *Clinica Chimica Acta.* 2007;377:1–13.

Facts and Comparisons. *Drug Facts and Comparisons.* St. Louis: Wolters Kluwer Health/Facts and Comparisons; 2007.

Gonzalez Castro LN, Milligan TA. Seizures in patients with cancer. *Cancer.* 2020;126:1379–1389.

Oberndorfer S, Piribauer M, Marosi C, Lahrmann H, Hitzenberger P, Grisold W. P-450 enzyme inducing and non-enzyme inducing antiepileptics in glioblastoma patients treated with standard chemotherapy. *J Neuro-Oncol.* 2005;72:255–260.

Patsalos PN, Froscher W, Pisani F, van Rijn CM. The importance of drug interactions in epilepsy therapy. *Epilepsia.* 2002;43:365–385.

Perucca E. Clinically relevant drug interactions with antiepileptic drugs. *Br J Clin Pharmacol.* 2005;61:246–255.

Perucca E. Optimizing antiepileptic drug treatment in tumoral epilepsy. *Epilepsia.* 2013;54(Suppl 9):97–104.

Rosche J, Froscher W, Abendorth D, Liebel J. Possible oxcarbazepine interaction with cyclosporine serum levels: A single case study. *Clin Neuropharmacol.* 2001;24:113–116.

Spina E, Pisani F, Perucca E. Clinically significant pharmacokinetic drug interactions with carbamazepine. *Clin Pharmacokinet.* 1996;31:198–214.

van Breemen MSM, Wilms EB, Vecht CJ. Epilepsy in patients with brain tumors: Epidemiology, mechanisms, and management. *Lancet Neurol.* 2007;6:421–430.

Vecht CJ, van Breemen M. Optimizing therapy of seizures in patients with brain tumors. *Neurology.* 2006;67:S10–S13.

Weller M, Stupp R, Wick W. Epilepsy meets cancer: When, why, and what to do about it? *Lancet Oncol.* 2012;13(9):e375–e382.

Yap KY, Chui WK, Chan A. Drug interactions between chemotherapeutic regimens and antiepileptics. *Clin Ther.* 2008;30(8):1385–1407.

Online Resources

Brivaracetam (Briviact). www.briviact.com/2020

Cannabidiol (Epidiolex). www.epidiolex.com/2020

Cenobamate (Xcopri). https://reference.medscape.com/drug/xcopri-cenobamate-1000328/2020

Eslicarbazine acetate (Aptiom). www.aptiom.com/2014

Ezogabine (Potiga). www.potiga.com/2014

Lacosamide (Vimpat). www.vimpat.com/2014

Perampanel (Fycompa). us.eisai.com/wps/wcm/connect/Eisai/Home/Our.../FYCOMPA/2014

Rufinamide (Banzel). www.banzel.com/2014

Vigabatrin (Sabril). www.lundbeck.com/upload/us/files/.../Sabril/2014

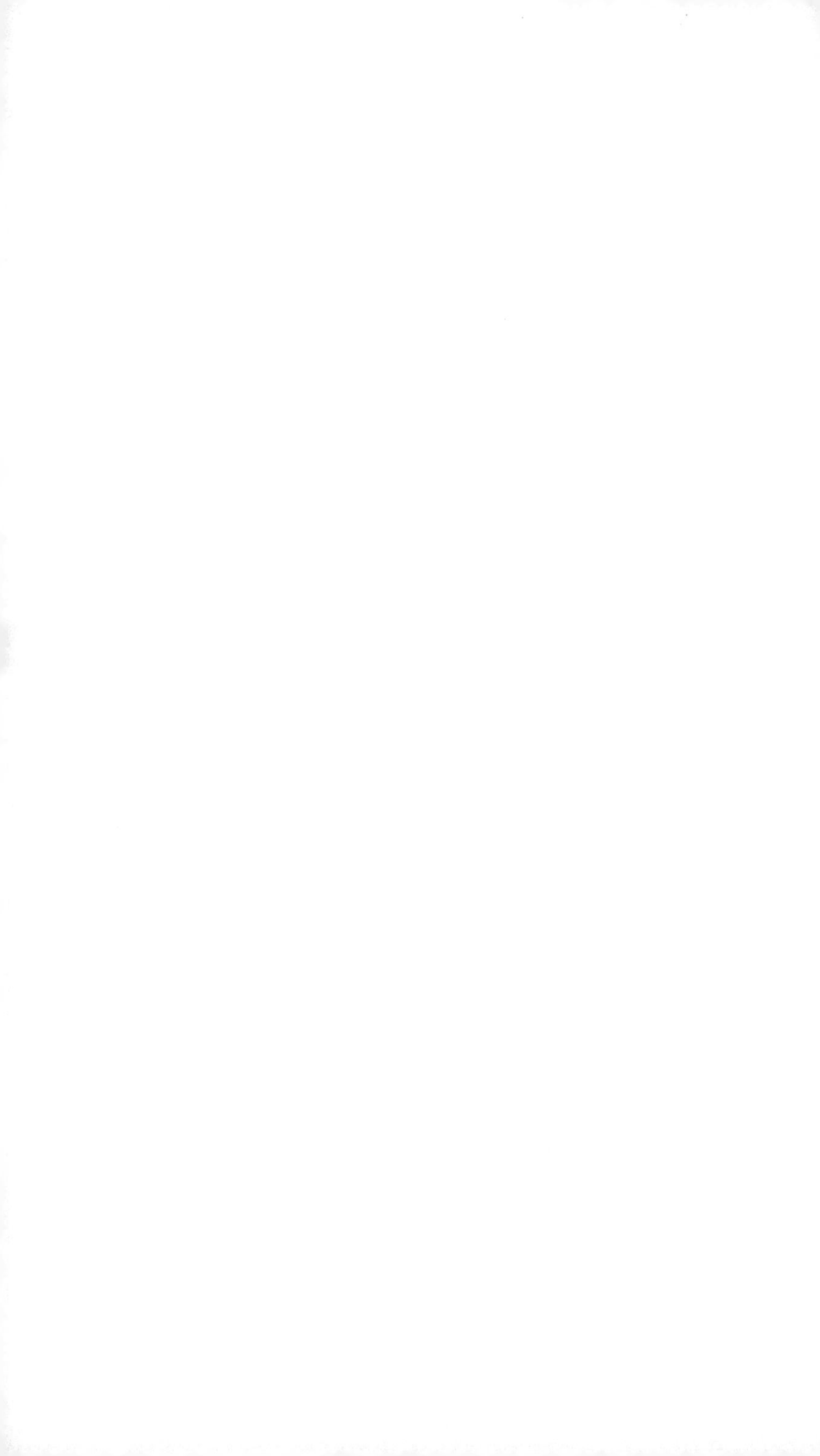

Chapter 20

Antiseizure Medications in Patients with Brain Tumors

Prophylactic anticonvulsant treatment is not advisable in brain tumor patients who have not experienced seizures. However, 30–50% of patients with brain tumors present with a seizure as their initial clinical manifestation and up to 30% more will later develop epileptic seizures. Management of seizures associated with brain tumors requires the consideration of several issues, including a relatively high rate of recurrence after a first seizure and, more importantly, the possibility of adverse interactions between antiseizure medications (ASMs) and anticancer agents (see Chapter 19) and the disease itself. Most of the available data on selecting ASMs in patients with epilepsy and brain tumors originate from uncontrolled studies, and no large-scale well-designed randomized trial has been performed in this population. Therefore, a fully evidence-based approach to ASM selection in patients with epilepsy secondary to brain tumors is not possible at present. Factors to be considered in making treatment selection include tolerability profile, comorbidities, drug interaction potential, and cost. In other words, drug choice relies on both the theoretical advantages of pharmacokinetic properties and clinical judgment (Perucca, 2013; Sperling and Ko, 2006).

There is no evidence that the efficacy ranking of currently available ASMs differs for patients with brain tumors compared with patients with focal seizures from other etiologies. However, limited evidence suggests that patients with brain tumors show increased susceptibility to the adverse effects of ASMs. This could be related to the underlying cerebral pathology or to an interaction with anticancer therapy. The risk of ASM-induced skin rashes, including Stevens-Johnson syndrome, is also increased in patients with brain tumors. The risk of interactions between ASMs and anticancer agents is a major concern (see Chapter 19). Although some anticancer drugs commonly used in primary brain tumors (such as temozolomide) do not seem to be susceptible to enzyme induction, with others, such as irinotecan, etoposide, and tyrosine kinase inhibitors (e.g., erlotinib and imatinib), the increase in clearance caused by enzyme-inducing ASMs (e.g., carbamazepine, phenobarbital, phenytoin, and primidone) can be considerable and may need to be compensated for by a corresponding increase in the dose of the anticancer agent (Perucca, 2013). Valproic acid may favorably influence prognosis in patients with glioblastoma. Valproic acid has been found to induce apoptosis, autophagy, growth arrest, and cell differentiation in tumor cells and also to inhibit tumor angiogenesis through inhibition of histone deacetylase and other mechanisms.

These actions could contribute to inhibit tumor growth and might explain the apparent prolongation of survival in brain tumor patients (particularly, glioblastoma) treated with valproic acid. On the other hand, valproic acid also has intrinsic hematologic toxicity, particularly on platelet function, and it inhibits a number of drug-metabolizing enzymes, causing an increase in the serum levels of some anticancer agents. Increased hematologic toxicity has been reported when valproic acid was given in combination with temozolomide and with other chemotherapeutic agents, including nitrosoureas, cisplatin, and etoposide. Valproic acid may cause thrombocytopenia, platelet dysfunction, and coagulation abnormalities, which represent a concern for patients in whom surgery is envisaged (see Chapter 18) (Perucca, 2013).

Levetiracetam, another potentially useful ASM, has low interaction potential and good tolerability; it can be up-titrated relatively rapidly and also has a parenteral formulation. In laboratory experiments, levetiracetam has been shown to enhance p53-mediated inhibition of O^6-methylguanine DNA methyltransferase (MGMT), a DNA repair protein that has an important role in tumor cell resistance to alkylating agents, and to sensitize glioblastoma cells to temozolomide; the clinical relevance of these findings is unknown. However, patients with glioma who are treated with levetiracetam may have an increased risk for drug-related anxiety compared with patients who do not receive levetiracetam (hazard ratio 2.8) (Knudsen-Baas et al., 2018). Brivaracetam has a parenteral formulation and is also a good choice for patients who require chemotherapy to minimize drug interactions. Switching from levetiracetam to brivaracetam can be considered for patients who have seizure control with levetiracetam but cannot tolerate its behavioral adverse effects. In this setting, an immediate switch from levetiracetam to brivaracetam at a 10:1 to 15:1 ratio without titration is possible (e.g., if taking levetiracetam 500 mg twice daily, may switch directly to brivaracetam 50 mg twice daily) (Feyissa, 2019). Lacosamide has a parenteral formulation and is a good choice for patients who require chemotherapy with regard to drug interactions. Brivaracetam and lacosamide have in vitro cytotoxic and anti-migration effects due to the modulation of several microRNAs, such as microRNA-195-5p and microRNA-107 (Rizzo et al., 2017).

Oxcarbazepine and eslicarbazepine acetate have a relatively low interaction potential with other drugs, but they do retain some enzyme-inducing and enzyme-inhibiting properties and may affect serum levels of certain anticancer drugs. Lamotrigine, perampanel, topiramate, and zonisamide need slow-dose titration, and they lack a parenteral formulation, which could be a disadvantage in patients with brain tumor (Perucca, 2013).

Recommended Antiseizure Medications in Patients with Brain Tumors

- *Generalized epilepsies*: Valproate, levetiracetam
- *Focal epilepsies*: Brivaracetam, lacosamide, levetiracetam, valproate

Antiseizure Medications and Cancer

There is considerable debate about the relationship between ASMs and cancer, in particular, whether ASMs promote or protect against cancer (Singh et al., 2005). Phenytoin and phenobarbital may induce carcinogenicity in rodent models. Phenobarbital promotes liver tumors in rats. Some early human epidemiological studies found an association between phenobarbital and hepatocellular carcinoma, and some subsequent studies suggested an association with lung cancer and brain tumor. Phenytoin causes lymphoid cell and liver tumors in rats. It has been associated with lymphoma, myeloma, and neuroblastoma in some human epidemiological studies (Murray et al., 1996). Carbamazepine results in a dose-related increase in the incidence of hepatocellular tumors in female rats and benign interstitial cell adenoma of testes in male rats. However, evidence for human carcinogenicity is inconsistent.

Valproate, in contrast, has been found to exert an antiproliferative effect on certain cancer cell lines both in vitro and in vivo (due to histone deacetylase inhibition). There are some reports of the use of valproate in human hematological and solid tumors (Kaiser et al., 2006; Olsen et al., 2004; Perucca, 2013).

Most new ASMs are probably safe with regard to carcinogenesis. There was no evidence of lacosamide related carcinogenicity in mice or rats. Vigabatrin showed no carcinogenic potential in mice or rats. There was no evidence of perampanel-related carcinogenicity in mice or rats. Oral administration of cenobamate to mice did not result in an increase in tumors. It is unknown whether gabapentin causes tumors in humans. A statistically significant increase in the incidence of pancreatic acinar cell adenomas and carcinomas has been found in male rats given gabapentin. However, in vitro testing has not shown mutagenic or clastogenic changes. In carcinogenicity studies of pregabalin in mice, an unexpectedly high incidence of hemangiosarcoma was identified. Clinical experience during pregabalin premarketing development provides no direct means to assess its potential for inducing tumors in humans. An increase in the incidence of hepatocellular adenomas and carcinomas was observed in mice with eslicarbazepine acetate. Increased incidences of tumors (benign bone tumors and/or hepatocellular adenomas and carcinomas) were observed in mice with rufinamide. Increased incidences of thyroid follicular adenomas were observed in rats with rufinamide. The incidence of hepatocellular adenoma in female rats and Leydig cell tumors in male rats was increased in a 2-year study with tiagabine. Oral administration of brivaracetam increased the incidence of liver tumors (hepatocellular adenoma and carcinoma) in male mice and thymus tumors (benign thymoma) in female rats. Finally, an increase in urinary bladder tumors was observed in mice given topiramate. Adequate studies of the carcinogenic potential of cannabidiol have not been conducted. The clinical significance of these findings in humans is unknown because mutagenesis is usually species-specific (Facts and Comparisons, 2007; Singh et al., 2005; see also individual drug websites listed in the Online Resources at the end of this chapter).

References

Facts and Comparisons. *Drug Facts and Comparisons*. Wolters Kluwer Health/ Facts and Comparisons, St. Louis; 2007.

Feyissa AM. Brivaracetam in the treatment of epilepsy: A review of clinical trial data. *Neuropsychiatr Dis Treat*. 2019;15:2587–2600.

Kaiser M, Zavrski I, Sterz J, et al. The effects of the histone deacetylase inhibitor valproic acid on cell cycle, growth suppression and apoptosis in multiple myeloma. *Haematology*. 2006;91:248–251.

Knudsen-Baas KM, Johannesen TB, Myklebust TÅ, et al. Antiepileptic and psychiatric medication in a nationwide cohort of patients with glioma WHO grade II-IV. *J Neuro-Oncol*. 2018;140:739–748.

Murray JC, Hill RM, Hegemier S, Hurwitz RL. Lymphoblastic lymphoma following prenatal exposure to phenytoin. *J Pediatr Hematol Oncol*. 1996;18(2):241–243.

Olsen CM, Meussen-Elholm ET, Roste LS, Tauboll E. Antiepileptic drugs inhibit cell growth in the human breast cancer cell line MCF7. *Mol Cell Endocrinol*. 2004;213:173–179.

Perucca E. Optimizing antiepileptic drug treatment in tumoral epilepsy. Epilepsia 2013;54(Suppl 9):97–104.

Rizzo A, Donzelli S, Girgenti V, et al. In vitro antineoplastic effects of brivaracetam and lacosamide on human glioma cells. *J Exp Clin Cancer Res*. 2017;36:76.

Singh G, Driever PH, Sander JW. Cancer risk in people with epilepsy: The role of antiepileptic drugs. *Brain*. 2005;128:7–17.

Sperling MR, Ko J. Seizures and brain tumors. *Semin Oncol*. 2006;33:333–341.

Online Resources

Brivaracetam (Briviact). www.briviact.com/2020

Cannabidiol (Epidiolex). www.epidiolex.com/2020

Cenobamate (Xcopri). https://reference.medscape.com/drug/xcopri-cenobamate-1000328/2020

Eslicarbazine acetate (Aptiom). www.aptiom.com/2014

Ezogabine (Potiga). www.potiga.com/2014

Lacosamide (Vimpat). www.vimpat.com/2014

Perampanel (Fycompa). us.eisai.com/wps/wcm/connect/Eisai/Home/Our.../FYCOMPA/2014

Rufinamide (Banzel). www.banzel.com/2014

Vigabatrin (Sabril). www.lundbeck.com/upload/us/files/.../Sabril/2014

Chapter 21

Antiseizure Medications in Patients with Stroke

Stroke and cerebrovascular lesions are the main cause of epilepsy in the elderly. The risk for development of epilepsy is 17-fold higher after stroke than in the age-matched general population; it is estimated that 10–15% of stroke patients develop epilepsy (Ferro and Pinto, 2004). Seizures can be a presenting feature of acute stroke or may be a late complication.

Many similarities exist between cerebral ischemia and epilepsy regarding brain damage and autoprotective mechanisms that are activated following the injurious insult. Therefore, drugs that are effective in minimizing seizure-induced brain damage may also be useful in minimizing ischemic injury. On the other hand, some antiseizure medications (ASMs) may have detrimental effects in stroke patients, and there is evidence that recovery is worse in patients treated with particular ASMs after stroke (Goldstein, 2000; Stepien et al., 2005).

There is no clinical evidence that prophylactic anticonvulsant treatment after stroke protects against the development of epilepsy. Transient ASM therapy may be needed after a seizure occurring in the setting of an acute stroke (seizure occurring within the first week after a stroke), but prolonged, usually life-long therapy is required after delayed seizures (seizure occurring more than 1 week after a stroke) due to a high probability of seizure recurrence. For the management of stroke-related seizures, no single ASM was found to be more effective than others, though some newer ASMs are associated with fewer adverse effects (Wang et al., 2017). When selecting an ASM for a patient with stroke, one should consider the impact of an ASM on comorbidity and comedications, its adverse effects, and its cost, among other factors (Gilad, 2012; Stepien et al., 2005; Ryvlin and Montavont, 2006).

On the other hand, concern has been raised recently that some ASMs might increase the levels of serologic markers associated with an increased risk of vascular diseases (see Chapter 15 and Chapter 17). The duration of exposure to some ASMs may also predict acceleration of atherosclerosis. Based on these mechanisms, patients exposed to some ASMs could have an increased risk of vascular diseases such as stroke. In a recent study, the authors found that exposure to phenytoin was associated with a higher stroke risk as compared to carbamazepine. In addition, a longer duration and higher dosage of phenytoin demonstrated a dose–response relationship to increased stroke risk. In addition, studies have found that patients with epilepsy have higher stroke-related morbidity and mortality, which is probably related to ASMs, at least in part (Hsieh et al., 2013).

Antiseizure Medications in Stroke

Benzodiazepines

Benzodiazepines may have potential detrimental effects in patients with stroke (Goldstein, 2000; Schallert et al., 1986). In addition, adverse effects of benzodiazepines are significant in the elderly (Facts and Comparisons, 2007; Levy et al., 2002). Thus, benzodiazepines are not recommended.

Brivaracetam

Due to its favorable pharmacokinetic profile and lack of significant drug interactions, this drug is a good choice for acute or chronic use in patients following stroke. The IV formulation can be used in patients with swallowing difficulty (brivaracetam; www.briviact.com/2020).

Carbamazepine

Carbamazepine has had some degree of neuroprotective activity in an ischemic/hypoxic model of neuronal injury (Willmore, 2005). However, due to enzyme induction and drug interactions, other ASMs may be a better choice (Facts and Comparisons, 2007; Levy et al., 2002; Parrish et al., 2006). Because it induces cytochrome P-450 enzymes, doses of warfarin and other drugs that are metabolized by the same system (e.g., statins) will need to be increased.

Cenobamate

There is insufficient data regarding cenobamate use in the elderly. Because of pharmacokinetic interactions with other drugs, this may be a suboptimal drug for early use in elderly patients with stroke.
(https://reference.medscape.com/drug/xcopri-cenobamate-1000328/2020).

Eslicarbazepine

Occurrence of hyponatremia is a potential problem. In addition, in vivo studies suggest that eslicarbazepine acetate can induce CYP3A4, thus decreasing plasma concentrations of drugs that are metabolized by this isoenzyme (e.g., simvastatin). Although the pharmacokinetics of eslicarbazepine are not affected by age independently, dose selection should take into consideration the greater frequency of renal impairment, medical comorbidities, and drug therapies in the elderly patient.

Gabapentin

This drug does not demonstrate significant interaction with anticoagulants, antiplatelet agents, or other medications commonly prescribed in stroke patients, and its safety profile is relatively favorable (Stepien et al., 2005). Low target dosages (900–1,200 mg/day) and slow titration over several weeks are appropriate in patients with stroke (Stepien et al., 2005).

Lacosamide

This drug does not demonstrate significant interaction with anticoagulants, antiplatelet agents, or other medications commonly prescribed in stroke patients, and its safety profile is relatively favorable, but cardiovascular adverse effects and the possibility of syncope should be kept in mind. The IV formulation can be used in patients with swallowing difficulty. Lacosamide treatment following status epilepticus attenuated neuronal cell loss and alterations in hippocampal neurogenesis in a rat electrical status epilepticus model (Licko et al., 2013).

Lamotrigine

This drug has fared well in randomized comparison trials in the elderly population (see Chapter 11) and is a good choice for stroke patients (Stepien et al., 2005). Lamotrigine also has had some degree of neuroprotective activity in an ischemic/hypoxic model of neuronal injury (Willmore, 2005). In addition, lamotrigine may help treat central poststroke pain (Frese et al., 2006; Vestergaard et al., 2001).

Levetiracetam

Due to its favorable pharmacokinetic profile and lack of drug interaction, this drug is a good choice for acute or chronic use. It is well-tolerated for the treatment of post-stroke seizures (Brigo et al., 2018). The IV formulation can be used in patients with swallowing difficulty. Levetiracetam may have some neuroprotective activity.

Oxcarbazepine

This drug is a reasonable choice, although the relatively common occurrence of hyponatremia is a potential problem. In dosages of less than 900 mg/day, this drug does not demonstrate significant interaction with anticoagulants, antiplatelet agents, or other medications commonly prescribed in stroke patients, and its safety profile is relatively favorable (Stepien et al., 2005).

Perampanel

This drug does not demonstrate significant interaction with anticoagulants, antiplatelet agents, or other medications commonly prescribed in stroke patients, and its safety profile is relatively favorable. Elderly patients had an increased risk of falls compared to younger adults.

Phenobarbital

This is a suboptimal drug for chronic use in patients with stroke. There are reports of delay in functional recovery in animal models of stroke or brain damage (Stepien et al., 2005). Phenobarbital may have potential detrimental effects in stoke patients (Goldstein, 2000). Importantly, due to adverse effects and drug interactions, use with precaution in elderly patients (Facts and Comparisons, 2007; Levy et al., 2002).

Phenytoin

This drug is suboptimal for acute and long-term use, although the IV formulation offers acute treatment advantages. Hepatic enzyme induction, drug interactions, and its zero-order kinetics all pose difficulties (Facts and Comparisons, 2007; Levy et al., 2002). Because it induces cytochrome P-450 enzymes, doses of warfarin and other drugs that are metabolized by the same system (e.g., statins) will need to be increased. Moreover, there are reports of alteration or delay in functional recovery in animal models of stroke or brain damage (Brailowsky et al., 1986; Stepien et al., 2005). Phenytoin may have detrimental effects in stroke patients as well (Goldstein, 2000). Likewise, prophylactic phenytoin may contribute to poor functional and cognitive outcomes in a dose-dependent manner after subarachnoid hemorrhage (Naidech et al., 2005). Phenytoin may also cause fever, which is associated with poor outcome and increased length of stay in direct proportion to the length of time the patient is febrile. However, phenytoin has demonstrated efficacy in treating central post-stroke pain (Frese et al., 2006).

Pregabalin

There are little data regarding the use of this agent after stroke, but it has a good pharmacological profile.

Tiagabine

This drug is rarely used after stroke.

Topiramate

This drug is a reasonable choice, although drug interactions and cognitive adverse effects must be carefully monitored. Topiramate has neuroprotective properties and also reduces hemorrhagic incidence in focal cerebral ischemia in animal models; however, the human benefit has not been shown (Ferro and Pinto, 2004; Willmore, 2005).

Valproic Acid, Valproate, Divalproex Sodium

This agent has significant drug interactions, inhibits cytochrome P-450 enzymes, and binds extensively to plasma proteins. For these reasons, it is not an especially good choice for post-stroke seizures.

Zonisamide

This drug has a favorable pharmacological profile and is a reasonable choice. Zonisamide is an anticonvulsant compound that reduced infarct volume in ischemia-induced neuronal damage. Neuroprotective efficacy of zonisamide pretreatment was also shown in hypoxic/ischemic damage in neonatal rats (Ferro and Pinto, 2004; Willmore, 2005). Adverse effects are sometimes important, and the potential for renal stones should be remembered.

Note: Direct oral anticoagulants (DOACs) (apixaban, dabigatran, edoxaban, and rivaroxaban) are increasingly prescribed among the general population because they are considered to be associated with lower bleeding risk than warfarin and they do not require monitoring. In addition, DOACs are increasingly concomitantly prescribed in patients with epilepsy who are taking ASMs. As a result, potential drug-drug interactions may cause an increased risk of DOAC-related bleeding or a reduced antithrombotic efficacy. Enzyme-inducing ASMs (such as phenobarbital, phenytoin, and carbamazepine) are more likely to significantly reduce the anticoagulant effect of

DOACs (especially rivaroxaban, apixaban, and edoxaban). Other ASMs not affecting CYP or P-glycoprotein significantly, such as lamotrigine, are not likely to affect DOACs efficacy. Lacosamide, which does not affect CYP activity significantly, likely has a safe profile even though its effects on P-glycoprotein are not well-known yet. Levetiracetam exerts only a potential effect on P-glycoprotein activity and thus appears safe (Galgani et al., 2018).

Recommended Antiseizure Medications in Patients with Stroke

Brivaracetam, lacosamide, lamotrigine, levetiracetam

References

Brailowsky S, Knight RT, Efron R. Phenytoin increases the severity of cortical hemiplegia in rats. *Brain Res.* 1986;376:71–77.

Brigo F, Lattanzi S, Zelano J, et al. Randomized controlled trials of antiepileptic drugs for the treatment of post-stroke seizures: A systematic review with network meta-analysis. *Seizure.* 2018;61:57–62.

Facts and Comparisons. *Drug Facts and Comparisons.* St. Louis: Wolters Kluwer Health/Facts and Comparisons; 2007.

Ferro JM, Pinto F. Poststroke epilepsy: epidemiology, pathophysiology and management. *Drugs Aging.* 2004;21:639–653.

Frese A, Husstedt IW, Ringelstein EB, Evers S. Pharmacologic treatment of central post-stroke pain. *Clin J Pain.* 2006;22:252–260.

Galgani A, Palleria C, Iannone LF, et al. Pharmacokinetic interactions of clinical interest between direct oral anticoagulants and antiepileptic drugs. *Front Neurol.* 2018;9:1067.

Gilad R. Management of seizures following a stroke: What are the options? *Drugs Aging.* 2012;29(7):533–538.

Goldstein LB. Rehabilitation and recovery after stroke. *Curr Treat Opt Neurol.* 2000;2:319–328.

Hsieh CY, Lai EC, Yang YH, Lin SJ. Comparative stroke risk of antiepileptic drugs in patients with epilepsy. *Epilepsia.* 2013;54(1):172–180.

Levy RH, Mattson RH, Meldrum BS, Perucca E. *Antiepileptic Drugs.* 5th ed. Philadelphia: Lippincott Williams and Wilkins; 2002.

Licko T, Seeger N, Zellinger C, Russmann V, Matagne A, Potschka H. Lacosamide treatment following status epilepticus attenuates neuronal cell loss and alterations in hippocampal neurogenesis in a rat electrical status epilepticus model. *Epilepsia.* 2013;54(7):1176–1185.

Naidech AM, Kreiter KT, Janjua N, et al. Phenytoin exposure is associated with functional and cognitive disability after subarachnoid hemorrhage. *Stroke.* 2005;36:583–587.

Parrish RH, Pazdur DE, O'Donnell PJ. Effect of carbamazepine initiation and discontinuation on antithrombotic control in a patient receiving warfarin: Case report and review of the literature. *Pharmacotherapy.* 2006;26:1650–1653.

Ryvlin P, Montavont A, Nighoghossian N. Optimizing therapy of seizures in stroke patients. *Neurology.* 2006;67:S3–S9.

Schallert T, Hernandez TD, Barth TM. Recovery of function after brain damage: Severe and chronic disruption by diazepam. *Brain Res* 1986;379:104–111.

Stepien K, Tomaszewski M, Czuczwar SJ. Profile of anticonvulsant activity and neuroprotective effects of novel and potential antiepileptic drugs: An update. *Pharmacol Rep*. 2005;57:719–733.

Vestergaard K, Andersen G, Gottrup H, et al. Lamotrigine for central poststroke pain: A randomized controlled trial. *Neurology*. 2001;23;56:184–190.

Wang JZ, Vyas MV, Saposnik G, Burneo JG. Incidence and management of seizures after ischemic stroke: Systematic review and meta-analysis. *Neurology*. 2017;89:1220–1228.

Willmore LJ. Antiepileptic drugs and neuroprotection: Current status and future roles. *Epilepsy Behav*. 2005;7(Suppl 3):S25–S28.

Online Resources

Brivaracetam (Briviact). www.briviact.com/2020

Cenobamate (Xcopri). https://reference.medscape.com/drug/xcopri-cenobamate-1000328/2020

Chapter 22

Antiseizure Medications in Patients with Multiple Sclerosis

Multiple sclerosis (MS) is a chronic disabling disease of the brain. Comorbid neurological disorders such as epilepsy are more common in patients with MS compared with that in the general population; the prevalence of epilepsy is about 3% in patients with MS (Marrie et al., 2015). Co-occurrence of a seizure in a patient with MS may complicate the management process and any person with MS, who experiences a seizure for the first time, should be investigated by an expert (Asadi-Pooya et al., 2019).

In one study of the assessment of risk of epilepsy after a single seizure in patients with MS (Mahamud et al., 2018), the authors observed that the 10-year risk of epilepsy was 46% (95% confidence interval (CI): 35–57) for patients with relapsing remitting MS (RRMS) and 61% (95% CI: 47–75) for patients with secondary progressive MS (SPMS). For patients with MS who experienced status epilepticus (SE), the 10-year risk of epilepsy was 86% (95% CI: 68–100) (Mahamud et al., 2018). The International League Against Epilepsy (ILAE) clinical definition of epilepsy allows a diagnosis of epilepsy after a single unprovoked seizure if the 10-year recurrence risk exceeds 60% (Fisher et al., 2014). Therefore, if a patient with RRMS experiences a seizure that could not be explained by any cause other than MS, starting a long-term antiseizure medication (ASM) regimen is not required. These patients have a similar risk as controls of developing epilepsy after a single seizure (Mahamud et al., 2018). However, if the seizure is considered to be related to relapse of MS in a patient with RRMS, one may want to prescribe an ASM until the acute phase is over, often for 4–6 weeks (Asadi-Pooya et al., 2019). A single seizure associated with RRMS relapse is generally transient, often carries a good prognosis, and therefore prolonged ASM treatment is not recommended due to the adverse effects of many ASMs (Mahamud et al., 2018; Moreau et al., 1998; Solaro et al., 2005). Patients with SPMS could run a greater risk of subsequent epilepsy (Burman and Zelano 2017; Mahamud et al., 2018), but the risk does not significantly exceed the threshold specified by the ILAE (Fisher et al., 2014; Mahamud et al., 2018); however, the authors are in favor of starting an appropriate ASM (long-term) for these patients. Patients with MS who experience SE that could not be explained by any cause other than MS have a high risk of subsequent epilepsy (Mahamud et al., 2018) that justifies the start of an appropriate ASM (for long-term) (Asadi-Pooya et al., 2019).

All patients with MS who experience epileptic seizures that could not be explained by any cause other than MS have focal epilepsy; these patients often responded well to ASM monotherapy (Benjaminsen et al., 2017). In one study of ASM utilization, often prescribed for neuropathic pain and paroxysmal symptoms, in a cohort of patients with MS (Solaro et al., 2005), carbamazepine was prescribed in 36 patients, with adverse effects reported in 20 (56%) patients. Gabapentin was prescribed in 94 patients, with adverse effects reported in 16 (17%). Lamotrigine was prescribed in 22 patients, with adverse effects reported in 4 (18%) patients (Solaro et al., 2005). Therefore, the adverse-effect profile of ASMs is a significant determining factor in the selection of an appropriate ASM to treat seizure(s) in a patient with MS (Asadi-Pooya et al., 2019). Consideration of possible adverse effects of ASMs, particularly in the context of the patient's symptoms (e.g., cerebellar symptoms, cognitive dysfunction, psychiatric problems), should guide the choice of the ASMs in these patients (Durmus et al., 2013).

Drug interaction is another significant determining factor in the selection of an appropriate ASM to treat seizure(s) in a patient with MS. Carbamazepine, phenobarbital, primidone, and phenytoin may decrease plasma levels of cyclophosphamide, cyclosporine, dexamethasone, methotrexate, methylprednisolone, and prednisolone. Oxcarbazepine may decrease cyclosporine plasma levels. Methotrexate may decrease valproic acid plasma levels. No significant interactions have been reported between ASMs and disease-modifying drugs in patients with MS (Asadi-Pooya et al., 2019; Atmaca and Gurses, 2018).

The third determining factor in the selection of an appropriate ASM to treat seizure(s) in a patient with MS is the existence of other neurological symptoms (e.g., neuropathic pain and paroxysmal demyelinating symptoms). Many ASMs have drug–disease interactions (e.g., gabapentin is also helpful for neuropathic pain, and carbamazepine is helpful for paroxysmal demyelinating symptoms) (Asadi-Pooya et al., 2019).

We favor four ASMs for use in patients with MS: brivaracetam, lamotrigine, levetiracetam, and lacosamide. Brivaracetam has no drug interactions with MS medications, has PO and IV formulations available (for use in emergency situations and rapid titration), and has a reasonable adverse drug profile (brivaracetam; www.briviact.com/2020). Lamotrigine has a favorable adverse-effect profile and no significant drug interactions with MS medications, but its slow titration schedule may hamper its use (Asadi-Pooya et al., 2019). Levetiracetam has no drug interactions with MS medications, has PO and IV formulations available (for use in emergency situations and rapid titration), and has a reasonable adverse drug profile. But in patients with suicidal ideation, depression, and behavioral problems (e.g., aggressive behavior) it is not an optimal option (considering the fact that depression is common in patients with MS) (Asadi-Pooya et al., 2019; Patten et al., 2017). Lacosamide has no drug interactions with MS medications, has PO and IV formulations available (for use in emergency situations and rapid titration), and has a reasonable adverse drug profile (Asadi-Pooya et al., 2019). Gabapentin has a favorable adverse-effect profile and no significant drug interactions with MS medications but is less efficacious than other agents (Marson et al., 2007).

Recommended Antiseizure Medications in Patients with MS

Brivaracetam, lacosamide, lamotrigine, levetiracetam

References

Asadi-Pooya AA, Stewart GR, Abrams DJ, Sharan A. Prevalence and incidence of drug-resistant mesial temporal lobe epilepsy in the United States. *World Neurosurg*. 2017;99:662–666.

Asadi-Pooya AA, Sahraian MA, Sina F, et al. Management of seizures in patients with multiple sclerosis: An Iranian consensus. *Epilepsy Behav*. 2019;96:244–248.

Atmaca MM, Gurses C. Status epilepticus and multiple sclerosis: A case presentation and literature review. *Clin EEG Neurosci*. 2018;49:328–334.

Benjaminsen E, Myhr KM, Alstadhaug KB. The prevalence and characteristics of epilepsy in patients with multiple sclerosis in Nordland county, Norway. *Seizure*. 2017;52:131–135.

Burman J, Zelano J. Epilepsy in multiple sclerosis: A nationwide population-based register study. *Neurology*. 2017;89:2462–2468.

Durmus H, Kurtuncu M, Tuzun E, et al. Comparative clinical characteristics of early- and adult-onset multiple sclerosis patients with seizures. *Acta Neurol Belg*. 2013;113:421–426.

Fisher RS, Acevedo C, Arzimanoglou A, et al. ILAE official report: A practical clinical definition of epilepsy. *Epilepsia*. 2014;55:475–482.

Mahamud Z, Burman J, Zelano J. The risk of epilepsy after a single seizure in multiple sclerosis. *Eur J Neurol*. 2018;25:854–860.

Marrie RA, Reider N, Cohen J, et al. A systematic review of the incidence and prevalence of sleep disorders and seizure disorders in multiple sclerosis. *Mult Scler*. 2015;21:342–349.

Marson AG, Al-Kharusi AM, Alwaidh M. The SANAD study of effectiveness of carbamazepine, gabapentin, lamotrigine, oxcarbazepine, or topiramate for treatment of partial epilepsy: An unblinded randomized controlled trial. *Lancet*. 2007;369:1000–1015.

Moreau T, Sochurkova D, Lemesle M, et al. Epilepsy in patients with multiple sclerosis: Radiological-clinical correlations. *Epilepsia*. 1998;39:893–896.

Patten SB, Marrie RA, Carta MG. Depression in multiple sclerosis. *Int Rev Psychiatry*. 2017;29:463–472.

Solaro C, Brichetto G, Battaglia MA, Messmer Uccelli M, Mancardi GL. Antiepileptic medications in multiple sclerosis: Adverse effects in a three-year follow-up study. *Neurol Sci*. 2005;25:307–310.

Online Resources

Brivaracetam (Briviact). www.briviact.com/2020

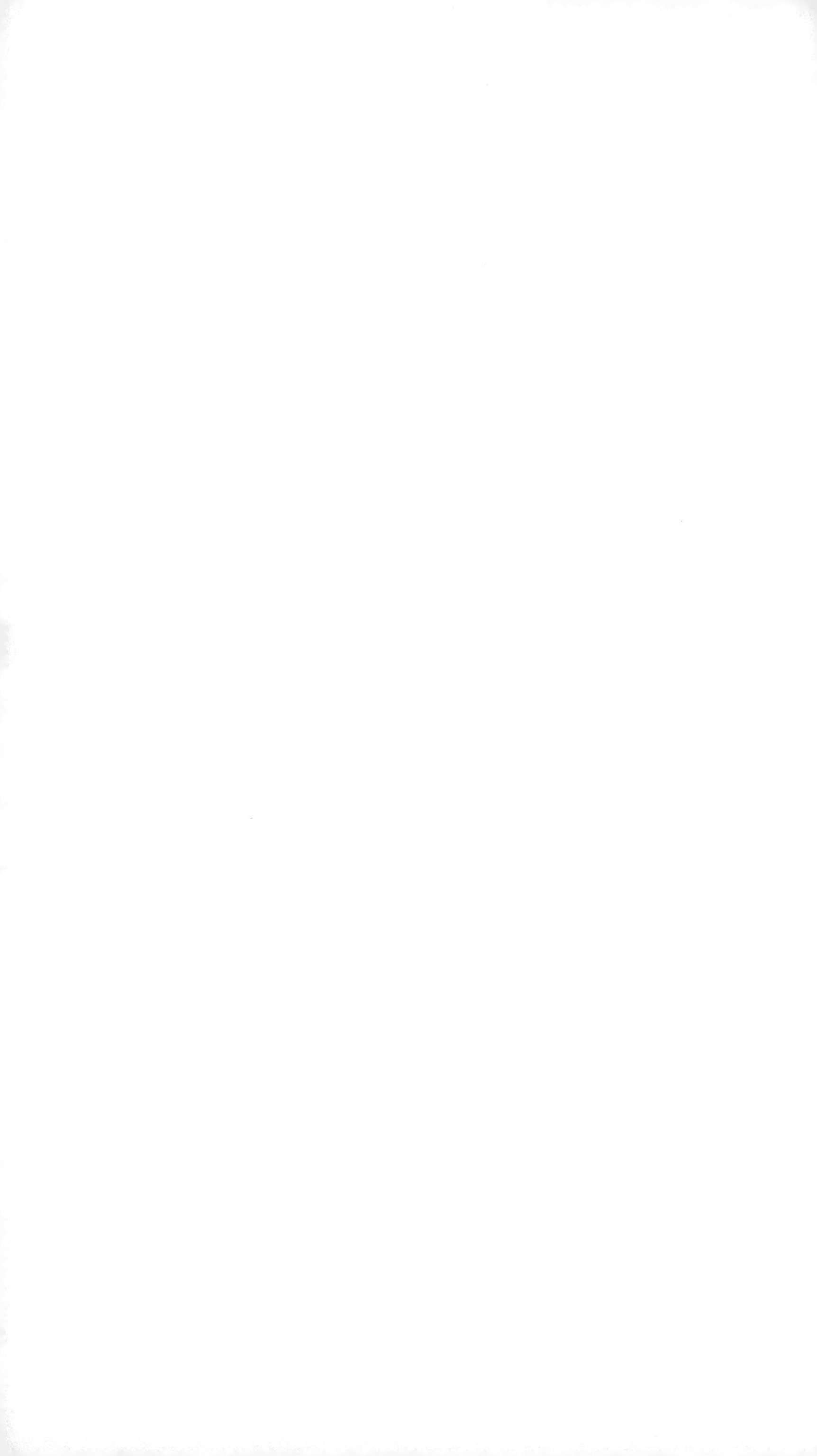

Chapter 23

Antiseizure Medications in Patients with Preexisting Psychiatric Problems

Although most people with epilepsy lead normal lives, neurobehavioral problems are found in a large proportion of patients. Higher rates of psychopathology are observed in people with epilepsy relative to the general population, to other neurological control groups, and to people with chronic non-neurological disorders. This largely reflects the effect of uncontrolled epilepsy and the underlying brain injury, which predispose patients to depression, anxiety, and other psychiatric symptoms. In particular, increased psychopathology is common in patients with temporal lobe epilepsy (TLE). Depression is the most frequent type of psychiatric disorder identified in patients with epilepsy, with community prevalence of about 25%, and higher in people with uncontrolled epilepsy (Fiest et al., 2013). Epidemiological studies have identified a variety of psychoses in up to 9% of patients with epilepsy. Likewise, patients with epilepsy commonly report anxiety and, finally, the risk of suicide in patients with epilepsy is estimated to be 4 to 5 times greater than that of the general population, with a higher risk is found in TLE (Kanner and Palac, 2002). The treatment of epilepsy is not limited solely to the achievement of a seizure-free state. It must also incorporate the management of comorbidities, including psychiatric comorbidities, which often have a significant impact on patients' lives at various levels (Kanner et al., 2018).

The causes of psychopathology in epilepsy are multifactorial and include genetic predisposition, biological risk factors, etiology of the epilepsy, iatrogenic causes (e.g., antiepileptic drugs), and other causes. A bidirectional relationship between psychosis or depression and epilepsy has been suggested in the literature. For example, similar neurotransmitter alterations may underlie both depression and epilepsy (Kanner et al., 2018; Yan et al., 1998). Although the clinical manifestations of psychiatric disorders in epilepsy are often indistinguishable from those of nonepileptic patients, certain types of depression and psychotic disorders may present with clinical characteristics that are particular to those of patients with epilepsy. These include postictal psychosis, alternate psychosis (or forced normalization), and certain forms of interictal depressive disorders.

Some antiseizure medications (ASMs) are also psychotropic agents with positive or negative effects. The psychotropic effects of ASMs in people with epilepsy are, however, variable and unpredictable. Unfortunately, a history

Table 23.1 Approved psychiatric indications for antiseizure medications

Benzodiazepines	Anxiety disorders, alcohol withdrawal, insomnia
Carbamazepine	Bipolar disorder, mania
Valproate	Bipolar disorder, mania and bipolar disorder, mixed
Lamotrigine	Bipolar disorder, maintenance
Pregabalin	Generalized anxiety disorder

Adapted from: Kaufman KR. Antiepileptic drugs in the treatment of psychiatric disorders. *Epilepsy Behav.* 2011;21(1):1–11.

of psychiatric illness may be a risk factor for a negative psychotropic effect by an ASM. Thus, the beneficial psychotropic effects seen with ASMs in the general nonepileptic population may be less apparent in patient with epilepsy. However, for example, it would be reasonable to prescribe an appropriate ASM with anxiolytic potential in a patient with preexisting anxiety disorder. For instance, pregabalin and, to a lesser extent, gabapentin are effective in anxiety disorders, and pregabalin is in fact licensed for the treatment of generalized anxiety disorder (Table 23.1). On the other hand, the treating physician should be aware of the possibility of aggravating anxiety symptomatology when prescribing certain ASMs to patients with epilepsy (Table 23.2).

Table 23.2 Psychiatric adverse effects of antiseizure medications in patients with preexisting psychopathologies

Preexisting psychopathology	Precautions in using antiseizure medications	Possible adverse effects
Dysthymia	Phenobarbital, tiagabine, levetiracetam, topiramate, vigabatrin, zonisamide	Major depression
Paranoia	Phenytoin, ethosuximide, topiramate, vigabatrin, zonisamide	Schizophrenic psychosis
Dysphoria	Levetiracetam, zonisamide	Aggression
Agitation	Lamotrigine	Insomnia, anxiety, hypomania
Anxiety	Levetiracetam, zonisamide	Agitation or aggression
Attention-deficit hyperactivity disorder	Phenobarbital, primidone, valproate, gabapentin, topiramate, lamotrigine, levetiracetam	Deterioration of attention and behavior
Hyperactivity	Benzodiazepines, phenobarbital (usually in children or elderly)	Paradoxical central nervous system stimulation
Learning disability	Phenobarbital, topiramate, zonisamide	Behavioral disorders, impaired cognition
Developmental disabilities with cognitive dysfunction	Phenobarbital, topiramate, benzodiazepines, gabapentin, zonisamide	Worsening of intellectual disabilities

From Tiffin and Perini (2001), Devinsky (2004), Schubert (2005), Schmitz (2006), Aldendamp et al. (2006), Brodtkorb and Mula (2006), and Smith (2006).

In addition, use of sedating doses and combinations of ASMs that can impair cognitive and behavioral functions should be avoided in all patients (Bialer, 2012; Kaufman, 2011; Kimiskidis and Valeta, 2012; Nadkarni and Devinsky, 2005; Schmitz, 2006). When prescribing an ASM for a patient with epilepsy, preexisting psychiatric problems, or learning disabilities, the drug-drug interactions and adverse effects of the ASM should be considered (Tables 23.2, 23.3, and 23.4). The treating physician should consider which ASM might best help the patient in maximizing seizure control and minimizing psychiatric symptoms.

Last, all ASMs have the potential to cause adverse psychiatric effects. Some antiseizure medications may increase the risk of suicidal thoughts or behavior in patients taking these drugs for any indication. An increased risk of suicidal thoughts or behavior with ASMs has been observed as early as 1 week after starting treatment and can persist for the duration of treatment. Patients treated with *any ASM for any indication* should be cautioned and monitored for the emergence or worsening of depression, suicidal thoughts or behavior, and any unusual changes in mood or behavior. However, in the authors' experience, some agents are more apt to do so than others. We have observed the greatest incidence of psychiatric adverse effects with phenobarbital, primidone, levetiracetam, topiramate, perampanel, and zonisamide. Patients and their families should be cautioned about potential psychiatric adverse effects when these agents are used so that problems can be promptly addressed should they occur (Table 23.3 and Table 23.4).

In addition, ASMs may cause sexual dysfunction, which may lead to psychiatric consequences.

1. Enzyme-inducing ASMs, such as carbamazepine, phenytoin, phenobarbital, primidone, and oxcarbazepine and topiramate in high doses, can increase sex hormone–binding globulin, reduce free (bioactive) testosterone, and thereby reduce libido and impair sexual function (Harden, 2006).

Table 23.3 Recommended antiseizure medications in patients with preexisting psychiatric, learning, and behavioral problems

Preexisting psychopathology	Recommended antiseizure medications
Depression	Carbamazepine, lamotrigine
Mania	Valproate, carbamazepine, oxcarbazepine
Bipolar disorder	Valproate, carbamazepine, lamotrigine, oxcarbazepine
Aggression and agitation	Valproate, carbamazepine, phenytoin
Anxiety disorders	Pregabalin (generalized anxiety disorder), gabapentin (social anxiety disorder)
Binge-eating disorder	Topiramate, zonisamide
Learning disability	Lamotrigine, levetiracetam
Attention-deficit-hyperactivity disorder	Lamotrigine, carbamazepine, oxcarbazepine

From Nadkarni and Devinsky (2005), Brodtkorb and Mula (2006), Schubert (2005), Schmitz (2006), Mula et al. (2007), Tassone et al. (2007), Kaufman (2011), Bialer (2012), Kimiskidis and Valeta (2012), and Kanner (2016).

Table 23.4 Psychiatric adverse effects of antiseizure medications in general

Antiseizure medication	Psychiatric adverse effects	Note
Acetazolamide	Irritability, libido decrease	—
Benzodiazepines	Depression, paradoxical central nervous system stimulation (hostility, nightmares, talkativeness, excitement, mania, tremors, sleep disturbances, increased muscle spasticity, acute rage reactions, anxiety, restlessness, euphoria, and hyperreflexia, particularly in psychiatric patients and hyperactive children), dependence, sexual dysfunction, and libido decrease	Most of the adverse effects are dose dependent. Tolerance may develop to these effects. Benzodiazepine therapy should be discontinued if any of the signs of paradoxical CNS excitement occur.
Brivaracetam	Irritability, anxiety, nervousness, aggression, depression, psychomotor hyperactivity, abnormal behaviour, psychotic disorder along with hallucination, paranoia, acute psychosis, and psychotic behavior	Reported in approximately 13% of patients.
Cannabidiol	Insomnia, irritability, agitation, aggression	—
Carbamazepine	Irritability, agitation, depression, talkativeness, sexual dysfunction	—
Cenobamate	Confusional state, suicidal ideation	—
Eslicarbazepine acetate	Depression, insomnia	—
Ethosuximide	Aggression, irritability, restlessness or hyperactivity, depression (with suicidal ideations), insomnia, euphoria, and rarely: nightmares, emotional lability, paranoia-type psychosis, libido increase	Rare adverse effects are more likely to occur in patients who have previously shown abnormal psychological reactions.
Ezogabine	Confusional state, psychotic symptoms, hallucinations, abnormal thinking, dependence	These effects are dose-related and generally appear within the first 8 weeks of treatment. Rapid titration at greater than the recommended doses appeared to increase the risk of psychosis and hallucinations.
Felbamate	Somnolence, insomnia, nervousness, aggression, anxiety, depression, abnormal thinking, hallucination, psychosis, emotional lability, euphoria, mania	Adverse psychiatric effects have caused discontinuance of the drug in about 2% of adults and 1% of children.

Table 23.4 *Continued*

Antiseizure medication	Psychiatric adverse effects	Note
Gabapentin	Irritability, agitation, anxiety and hostility, hyperkinesia, abnormal thinking	All more common in children with disabilities. Pediatric patients should be monitored closely for central nervous system adverse effects.
Lacosamide	Depression, confusional state, aggression, agitation, hallucination, insomnia, psychotic disorder	—
Lamotrigine	Insomnia, irritability (usually in children with disabilities), depression, anxiety, emotional lability	—
Levetiracetam	Anxiety, depression, irritability, agitation, aggression, anger, insomnia, apathy, depersonalization, emotional lability, hyperkinesia, hallucinations, hostility, personality disorders, psychosis, psychotic depression	May be seen at any dose. Counsel patients and caregivers of the need to monitor for the emergence of anger, aggression, hostility, unusual changes in mood, personality, or behavior.
Oxcarbazepine	Emotional lability, insomnia, abnormal thinking	Usually occurs with dosages >1,200 mg/day
Perampanel	Hostility, aggression, irritability, anger, anxiety, paranoia, mood changes, confusional state	These effects are dose-related and generally appear within the first 6 weeks of treatment. Counsel patients and caregivers of the need to monitor for the emergence of anger, aggression, hostility, unusual changes in mood, personality, or behavior.
Phenobarbital	Aggression, depression, emotional lability, irritability, anxiety, sexual dysfunction and libido decrease, dependence, paradoxical CNS stimulation (adverse behavioral reactions, hyperactivity, nightmares, insomnia), or exacerbation of preexisting hyperactivity in some children	Geriatric patients have experienced agitation, excitation, or depression.
Phenytoin	Depression, sexual dysfunction including libido decrease, impotence	The severity of these adverse reactions increases as serum concentrations of phenytoin increase.

(*continued*)

Table 23.4 (Continued)

Antiseizure medication	Psychiatric adverse effects	Note
Pregabalin	Abnormal thinking, euphoria, impotence, libido decrease, insomnia, dependence	The majority of these adverse events are mild to moderate in intensity and dose dependent.
Rufinamide	Psychomotor hyperactivity, anxiety, aggression, behavioral disturbance, depression	—
Tiagabine	Depression, irritability, hostility, anxiety, abnormal thinking, insomnia	Slow initial titration may help to minimize these central nervous system effects.
Topiramate	Depression, psychomotor impairment, irritability, nervousness, anxiety, emotional lability, depersonalization, insomnia, hallucinations, euphoria, psychosis, impotence, libido decrease	Most psychiatric adverse effects usually occur with dosages >200 mg/day.
Valproate	Depression, agitation, nervousness, hallucinations, euphoria	Mental status changes (e.g., depression, agitation) are most likely to occur in children.
Vigabatrin	Insomnia, irritability, depression, confusional state, abnormal behaviour, abnormal thinking, abnormal dream	—
Zonisamide	Aggression, irritability, nervousness, anxiety, depression, insomnia, emotional lability, schizophrenic/schizophreniform behaviour	Most psychiatric adverse effects usually occur with dosages >300 mg/day.

All antiseizure medications may increase the risk of suicidal thoughts or behavior in patients taking these drugs for any indication.

From: Levy et al. (2002); Facts and Comparisons (2007); Kaufman (2011); see also individual drug websites listed in the Online Resources section at the end of this chapter.

2. Other ASMs, including acetazolamide, benzodiazepines, and pregabalin may cause sexual dysfunction as well.
3. Sexual dysfunction is not common with ethosuximide, gabapentin, lamotrigine, levetiracetam, tiagabine, valproate, and zonisamide (Facts and Comparisons, 2007).

Note: There is almost no evidence-based data on the efficacy of psychotropic drugs for the treatment of psychiatric comorbidities in patients with epilepsy. Therefore, physicians have followed the treatment strategies used in primary psychiatric disorders for the treatment of psychiatric comorbidities in patients with epilepsy (Table 23.5) (Kanner 2016).

Table 23.5 Efficacy of psychiatric drugs in primary depression and anxiety disorders

Antidepressant	Depression	Panic disorder	Generalized anxiety	Starting dose (mg daily)	Maximum dose (mg daily)
Paroxetine*	++	++	++	10	60
Sertraline*	++	++	+	25	200
Fluoxetine*	++	++	–	10	80
Citalopram*	++	+	++	10	60
Escitalopram*	++	+	+	5	30
Fluvoxamine	+	+	+	50	300
Venlafaxine‡	++	+	+	37.5	300
Duloxetine‡	++	+	+	20	120

+, The drug is used for the treatment of this condition; ++, the drug has approval from the US Food and Drug Administration (FDA) for this condition; –, the drug is not used to treat this condition.

From: Kanner AM. Management of psychiatric and neurological comorbidities in epilepsy. *Nat Rev Neurol*. 2016; 12: 106–116.

References

Aldenkamp AP, Arzimanoglou A, Reijs R, Van Mil S. Optimizing therapy of seizures in children and adolescents with ADHD. *Neurology*. 2006;67:S49–S51.

Fiest KM, Dykeman J, Patten SB, et al. Depression in epilepsy. *Neurology*. 2013;80:590–599.

Bialer M. Why are antiepileptic drugs used for nonepileptic conditions? *Epilepsia*. 2012;53(Suppl 7):26–33.

Brodtkorb E, Mula M. Optimizing therapy of seizures in adult patients with psychiatric comorbidity. *Neurology*. 2006;67:S39–S44.

Devinsky O. Therapy for neurobehavioral disorders in epilepsy. *Epilepsia*. 2004;45(Suppl 2):34–40.

Facts and Comparisons. *Drug Facts and Comparisons*. St. Louis: Wolters Kluwer Health/Facts and Comparisons; 2007.

Harden CL. Sexuality in men and women with epilepsy. *CNS Spectrums*. 2006;11(8 Suppl 9):13–18.

Kanner AM, Palac S. Neuropsychiatric complications of epilepsy. *Curr Neurol Neurosci Rep*. 2002;2:365–372.

Kanner AM. Management of psychiatric and neurological comorbidities in epilepsy. *Nat Rev Neurol*. 2016;12:106–116.

Kanner AM, Ribot R, Mazarati A. Bidirectional relations among common psychiatric and neurologic comorbidities and epilepsy: Do they have an impact on the course of the seizure disorder? *Epilepsia Open*. 2018;3(Suppl 2):210–219.

Kaufman KR. Antiepileptic drugs in the treatment of psychiatric disorders. *Epilepsy Behav*. 2011;21(1):1–11.

Kimiskidis VK, Valeta T. Epilepsy and anxiety: Epidemiology, classification, aetiology, and treatment. *Epileptic Disord*. 2012;14(3):248–256.

Levy RH, Mattson RH, Meldrum BS, Perucca E. *Antiepileptic Drugs*. 5th ed. Philadelphia: Lippincott Williams and Wilkins; 2002.

Mula M, Pini S, Cassano GB. The role of anticonvulsant drugs in anxiety disorders: A critical review of the evidence. *J Clin Psychopharmacol*. 2007;27:263–272.

Nadkarni S, Devinsky O. Psychotropic effects of antiepileptic drugs. *Epilepsy Curr*. 2005;5(5):176–181.

Schmitz B. Effects of antiepileptic drugs on mood and behavior. *Epilepsia*. 2006;47(Suppl 2):28–33.

Schubert R. Attention deficit disorder and epilepsy. *Pediatr Neurol*. 2005;32:1–10.

Smith MC. Optimizing therapy of seizures in children and adolescents with developmental disabilities. *Neurology*. 2006;67:S52–S55.

Tassone DM, Boyce E, Guyer J, Nuzum D. Pregabalin: A novel gamma aminobutyric acid analogue in the treatment of neuropathic pain, partial-onset seizures, and anxiety disorders. *Clin Therap*. 2007;29:26–48.

Tiffin PA, Perini AF. The use of antiepileptic drugs in learning disabled people with epilepsy: An audit of adult in-patients in a treatment and continuing care service. *Seizure*. 2001;10:500–504.

Yan QS, Dailey JW, Steenbergen JL, et al. Anticonvulsant effect of enhancement of noradrenergic transmission in the superior colliculus in genetically epilepsy-prone rats (GEPRs): A microinjection study. *Brain Res*. 1998;780:199.

Online Resources

Brivaracetam (Briviact). www.briviact.com/2020

Cannabidiol (Epidiolex). www.epidiolex.com/2020

Cenobamate (Xcopri). https://reference.medscape.com/drug/xcopri-cenobamate-1000328/2020

Eslicarbazine acetate (Aptiom). www.aptiom.com/2014

Ezogabine (Potiga). www.potiga.com/2014

Lacosamide (Vimpat). www.vimpat.com/2014

Perampanel (Fycompa). us.eisai.com/wps/wcm/connect/Eisai/Home/Our.../FYCOMPA/2014

Rufinamide (Banzel). www.banzel.com/2014

Vigabatrin (Sabril). www.lundbeck.com/upload/us/files/.../Sabril/2014

Chapter 24

Antiseizure Medications and Cognition

Cognition comprises a broad range of functions, such as attention, intelligence, visual memory, and language skills, among others. Problems with cognition can be manifested as reductions in attention, IQ, language and perceptual skills, executive functions including problem-solving, verbal and visual memory, and motor speed. Treating a patient with epilepsy involves more than just treating seizures. Many patients have associated learning and cognitive problems that may lead to significant difficulties at school or work. Educational underachievement is considered to be the greatest academic complication in a child with epilepsy. Children with epilepsy, even those with normal intelligence, often experience educational difficulties more often than unaffected children. These educational problems tend to persist into adulthood and are sometimes manifested as underemployment (Hermann et al., 2010; Vinayan, 2006).

The causes of cognitive impairment in patients with epilepsy include effects of ongoing seizures and interictal epileptiform activity, underlying structural brain lesions, and the adverse effects of antiseizure medications (ASMs) (Ortinski and Meador, 2004; Park and Kwon, 2008). The effect of ASMs on the learning process and cognitive function in a patient with epilepsy is double-edged. ASMs can control epileptic seizures, thus leading to improvement in cognitive functions and other learning processes. On the other hand, ASMs can adversely affect learning processes and cognition. Although the cognitive effects of ASMs are generally modest, these effects at times have clinical significance (Brunbech and Sabers, 2002; Meador, 2006; Vinayan, 2006).

Therefore, two considerations are important when treating someone with epilepsy. Seizures must be prevented, but adverse effects, especially cognitive ones, should be avoided. This is especially important for children who are in a critical period of brain development, whose major "occupation" is learning. Maintaining cognitive abilities is important for everyone else as well because everyone requires good mental function; this is especially important for people whose vocations require high-level cognitive processing. All ASMs have the potential for detrimentally affecting cognitive function. These effects are especially common with higher doses of ASMs or with polytherapy. In addition, cognitive effects exerted by an

ASM could vary depending on factors linked to patient characteristics and individual susceptibility. Of the older ASMs, phenobarbital, primidone, and benzodiazepines produce the greatest degree of learning and cognitive impairments. Phenobarbital may influence IQ and have deleterious effects on attention; it can reduce processing efficiency. Phenobarbital is considered to have worse cognitive effects than valproate or carbamazepine. Phenytoin and high doses of valproate have also been reported to cause impairment in memory and learning processes. The cognitive effects associated with phenytoin may be more obvious but are generally restricted to visually guided motor functions. Valproate has been suggested to be preferable to carbamazepine, phenobarbital, and topiramate. However, attention dysfunction was more common with valproic acid than ethosuximide. Cognitive problems due to carbamazepine are not common, but high doses can impair functions. Carbamazepine has a cognitive profile that is worse than levetiracetam and lamotrigine but better than phenytoin. Oxcarbazepine, lamotrigine, and levetiracetam have favorable cognitive profiles in comparison with other ASMs. Among newer ASMs, topiramate and zonisamide have the greatest potential to impair cognition, but, with high doses, all drugs can cause problems (Brunbech and Sabers, 2002; Eddy et al., 2011; Facts and Comparisons, 2007; Kothare and Kaleyias, 2007; Meador, 2006; Ulate-Campos and Fernández, 2017; Vinayan, 2006).

It should be emphasized that cognition is only one consideration when choosing an ASM. Efficacy, the patient's profile, other adverse effects, and even cost must also be taken into account. Whenever possible, it is prudent to use the lowest effective dose of the ASM, titrate upward slowly, and employ monotherapy. Keep in mind, however, that a patient's perception of cognitive adverse effects of therapy might be more related to mood than to actual cognitive performance. Patients who report having trouble with memory or learning might actually be depressed. If there is evidence of a mood disorder, its treatment should be considered (see Chapter 23). It is also important to reassess the frequency and severity of the seizures and the efficacy of the ASMs in use, as well as to assess the adverse effects of the disease in addition to the adverse effects of treatment at each visit (Hermann et al., 2010) (Table 24.1).

- **Antiseizure medications that are not ideal in people with cognitive impairment:** Phenobarbital, cenobamate, topiramate, zonisamide, primidone, and benzodiazepines
- **Antiseizure medications that are reasonable in people with cognitive impairment:** Levetiracetam, brivaracetam, ethosuximide, lacosamide, lamotrigine, and oxcarbazepine

Table 24.1 Cognitive adverse effects of antiseizure medications		
Antiseizure medication	**Cognitive adverse effects**	**Note**
Acetazolamide	Drowsiness, confusion	Uncommon
Benzodiazepines	Drowsiness, confusion, paradoxical central nervous system stimulation	Most of these side effects are dose dependent. Clobazam has a more acceptable adverse effect profile than other benzodiazepines.
Brivaracetam	Drowsiness	
Cannabidiol	Drowsiness	
Carbamazepine	Drowsiness, confusion, impaired attention, impaired motor tasks	Seen mainly with high levels.
Cenobamate	Drowsiness, disturbance in attention, slowness of thought, and psychomotor retardation	Often not serious.
Eslicarbazepine acetate	Memory impairment, disturbance in attention, amnesia, aphasia, speech disorder, slowness of thought, disorientation, and psychomotor retardation	These side effects are dose-dependent.
Ethosuximide	Drowsiness, confusion, and rarely impaired cognition	
Ezogabine	Memory impairment, disturbance in attention, aphasia, amnesia	
Felbamate	Drowsiness, confusion	Often makes patients more alert with improvement in cognition.
Gabapentin	Amnesia, mental depression, drowsiness, impaired cognition	Minimal or some cognitive adverse effects. All are more common in children with disabilities.
Lacosamide	Memory impairment, disturbance in attention	Often, not severe.
Lamotrigine	Confusion, drowsiness	Minimal cognitive adverse effects except at high dosages >400–500 mg/day.
Levetiracetam	Drowsiness, amnesia	Cognitive adverse effects are minimal with dosages of 1,000–3,000 mg/day.
Oxcarbazepine	Confusion, drowsiness, impaired concentration and cognition, speech problems	Most adverse effects occur with dosages >1,200 mg/day.
Perampanel	Memory impairment, dysarthria	

(*continued*)

Table 23.4 (Continued)

Antiseizure medication	Cognitive adverse effects	Note
Phenobarbital	Impaired cognition, memory and attention, mental slowing, drowsiness, confusion, paradoxical CNS stimulation or exacerbation of preexisting hyperactivity in some children	Potentially significant cognitive adverse effects. Children treated chronically with phenobarbital may experience subtle cognitive decline. Geriatric patients have experienced agitation, excitation, depression, or confusion.
Phenytoin	Drowsiness, confusion, impaired attention, reduction in motor speed and problem solving	Some cognitive adverse effects. The severity of these adverse reactions increases as serum concentrations of phenytoin increase.
Pregabalin	Difficulty with concentration/attention, drowsiness, confusion, amnesia	Some cognitive adverse effects. The majority of these adverse events are mild to moderate in intensity and dose-dependent.
Rufinamide	Rare (not specified)	
Tiagabine	Impaired cognition, impaired concentration, drowsiness, confusion, amnesia	Minimal cognitive adverse effects. Slow initial titration may minimize these effects.
Topiramate	Psychomotor impairment, impaired cognition and language (word finding difficulty, memory impairment), drowsiness, confusion	Potentially significant cognitive adverse effects. Most adverse effects usually occur with dosages >200 mg/day, but can be seen with low doses. Slow titration minimizes these effects.
Valproate	Drowsiness	Some cognitive adverse effects. Mental status changes are most likely to occur in children.
Vigabatrin	Memory impairment, disturbance in attention, expressive language disorder	
Zonisamide	Confusion, drowsiness, difficulty concentrating, impaired cognition (memory), mental slowing and psychomotor impairment, speech impairment (speech abnormalities and difficulty in verbal expression)	Some cognitive adverse effects. Most adverse effects usually occur with dosages >300 mg/day.

From Mendez et al. (1986), Yan et al. (1998), Kanner and Palac (2002), Nadkarni and Devinsky (2005); see also individual drug websites listed in the Online Resources section at the end of this chapter.

References

Brunbech L, Sabers A. Effect of antiepileptic drugs on cognitive function in individuals with epilepsy. *Drugs*. 2002;62:593–604.

Eddy CM, Rickards HE, Cavanna AE. The cognitive impact of antiepileptic drugs. *Ther Adv Neurol Disord*. 2011;4(6):385–407.

Facts and Comparisons. *Drug Facts and Comparisons*. St. Louis: Wolters Kluwer Health/Facts and Comparisons; 2007.

Hermann B, Meador KJ, Gaillard WD, Cramer JA. Cognition across the lifespan: Antiepileptic drugs, epilepsy, or both? *Epilepsy Behav*. 2010;17(1):1–5.

Kanner AM, Palac S. Neuropsychiatric complications of epilepsy. *Curr Neurol Neurosci Rep*. 2002;2:365–372.

Kothare SV, Kaleyias J. The adverse effects of antiepileptic drugs in children. *Exp Opin Drug Safety*. 2007;6:251–265.

Meador KJ. Cognitive and behavioral effects of AEDs. *Epilepsy Res*. 2006;68:63–67.

Mendez MF, Cummings JL, Benson DF. Depression in epilepsy: significance and phenomenology. *Arch Neurol*. 1986;43:766–770.

Nadkarni S, Devinsky O. Psychotropic effects of antiepileptic drugs. *Epilepsy Curr*. 2005;5(5):176–181.

Ortinski P, Meador KJ. Cognitive side effects of antiepileptic drugs. *Epilepsy Behav*. 2004;5:S60–S65.

Park S-P, Kwon S-H. Cognitive effects of antiepileptic drugs. *J Clin Neurol*. 2008;4:99–106.

Ulate-Campos A, Fernández IS. Cognitive and behavioral comorbidities: An unwanted effect of antiepileptic drugs in children. *Semin Pediatr Neurol*. 2017;24:320–330.

Vinayan KP. Epilepsy, antiepileptic drugs and educational problems. *Indian Pediatr*. 2006;43:786–794.

Yan QS, Dailey JW, Steenbergen JL, et al. Anticonvulsant effect of enhancement of noradrenergic transmission in the superior colliculus in genetically epilepsy-prone rats (GEPRs): A microinjection study. *Brain Res*. 1998;780:199.

Online Resources

Brivaracetam (Briviact). www.briviact.com/2020

Cannabidiol (Epidiolex). www.epidiolex.com/2020

Cenobamate (Xcopri). https://reference.medscape.com/drug/xcopri-cenobamate-1000328/2020

Eslicarbazine acetate (Aptiom). www.aptiom.com/2014

Ezogabine (Potiga). www.potiga.com/2014

Lacosamide (Vimpat). www.vimpat.com/2014

Perampanel (Fycompa). us.eisai.com/wps/wcm/connect/Eisai/Home/Our.../FYCOMPA/2014

Rufinamide (Banzel). www.banzel.com/2014

Vigabatrin (Sabril). www.lundbeck.com/upload/us/files/.../Sabril/2014

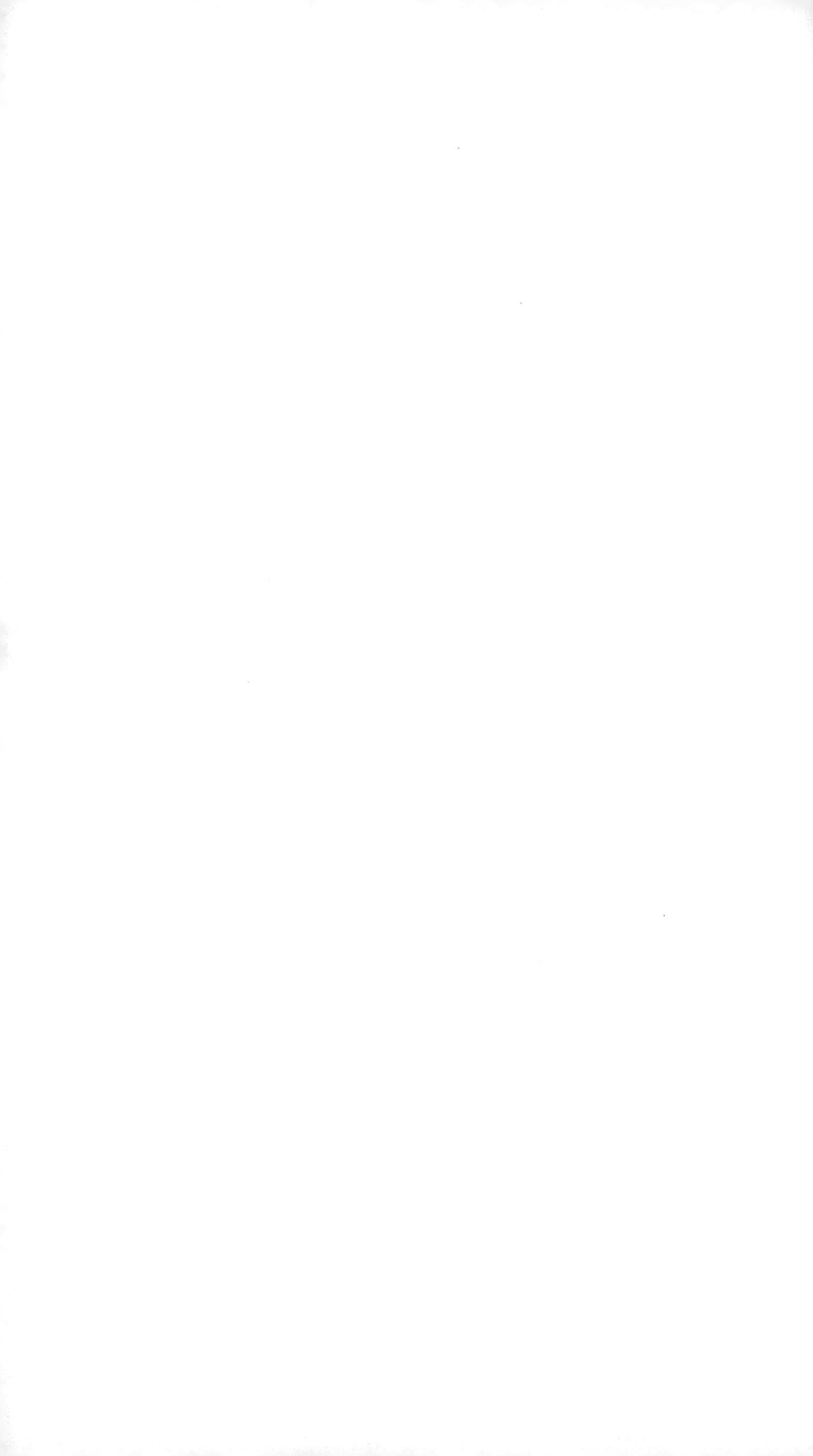

Chapter 25

Antiseizure Medications in Patients with Migraine Headaches

Two disorders are comorbid if they occur in the same person more frequently than by chance alone. Headache and epilepsy appear to be comorbid (Figure 25.1). The prevalence of epilepsy in persons with migraine headaches ranges from 1% to 17% with a median of 5.9%, substantially higher than the general population prevalence of epilepsy (Andermann and Andermann, 1987). The reported frequency of migraine in epileptic populations ranges from 15% to 45% (Caminero and Manso-Calderón 2014; Marks and Ehrenberg, 1993; Ottman and Lipton, 1996; Stevenson, 2006).

Migraine and epilepsy share several clinical features and also share some common pathophysiological mechanisms. Both are considered to be disorders of neuronal hyperexcitability. An initial excessive neuronal activity in migraine leads to cortical spreading depression and aura, with the subsequent recruitment of the trigeminal nucleus leading to central sensitization and pain. In epilepsy, neuronal overactivity leads to the recruitment of larger populations of neurons firing in a rhythmic manner that constitutes an epileptic seizure (Nye and Thadani, 2015). In addition, similar triggering factors have been identified for both migraine and epilepsy (e.g., menses, alcohol, and sleep deprivation). An imbalance between excitatory glutamate-mediated transmission and γ-aminobutyric acid (GABA)-mediated inhibition in specific brain areas has been postulated in both conditions. Moreover, abnormal activation of voltage-operated ionic channels has been implicated in both migraine and epilepsy (Aurora et al., 1999; Calabresi et al., 2007; Koch et al., 2005). Finally, genetic links are also evident between the two conditions and are particularly apparent in familial hemiplegic migraine, where different mutations can cause either migraine, epilepsy, or both (Nye and Thadani, 2015; Zangaladze et al., 2010).

Some antiseizure medications (ASMs) are effective in reducing migraine frequency. The ASMs that are most effective therapies for migraine prophylaxis in adults include valproate and topiramate. Indeed, these agents are prescribed as first-line agents for prophylactic treatment of migraine headaches, whether epilepsy is comorbid or not. Gabapentin is also somewhat effective and may be considered a second-line therapy in migraine prophylaxis (Calabresi et al., 2007; D'Amico, 2007; Modi and Lowder, 2006). On the other hand, some ASMs have no demonstrable effect on migraine, and

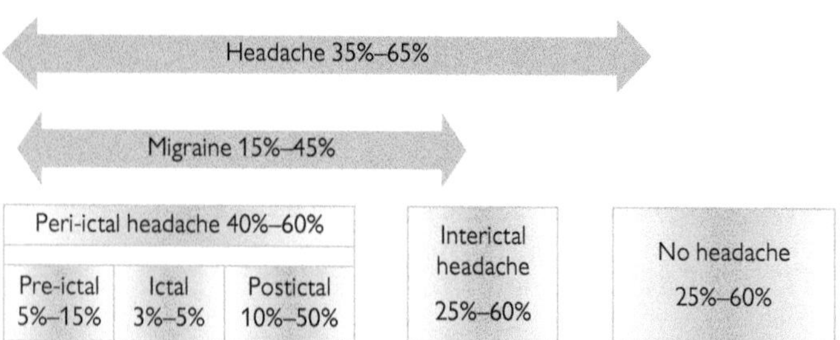

Figure 25.1 The numbers represent headache prevalence in people with epilepsy.
Modified from: Caminero A, Manso-Calderón R. Links between headaches and epilepsy: current knowledge and terminology. *Neurologia*. 2014; 29: 453–463.

others may be associated with increase in headache as an adverse effect (e.g., carbamazepine or oxcarbazepine). Therefore, caution should be exercised before overrelating epilepsy and migraines; while some features are shared, the differences probably outweigh the similarities.

Antiseizure Medications in Migraine Headaches

Gabapentin

Gabapentin has been evaluated in controlled trials and demonstrated conflicting results for migraine prophylaxis (Buchanan and Ramadan, 2006; Calabresi et al., 2007; D'Amico, 2007; Linde et al., 2013a; Mathew et al., 2001; Modi and Lowder, 2006; Pierangeli et al., 2006).

Lamotrigine

The efficacy of lamotrigine in migraine prevention is uncertain. Open-label studies suggest that it may be efficacious in migraine with aura (Buchanan and Ramadan, 2006; D'Amico, 2007), but one controlled double-blind study did not show efficacy in migraine prophylaxis (Steiner et al., 1997). It seems that lamotrigine is effective in treating the aura of migraine patients, although it is less effective against the pain (Caminero and Manso-Calderón, 2014).

Levetiracetam

A systematic review found that levetiracetam offered some benefit in episodic migraine compared with placebo but failed to find consistent support for benefit in chronic migraine (Watkins et al., 2018).

Pregabalin

Pregabalin is one of the gabapentinoids and may have some efficacy and safety for migraine prophylaxis (Buchanan and Ramadan, 2006) but more research is needed (Linde et al., 2013a).

Topiramate

Topiramate is efficacious and safe in migraine prevention. It is considered the best ASM for migraine treatment and has been shown in double-blind placebo-controlled trials to be effective for migraine prevention (Buchanan and Ramadan, 2006; Calabresi et al., 2007; D'Amico, 2007; Diener et al., 2007; Modi and Lowder, 2006; Pierangeli et al., 2006). In one study, the responder rate among patients with migraine was significantly greater with topiramate at 50 mg/day (39%, $P = 0.01$), 100 mg/day (49%, $P < 0.001$), and 200 mg/day (47%, $P < 0.001$) versus placebo (23%). Reductions in number of migraine days were significant for the 100 mg/day ($p = 0.003$) and 200 mg/day ($p < 0.001$) topiramate groups (Brandes et al., 2004). A meta-analysis demonstrated that topiramate in a 100 mg/day dosage is effective in reducing headache frequency and reasonably well-tolerated (Linde et al., 2013b). The extended-release (XR) topiramate has significantly fewer cognitive effects, improved adherence, and overall better outcomes of migraine prophylaxis than immediate-release (IR) topiramate (Silberstein, 2017). Caution should be exercised in its use in women of childbearing age, particularly those who may wish to become pregnant, due to potential teratogenic risks.

Valproic Acid, Valproate, Divalproex Sodium

Valproate has been studied in migraine as well, and its efficacy has been established. In one study, the mean reductions in 4-week migraine headache rate were 1.2 headaches per 4 weeks (from a baseline mean of 4.4) in the extended-release divalproex sodium group and 0.6 headache per 4 weeks (from a baseline mean of 4.2) in the placebo group ($p = 0.006$); reductions with extended-release divalproex sodium were significantly greater than with placebo in all three 4-week segments of the treatment period (Freitag et al., 2002). This result is not striking, but it is significant. This drug is a good choice for patients with migraine and comorbid bipolar disease or epilepsy (Buchanan and Ramadan, 2006; Calabresi et al., 2007; D'Amico, 2007; Modi and Lowder, 2006; Pierangeli et al., 2006).

Zonisamide

Data suggest that zonisamide may be effective for headache prophylaxis (Ashkenazi et al., 2006). One trial examined zonisamide (200 mg/day) versus topiramate (100 mg/day) and found no significant differences between them in reduction of headache frequency. Headache severity was reduced significantly better by zonisamide (Mohammadianinejad et al., 2011).

It is worth mentioning that evidence suggests that there may be a role for ASMs, especially valproate, topiramate, and gabapentin, in the prevention of cluster headaches as well as migraines (D'Amico, 2007; Pascual et al., 2007).

Some preventive treatments for migraine or other headaches, such as tricyclic antidepressants and neuroleptic drugs, may be used in people with epilepsy. While there is a theoretical risk of provoking seizures, this effect is rarely seen in the clinics. It is exceedingly rare in our experience for postictal headache to respond to analgesic treatment although this has been advocated by some (Caminero and Manso-Calderón, 2014).

Finally, it should be mentioned that chronic headache may occur in some patients treated with carbamazepine or oxcarbazepine (Palmieri, 2007). The cause is uncertain. In the authors' experience, this is occasionally dose-related, but usually use of the drug must discontinue for the headache to disappear.

Recommended Antiseizure Medications in Patients with Migraine Headaches

- *Generalized epilepsies*: Levetiracetam, topiramate, valproate, zonisamide
- *Focal epilepsies*: Levetiracetam, topiramate, valproate, zonisamide

References

Andermann E, Andermann FA. Migraine-epilepsy relationship: Epidemiological and genetic aspects. In Andermann FA, Lugaresi E, eds., *Migraine and Epilepsy*. Boston: Butterworths; 1987:281–291.

Ashkenazi A, Benlifer A, Korenblit J, Silberstein SD. Zonisamide for migraine prophylaxis in refractory patients. *Cephalalgia*. 2006;26:1199–1202.

Aurora SK, Cao Y, Bowyer SM, et al. The occipital cortex is hyperexcitable in migraine: Experimental evidence. *Headache*. 1999;39:469–476.

Brandes JL, Saper JR, Diamond M, et al. Topiramate for migraine prevention: A randomized controlled trial. *JAMA*. 2004;291965–973.

Buchanan TM, Ramadan NM. Prophylactic pharmacotherapy for migraine headaches. *Semin Neurol*. 2006;26:188–198.

Calabresi P, Galletti F, Rossi C, Sarchielli P, Cupini LM. Antiepileptic drugs in migraine: From clinical aspects to cellular mechanisms. *Trends Pharmacol Sci*. 2007;28:188–195.

Caminero A, Manso-Calderón R. Links between headaches and epilepsy: Current knowledge and terminology. *Neurologia*. 2014;29:453–463.

D'Amico D. Antiepileptic drugs in the prophylaxis of migraine, chronic headache forms and cluster headache: A review of their efficacy and tolerability. *Neurol Sci*. 2007;28:S188–S197.

Diener HC, Bussone G, Van Oene JC, et al. Topiramate reduces headache days in chronic migraine: A randomized, double-blind, placebo-controlled study. *Cephalalgia*. 2007;27:814–823.

Freitag FG, Collins SD, Carlson HA, et al. A randomized trial of divalproex sodium extended-release tablets in migraine prophylaxis. *Neurology*. 2002;58:1652–1659.

Koch UR, Musshoff U, Pannek HW, et al. Intrinsic excitability, synaptic potentials, and short-term plasticity in human epileptic neocortex. *J Neurosci Res*. 2005;80:715–726.

Linde M, Mulleners WM, Chronicle EP, McCrory DC. Gabapentin or pregabalin for the prophylaxis of episodic migraine in adults. *Cochrane Database Syst Rev*. 2013 Jun 24;6:CD010609.a

Linde M, Mulleners WM, Chronicle EP, McCrory DC. Topiramate for the prophylaxis of episodic migraine in adults. *Cochrane Database Syst Rev*. 2013 Jun 24;6:CD010610.b

Marks DA, Ehrenberg BL. Migraine related seizures in adults with epilepsy, with EEG correlation. *Neurology*. 1993;43:2476–2483.

Mathew NT, Rapoport A, Saper J, et al. Efficacy of gabapentin in migraine prophylaxis. *Headache*. 2001;41:119–128.

Modi A, Lowder DM. Medications for migraine prophylaxis. *Am Fam Phys*. 2006;73:72–78.

Mohammadianinejad SE, Abbasi V, Sajedi SA, Majdinasab N, Abdollahi F, Hajmanouchehri R, Faraji A. Zonisamide versus topiramate in migraine prophylaxis: A double-blind randomized clinical trial. *Clin Neuropharmacol*. 2011;34(4):174–177.

Nye BL, Thadani VM. Migraine and epilepsy: Review of the literature. *Headache*. 2015;55:359–380.

Ottman R, Lipton RB. Is the comorbidity of epilepsy and migraine due to a shared genetic susceptibility? *Neurology*. 1996;47:918–924.

Palmieri A. Oxcarbazepine-induced headache. *Cephalalgia*. 2007;27:91–93.

Pascual J, Lainez MJA, Dodick D, Hering-Hanit R. Antiepileptic drugs for the treatment of chronic and episodic cluster headache: A review. *Headache*. 2007;47:81–89.

Pierangeli G, Cevoli S, Sancisi E, Grimaldi D, Zanigni S, Montagna P, Cortelli P. Which therapy for which patient? *Neurological Sci*. 2006;27:S153–S158.

Silberstein SD. Topiramate in migraine prevention: A 2016 perspective. *Headache*. 2017;57:165–178.

Steiner TJ, Findley LJ, Yuen AWC. Lamotrigine versus placebo in the prophylaxis of migraine with and without aura. *Cephalalgia*. 1997;17:109–112.

Stevenson SB. Epilepsy and migraine headache: Is there a connection? *J Pediatr Health Care*. 2006;20:167–171.

Watkins AK, Gee ME, Brown JN. Efficacy and safety of levetiracetam for migraine prophylaxis: A systematic review. *J Clin Pharm Ther*. 2018;43:467–475.

Zangaladze A, Asadi-Pooya AA, Ashkenazi A, Sperling MR. Sporadic hemiplegic migraine and epilepsy associated with CACNA1A gene mutation. *Epilepsy Behav*. 2010;17:293–295.

Chapter 26

Antiseizure Medications in Patients with Neuropathic Pain Syndromes

Neuropathic pain is defined as pain caused by the dysfunction of or a primary lesion in the central or peripheral nervous system. Examples of neuropathic pain syndromes include postherpetic neuralgia, painful diabetic neuropathy, central poststroke pain syndrome, trigeminal neuralgia, and HIV infection–associated neuralgia. Patients have described dull, throbbing, burning, or lancinating pain with these conditions (Vinik, 2005; Zaremba et al., 2006). These pains are often paroxysmal, especially trigeminal neuralgia. Neuropathic pain affects between 3% and 8% of the world's population, with unpleasant consequences on the patient's quality of life, mood, and occupational functioning (Bialer, 2012; Gilron and Coderre 2007).

Some antiseizure medications (ASMs) can suppress or attenuate pain in these conditions. It is assumed that both epilepsy and neuropathic pain share an underlying common pathophysiology, enabling some ASMs to be useful for the treatment of several neuropathic pain conditions. Most ASMs reduce neuronal hyperexcitability by inhibiting ion channels, and they may act on different parts of the nociceptive pathway (Ardeleanu et al., 2020; Bialer, 2012; Khdour, 2020; Vinik, 2005). Carbamazepine was first approved for the treatment of trigeminal neuralgia, years before approval was granted to treat epilepsy, and other agents have also found use in treating various neuropathic pain syndromes. Carbamazepine, gabapentin, and pregabalin are currently the only three ASMs approved for the treatment of neuropathic pain syndromes.

Antiseizure Medications in Neuropathic Pain Syndromes

Carbamazepine

This drug is the most extensively investigated ASM used in the management of trigeminal neuralgia. Carbamazepine often successfully treats trigeminal neuralgia and may at times help symptoms of painful diabetic neuropathy (Maizels and McCarberg, 2005; Vinik, 2005). However, efficacy may be limited over many years. One study evaluated the efficacy of carbamazepine over 16 years in 146 patients. The authors reported initial success in 60% of participants, but only 22% of participants still found carbamazepine effective after 5–16 years (Taylor et al., 1981).

Gabapentin

Gabapentin is probably the best ASM for the treatment of neuropathic pain, especially painful diabetic neuropathy and postherpetic neuralgia. Gabapentin should be used as one of the first-line drugs in painful diabetic neuropathy and postherpetic neuralgia even in patients without epilepsy (Caraceni et al., 2004; Maizels and McCarberg, 2005; Serpell, 2002; Vinik, 2005; Wiffen et al., 2005; Zaremba et al., 2006). The recommended daily dosage usually ranges from 900 to 3,600 mg/day (Ardeleanu et al., 2020) although many people, particularly older individuals, may respond to doses as low as 300 mg/day. Combination with venlafaxine sometimes seems to provide additional benefit (Ardeleanu et al., 2020).

Lacosamide

Lacosamide has doubtful efficacy in treating peripheral diabetic neuropathy, but has possible limited beneficial effect at higher doses. Results from various studies were of low quality, producing moderate-quality evidence for some efficacy outcomes of lacosamide (400 mg/day) (Bialer, 2012). In the authors' experience, lacosamide may help patients with trigeminal neuralgia.

Lamotrigine

This agent has not been demonstrated to be effective for neuropathic pain. While it has been advocated by some for the management of trigeminal neuralgia, painful diabetic neuropathy, HIV-associated neuropathy, and post-stroke pain syndrome (Maizels and McCarberg, 2005; Vinik, 2005; Zaremba et al., 2006), randomized, double-blind, placebo-controlled studies were unable to demonstrate efficacy for pain associated with diabetic neuropathy (Vinik et al., 2007).

Oxcarbazepine

This ASM has been reported to be effective in patients with trigeminal neuralgia, painful radiculopathy, and painful diabetic neuropathy (Beydoun et al., 2007; Jorns and Zakrzewska, 2007; Zaremba et al., 2006).

Phenytoin

This drug is useful in the treatment of trigeminal neuralgia (Zaremba et al., 2006).

Pregabalin

This drug is efficacious in the management of painful diabetic neuropathy and postherpetic neuralgia. In four clinical trials in a total of 1,068 patients with diabetic peripheral neuropathy, patients receiving pregabalin at 300–600 mg/day had significantly greater improvement in mean pain scores than did placebo recipients. Patients with postherpetic neuralgia receiving pregabalin 450–600 mg/day had also significantly greater improvement in relief of pain and pain-related sleep interference than did placebo recipients (Maizels and McCarberg, 2005; Tassone et al., 2007; Vinik, 2005; Zaremba et al., 2006).

Dosage ranges from 150 to 300 mg/day have also been recommended (Ardeleanu et al., 2020). How pregabalin compares with gabapentin is uncertain. Pregabalin treatment does not appear to be associated with loss of glycemic control. However, as the thiazolidinedione class of antidiabetic drugs can cause weight gain and/or fluid retention, possibly exacerbating or leading to heart failure, care should be taken when coadministering pregabalin and these agents in diabetic patients.

Topiramate

Topiramate may help painful diabetic neuropathy (Vinik, 2005), but it often causes unpleasant tingling in the fingers and toes, so it is not particularly desirable for the treatment of neuropathy and is generally best avoided in this condition.

Valproic Acid, Valproate, Divalproex Sodium

Valproate is of uncertain efficacy for treating neuropathic pain syndromes (Vinik, 2005; Zaremba et al., 2006).

Zonisamide

No satisfactory evidence exists at present supporting the use of zonisamide for the treatment of neuropathic pain (Atli and Dogra, 2005; Krusz, 2003).

Summary

In a recent systematic review of the treatment of painful diabetic neuropathy, pregabalin was ranked as the only level A drug for the relief of this condition. Gabapentin was considered a level B drug for the treatment of painful diabetic neuropathy. Lacosamide, lamotrigine, and oxcarbazepine were not recommended for painful diabetic neuropathy treatment (Brill et al., 2011). There are insufficient data in the literature to evaluate the role of the other ASMs, including phenobarbital, felbamate, tiagabine, and vigabatrin, in the treatment of neuropathic pain syndromes.

Recommended Antiseizure Medications in Patients with Neuropathic Pain Syndromes

- *Generalized epilepsies*: Valproate
- *Focal epilepsies*: Carbamazepine, gabapentin, pregabalin; for patients with trigeminal neuralgia, these drugs as well as oxcarbazepine and lacosamide

Note: Valproate, carbamazepine, gabapentin, and pregabalin may cause weight gain. Weight should be monitored in diabetic patients.

References

Ardeleanu V, Toma A, Pafili K, et al. Current pharmacological treatment of painful diabetic neuropathy: A narrative review. *Medicina (Kaunas)*. 2020;56:25.

Atli A, Dogra S. Zonisamide in the treatment of painful diabetic neuropathy: A randomized, double-blind, placebo-controlled pilot study. *Pain Medicine*. 2005;6:225–234.

Beydoun S, Alarcon F, Mangat S, Wan Y. Long-term safety and tolerability of oxcarbazepine in painful diabetic neuropathy. *Acta Neurologica Scand*. 2007;115:284–288.

Bialer M. Why are antiepileptic drugs used for nonepileptic conditions? *Epilepsia*. 2012;53(Suppl. 7):26–33.

Brill V, England J, Franklin GM, et al. Evidence-based guideline: Treatment of painful diabetic neuropathy. *Neurology*. 2011;76:1758–1765.

Caraceni A, Zecca E, Bonezzi C, et al. Gabapentin for neuropathic cancer pain: A randomized controlled trial from the Gabapentin Cancer Pain Study Group. *J Clin Oncol*. 2004;22:2909–2917.

Gilron I, Coderre TJ. Emerging drugs in neuropathic pain. *Expert Opin Emerg Drugs*. 2007;12:113–126.

Jorns TP, Zakrzewska JM. Evidence-based approach to the medical management of trigeminal neuralgia. *Br J Neurosurg*. 2007;21:253–261.

Khdour MR. Treatment of diabetic peripheral neuropathy: A review. *J Pharm Pharmacol*. 2020 Feb 17. doi:10.1111/jphp.13241. [Epub ahead of print.]

Krusz JC. Treatment of chronic pain with zonisamide. *Pain Pract*. 2003;3:317–320.

Maizels M, McCarberg B. Antidepressants and antiepileptic drugs for chronic non-cancer pain. *Am Fam Phys*. 2005;71:483–490.

Serpell MG; Neuropathic Pain Study Group. Gabapentin in neuropathic pain syndromes: A randomised, double-blind, placebo-controlled trial. *Pain*. 2002;99:557–566.

Tassone DM, Boyce E, Guyer J, Nuzum D. Pregabalin: A novel gamma aminobutiric acid analogue in the treatment of neuropathic pain, partial-onset seizures, and anxiety disorders. *Clin Ther*. 2007;29:26–48.

Taylor JC, Brauer S, Espir MLE. Long-term treatment of trigeminal neuralgia. *Postgrad Med J*. 1981;57:16–18.

Vinik A. Use of antiepileptic drugs in the treatment of chronic painful diabetic neuropathy. *J Clin Endocrinol Metab*. 2005;90:4936–4945.

Vinik AI, Tuchman M, Safirstein B, et al. Lamotrigine for treatment of pain associated with diabetic neuropathy: Results of two randomized, double-blind, placebo-controlled studies. *Pain*. 2007;128:169–179.

Wiffen PJ, Mcquay HJ, Edwards JE, Moore RA. Gabapentin for acute and chronic pain. *Cochrane Database Syst Rev*. 2005;3:CD005452.

Zaremba PD, Bialek M, Blaszczyk B, Cioczek P, Czuczwar SJ. Non-epilepsy uses of antiepileptic drugs. *Pharmacol Rep*. 2006;58:1–12.

Chapter 27

Antiseizure Medications and Cutaneous Reactions

Idiosyncratic drug reactions are unexpected and unpredictable adverse reactions, fundamentally different from the dose-related adverse effects of drugs. A variety of idiosyncratic reactions may be seen, such as aplastic anemia, acute liver failure, and rash. Genetic factors are important in many of these events (Ihtisham et al., 2019; Pirmohamed and Park, 2001).

Drug-induced rashes are the most common type of idiosyncratic reactions due to the use of antiseizure medications (ASMs). The most common presentation is a maculopapular (Figure 27.1) or erythematous pruritic rash appearing within 4 weeks of initiating therapy with a new ASM. Systemic symptoms are usually absent, although fever may occur. The rash usually disappears within several days of discontinuing the drug. Other therapeutic measures are rarely needed, although diphenhydramine may help suppress itching, and a brief course of steroids may be helpful for severe rash, particularly when fever is present. Occasionally, the rash can be severe and present as erythema multiforme, Stevens-Johnson syndrome, or toxic epidermal necrolysis (Lyell syndrome) (Alvestad et al., 2007; Asconapé, 2002).

The ASM hypersensitivity syndrome (AHS), also known as *drug reaction with eosinophilia and systemic symptoms* (DRESS), is not common but is important and potentially life-threatening. A triad of fever, skin rash, and internal organ involvement characterizes AHS. It usually starts within the first 2–8 weeks after initiation of therapy. The initial symptoms include a low-grade fever followed by rash, lymphadenopathy, and pharyngitis. This is followed by internal organ involvement (e.g., eosinophilia, hepatitis, and less commonly, nephritis, carditis, pneumonitis, myositis, or blood dyscrasias). Facial edema is a striking feature of AHS, particularly in the periorbital area (Figure 27.2). The reported rate of liver involvement ranges from 34% to 94%, and fulminant hepatic necrosis may be seen. The presence of hepatitis worsens prognosis. Prompt recognition is the mainstay of treatment of AHS. To establish whether a drug is the cause of an immune-mediated reaction such as AHS, alternative causes, latency of a reaction after drug intake, and improvement after drug cessation should be considered. The causative drug should be immediately discontinued. The patient should never be rechallenged with the offending agent, as the relapse rate is extremely high. Sometimes, even after discontinuation of the offending agent, the disease activity can persist for 2–16 weeks. Cross-reactivity among the aromatic ASMs may explain these prolonged symptoms after switching to another aromatic ASM. The most

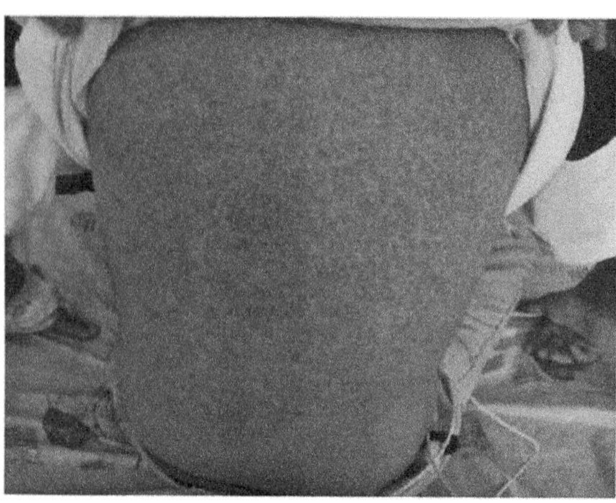

Figure 27.1 Generalized maculopapular rash on back.
Adapted from: Kocaoglu C, Cilasun C, Solak ES, Kurtipek GS, Arslan S. Successful treatment of antiepileptic drug-induced DRESS syndrome with pulse methylprednisolone. *Case Rep Pediatr.* 2013; 928910.

controversial issue in the management of AHS is the use of systemic corticosteroids. Although the role of corticosteroids is controversial, we advise prescribing prednisone, starting at a dosage of 1–2 mg/kg/day if symptoms are severe (e.g., hepatic involvement). Because stopping the offending ASM increases the risk of having seizures, a new ASM must be immediately started. In choosing a new drug, it is important to consider potential cross-reactivity. Valproate should be avoided if significant hepatic involvement has developed. Brivaracetam, levetiracetam, gabapentin, and topiramate are reasonably safe options and can be immediately begun at therapeutic doses. Use of intermittent benzodiazepine therapy can help manage breakthrough seizure clusters during the transition. However, the structure of benzodiazepines contains aromatic rings, and part of their metabolism involves cytochrome P-450 isoforms. Therefore, there is still potential for cross-reactivity (Alvestad et al., 2007; Asconapé, 2002; Knowles et al., 1999; Kwong et al., 2006).

Stevens-Johnson and other severe syndromes have been reported in patients taking ASMs. It is possible that lamotrigine is associated with a higher risk of developing a severe skin eruption than other drugs. Unfortunately, there is no reliable way to determine early in the clinical course of a rash if it will remain as a benign maculopapular rash or evolve into a severe skin reaction. Therefore, the offending drug should usually be discontinued as soon as possible. Signs and symptoms that may indicate the presence of a more severe reaction include a painful rash, mucosal involvement (Figure 27.3), fever, and other systemic symptoms (Asconapé, 2002). There are occasions, however, when it may be undesirable to stop a particular ASM that has just caused a rash. In these circumstances, provided there are no signs of a more severe problem, one can continue that ASM while observing the patient

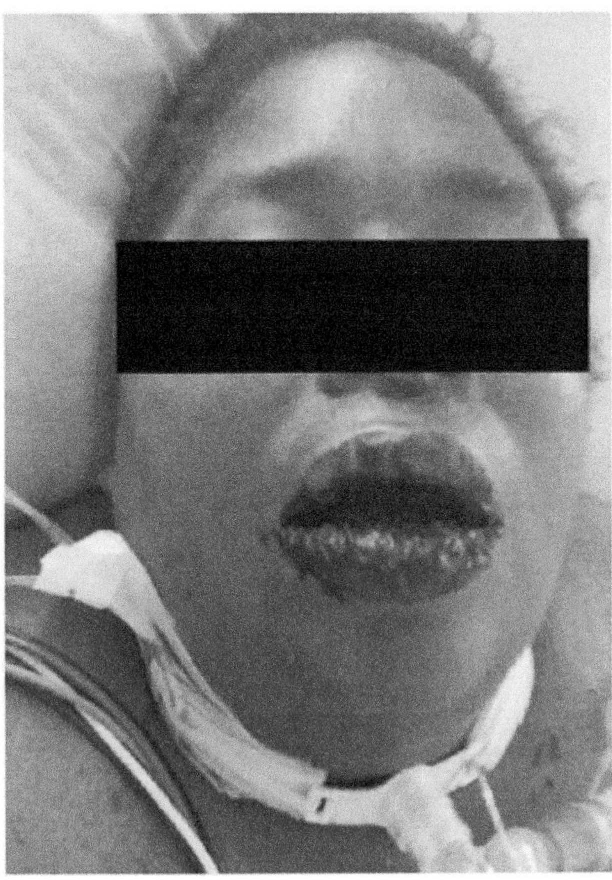

Figure 27.2 Severe facial edema in a patient with anticonvulsant hypersensitivity syndrome (AHS) or drug reaction with eosinophilia and systemic symptoms (DRESS).

Adapted from: Fleming P, Marik PE. The DRESS syndrome: The great clinical mimicker. *Pharmacotherapy*. 2011; 31(3): 45e–49e.

closely and treating symptoms such as itching with an antihistamine. Provided more severe symptoms do not appear, in many cases, the rash will prove to be transient and disappear. This course of action should be carried out only when there are compelling reasons to continue an ASM or there is a strong presumption that the next drug will likely provoke a similar initial rash.

The aromatic (Figure 27.4) ASMs—phenytoin, carbamazepine, oxcarbazepine, eslicarbazepine acetate, phenobarbital, primidone, zonisamide, and lamotrigine—are more frequently associated with cutaneous eruptions and other signs or symptoms of drug hypersensitivity. There is a high degree of cross-reactivity (40–80%) in patients with hypersensitivity or allergic

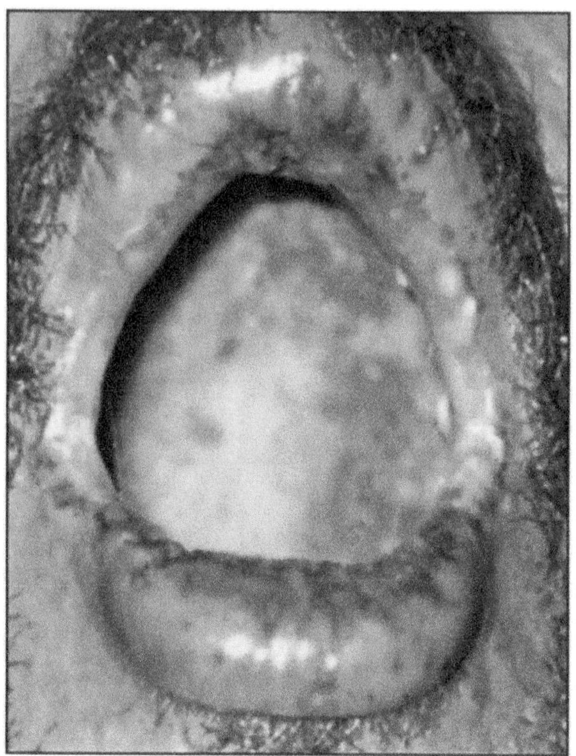

Figure 27.3 Multiple oral ulcers in a patient with Stevens-Johnson syndrome.

Adapted from: Reddy RB, Shekar PC, Chandra KL, Aravind R. Oral lesions associated with Nevirapine-induced Stevens-Johnson syndrome and toxic epidermal necrolysis: A report of 10 cases. *J Oral Maxillofac Pathol*. 2013; 17: 431–435.

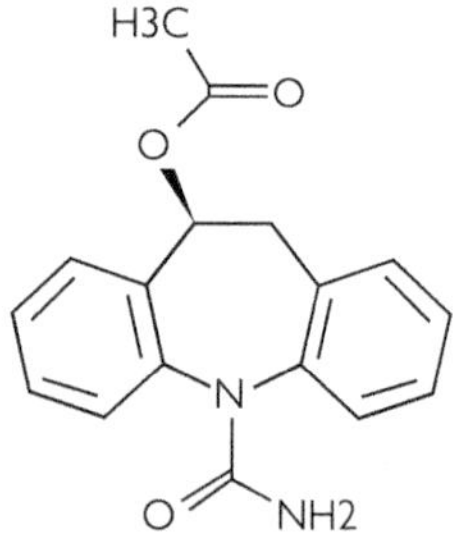

Figure 27.4 The aromatic chemical structure of eslicarbazepine acetate.

Adapted from: www.aptiom.com/2014.

reactions to phenytoin, phenobarbital, primidone, and carbamazepine. These drugs are all metabolized to hydroxylated aromatic compounds via the cytochrome P-450 hepatic enzymes. Arene oxide intermediates are formed during metabolism and are thought to be responsible for cross-sensitivity among these ASMs in susceptible individuals. Some individuals may have a reduced ability to detoxify the intermediate toxic metabolites (e.g., arene oxides) of these ASMs, a situation that may be genetically mediated. However, there is no way to predict with certainty which patients will exhibit cross-sensitivity (Alvestad et al., 2007; Asconapé, 2002; Knowles et al., 1999; Kwong et al., 2006; Levy et al., 2002). Whether drugs such as lacosamide, lamotrigine, and zonisamide will also show a similar risk of cross-reactivity has not been properly evaluated, but this is likely due to the aromatic structure of these drugs. Nonaromatic ASMs (e.g., brivaracetam, levetiracetam, topiramate) are safe alternatives for patients with severe, aromatic ASM-induced cutaneous adverse drug reactions.

The rate of an ASM-induced rash is often greater in patients with another ASM rash (8.8%) versus in those without (1.7%) (odds ratio 3:1) (Arif et al., 2007; Fowler et al., 2019) (Figure 27.5). Therefore, patients with a history of an ASM-induced rash should be treated with drugs with a lower risk for allergic reactions (e.g., brivaracetam, gabapentin, topiramate, levetiracetam). The rate of dose titration is also an important issue. The risk of allergic reaction I s decreased when a drug is begun at a low dose and gradually increased; slow titration may allow desensitization to occur. A relation between starting dose and titration rate and the incidence of skin reactions is particularly evident for lamotrigine, carbamazepine, and phenytoin (Zaccara et al., 2007). Female gender may also be associated with a higher risk of ASM-induced rash (Alvestad et al., 2007). Table 27.1 shows the clinical characteristics of common cutaneous skin reactions and their management strategies (Fowler et al., 2019).

Skin testing, in particular the patch test, may be a useful screening method to discover the specific cause of an exanthematous cutaneous reaction if several drugs are possible offenders (Lammintausta and Kortekangas-Savolainen, 2005). In the unusual patient considered to be at high risk for a hypersensitivity reaction, skin tests to predict individual reactivity may be helpful (Zaccara et al., 2007).

Recent studies have shown that different ethnic populations may have dissimilar risks regarding the development of severe, ASM-induced cutaneous adverse drug reactions due to various genetic backgrounds (Ihtisham et al., 2019; Neuman et al., 2012; Yang et al., 2011). Genetic markers, such as the human leukocyte antigen (HLA), are useful in predicting an individual's predisposition to ASM hypersensitivity reactions. Ever since it was first linked with carbamazepine-related Stevens-Johnson syndrome in Han Chinese, HLA allele B*1502 (HLA-B*1502) has become the strongest HLA correlation known among human diseases. This association holds true for certain ethnic groups only, in particular Han Chinese, Thai, Malay, and to a lesser degree, Indians. Regardless of ethnicity, a hypersensitivity reaction predisposition can be predicted by in vitro lymphocyte toxicity assay (LTA) as well. LTA is a good

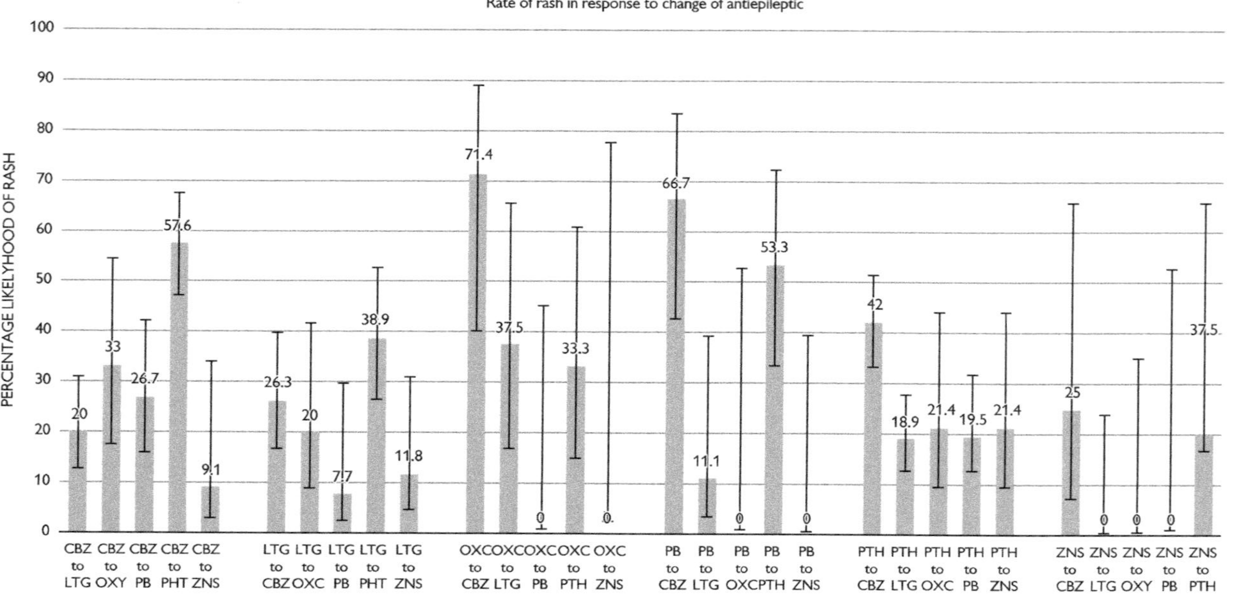

Figure 27.5 Risk of allergic rash/hypersensitivity with new antiseizure medication in patients with history of skin reaction to a previous medication.

Adapted from: Fowler T, Bansal AS, Lozsádi D. Risks and management of antiepileptic drug induced skin reactions in the adult out-patient setting. *Seizure*. 2019; 72: 61–70.

Table 27.1 Common cutaneous skin reactions due to antiseizure medications.

Reaction	maculopapular	Urticaria	Fixed Drug reaction	SJS/TEN	DRESS	AGEP
Picture						
Incidence	Some data suggests 1.7/100,000 of the total population. Of these 0.05/100,000 from antiepileptics.	Some data suggests 1.7/100,000 of the total population. Of these 0.01/100,000 from antiepileptics.	No good statistics on incidence.	Around 0.1/100,000 of the total population.For incidence among new users of CBZ, LTG, PB, PHT, the incidence is around 0.1-0.01% Rapid titration.	Good data is lacking, however estimated to be 0.1-0.01% of patients exposed to potentially causative drugs.	0.1-0.5/100,000 of the total population.

(*continued*)

Table 27.1 *Continued*

Reaction	maculopapular	Urticaria	Fixed Drug reaction	SJS/TEN	DRESS	AGEP
Risk Factors	Commonly associated with CBZ and PHT CFHR4 has an association with Phenytoin induced maculopapular exanthema. HLA-A*3101 has an association with CBZ induced maculopapular exanthema.	Most common in children and young adults, and in those with a history of allergy or atopy	HLA-B*22	Genetic risk factors include; HLA-B*1502, and HLA-A*2402 in Han Chinese populations. HLA-A*3101 for CBZ in European populations.	HLA-A*3101	More frequent in women. Genetic risk factors include IL-36RN
Rash onset	Under 2 weeks	Days	Days	2-8 weeks	2-8 weeks	Within 11 days
Preceding features	Usually none, however some complain of malaise	Usually no preceding symptoms	Usually no preceding symptoms	Fever, headache, rhinitis and myalgia, preceding exposure by 1-3 days	Fever over 38.5, in 90% of patients. Also dysphagia, Lymphadenopathy, puritis and pain.	Preceding symptoms are vague with malaise and sometimes low grade fever.
Associated features	Itch (excoriation)	Lesions fluctuate, may be confluent and itchy	Locally pruritis, burning and pain. Systemic symptoms are uncommon.	Mucosal blistering, fever, fatigue, flu-like symptoms desquamation and bullae	Eosinophilia, abnormal liver function tests, gastrointestinal and pulmonary involvement	Oedema of the face, sometimes mild oral mucous membrane involvement, fever and leucoytosis.
Resolution	Under 2 weeks	Rarely lasts more than a few days, chronic urticaria if over 6 weeks.	Days to weeks	Re-epithelialisation occurs within 3 weeks. Further complications take longer to resolve	May begin to resolve within 1 month, but still at risk of complications after several months	Days

Reaction	maculopapular	Urticaria	Fixed Drug reaction	SJS/TEN	DRESS	AGEP
Differential diagnoses	Measles, scarlet fever, viral exanthema.	Eczema, maculopapular, erythema multiforme, pityriasis rosea.	Spider bite, bullous pemphigoid	Staphylococcal scalded skin syndrome, disseminated fixed bullous drug eruption, graft vs host disease, EMM	At onset it may be difficult to differentiate from maculopapular exanthema or AGEP.	AGEP, corneal pustular dermatosis, IgA pemphigus, Bullous Impetigo.
Treatment	Purely symptomatic. Some prescribe topical corticosteroids or oral antihistamines.	Antihistamines or oral Steroids.	Top steroid, oral treatment rarely required	Supportive care, consult dermatology, burn unit if over 25% BSA involve	Supportive therapy, including antipyretics, antihistamines, topical corticosteroids. If internal organ involvement, corticosteroids, can be considered	Admission, and treatment with moisturisers, topical corticosteroids, oral antihistamines.
Desensitize / rechallenge	Desensitisation possible	Desensitisation possible	Desensitisation possible.	No	No	Possible with caution
mortality	N/A	Rare unless angioedema develops	N/A	Up to 30%	10%	4%

AGEP=Acute generalized exanthematous pustulosis, CBZ=Carbamazepine, HLA=human leukocyte antigen, LTG=Lamotrigine, PB=Phenobarbital, PHT=Phenytoin.

Adapted from: Fowler T, Bansal AS, Lozsádi D. Risks and management of antiepileptic drug induced skin reactions in the adult out-patient setting. *Seizure*. 2019; 72: 61–70.

predictor tool for possible hypersensitivity reactions in patients with epilepsy (Neuman et al., 2012).

Another potential adverse effect of ASMs is *photosensitivity*, which describes either a phototoxic response or a less frequent photoallergic reaction. A phototoxic reaction is immediate and resembles exaggerated sunburn. In comparison, a photoallergic reaction has an immunological basis and requires previous exposure to the photosensitizing agent. Patients who experience photoallergic responses typically present 1–14 days after exposure to sunlight with a papulovesicular eruption, pruritus, and eczematous dermatitis (Dubakiene and Kupriene, 2006). Photosensitivity reactions are not predictable and can occur at any age. Many medications, including ASMs, are associated with photosensitivity reactions (Dubakiene and Kupriene, 2006; Facts and Comparisons, 2007; Moore, 2002). Protection from sunlight often prevents photosensitivity reactions. Avoidance of direct sunlight and sun-tanning facilities, using protective clothing and eyewear, application of an appropriate sunscreen with a high UV protection rating, and evening dosing of the drug are measures that can minimize the risk of photosensitivity effects from most drugs (Dubakiene and Kupriene, 2006; Moore, 2002). Treatment is necessary when a severe burning reaction occurs. In the case of a phototoxic reaction, the treatment is the same as for sunburn. Avoidance of the offending photosensitizing agent or sunlight exposure is required, but sometimes an offending ASM may not be avoidable. Therefore, preventive measures are of great significance. Antihistamines and corticosteroids may be required to treat the inflammation arising from photoallergic reactions (Moore, 2002). Should preventative measures be impractical or ineffective, then a new drug should be chosen. Photosensitivity has been reported with lamotrigine treatment in 2% of patients. Other ASMs associated with photosensitivity include carbamazepine, felbamate, gabapentin, oxcarbazepine, phenobarbital, phenytoin, tiagabine, topiramate, and valproic acid. The incidence of photosensitivity in patients taking these ASMs is less than 1%. Insufficient data are available for accurate estimates of incidence in most ASMs.

Note: Avoid lamotrigine and acetazolamide in patients with known photosensitivity to multiple drugs.

Antiseizure Medications and Cutaneous Reactions

Acetazolamide

Acetazolamide is a sulfonamide. Acetazolamide has been associated with Stevens-Johnson syndrome, toxic epidermal necrolysis, and acute generalized exanthematous pustulosis. The nonfollicular, pustular, erythematous rash starts 2–3 weeks after starting the drug and is associated with fever. Re-exposure may cause a second episode within 2 days. Acetazolamide is contraindicated in any patient with sulfonamide sensitivity (Facts and Comparisons, 2007; Levy et al., 2002).

Like other sulfonamide derivatives, photosensitivity may occur with carbonic anhydrase inhibitors, including acetazolamide. Some patients may be more sensitive to sunlight (UV) exposure while receiving acetazolamide.

Benzodiazepines

Drug-induced rashes and allergic reactions are not frequent with benzodiazepines (Facts and Comparisons, 2007; Levy et al., 2002). Approximately 2% of patients taking clobazam develop a skin rash (Arif et al., 2007).

Brivaracetam

Drug-induced rashes have not been reported with this drug yet. But, as with any other agent, rashes may occur (brivaracetam; www.briviact.com/2020).

Cannabidiol

Drug-induced rashes may happen with an incidence of at least 10% (cannabidiol; www.epidiolex.com/2020).

Carbamazepine

Some dermatological effects of carbamazepine include photosensitivity, alopecia, urticaria, alterations in skin pigmentation, exfoliative dermatitis, erythema multiforme, and erythema nodosum. Approximately 4–11% of patients develop a skin rash (Alvestad et al., 2007; Arif et al., 2007). The rash usually develops during the first 2–8 weeks of therapy. Serious dermatologic reactions including Stevens-Johnson syndrome, toxic epidermal necrolysis, and angioedema have been reported. Carbamazepine has also been associated with acute generalized exanthematous pustulosis. Multiorgan hypersensitivity reactions (AHS) occurring days to weeks or months after initiating treatment are rare (Facts and Comparisons, 2007; Levy et al., 2002).

Cenobamate

Drug-induced rashes may occur with cenobamate. DRESS, also known as multiorgan hypersensitivity, was reported in patients taking cenobamate in phase II trials starting at doses of 50 mg/day or 100 mg/day with weekly increases in dose. No cases were reported in a phase III trial of 1,339 patients starting at doses of 12.5 mg/day and 2-week intervals of slow titration (Sperling et al., 2020) nor in the first year after general availability (https://reference.medscape.com/drug/xcopri-cenobamate-1000328/2020).

Eslicarbazepine Acetate

Serious dermatologic reactions including Stevens-Johnson syndrome and also AHS have been reported in association with eslicarbazepine acetate. This drug is chemically similar to carbamazepine and oxcarbazepine. Patients with a prior dermatologic reaction, AHS, or other serious reactions to either oxcarbazepine or eslicarbazepine acetate should not be treated with this drug.

Ethosuximide

Dermatological side effects during ethosuximide therapy include erythematous skin rash, pruritus, and urticaria. More serious reactions, which may be accompanied by fever, lymphadenopathy, pharyngitis, and muscle pain, are uncommon but can develop, including erythema multiforme and Stevens-Johnson syndrome. Ethosuximide should not be used in patients with a history of succinimide hypersensitivity (Facts and Comparisons, 2007; Levy et al., 2002).

Ezogabine

Ezogabine can cause skin discoloration (blue, gray-blue, or brown). This discoloration occurs predominantly on or around the lips or in the nail beds of the fingers or toes but more widespread involvement has also been reported. Approximately 10% of patients in long-term clinical trials developed skin discoloration, generally after 2 or more years of treatment and at high doses. The possibility of more extensive systemic involvement has not been excluded. If a patient develops skin discoloration, serious consideration should be given to changing to an alternate medication.

Felbamate

Acne, rash, and pruritus have occurred with felbamate therapy. Approximately 1–2% of patients develop a skin rash (Arif et al., 2007). Toxic epidermal necrolysis due to felbamate has been reported (Facts and Comparisons, 2007; Levy et al., 2002).

Gabapentin

Fewer than 1% of patients develop a skin rash (Arif et al., 2007).

Lacosamide

Mild (e.g., pruritus) and severe (e.g., AHS) reactions have rarely been reported in patients taking lacosamide. Large studies of lacosamide, which is an aromatic ASM, report risk of rash comparable to that of placebo (Fowler et al., 2019).

Lamotrigine

Rash is the most common cause for discontinuation of lamotrigine therapy. Approximately 10% of patients develop erythema and a maculopapular rash, although the incidence is lower when slow titration schedules are used, with a starting dose of 25 mg/day (Arif et al., 2007). The rash usually develops during the first 2–8 weeks of therapy. Serious dermatological reactions including Stevens-Johnson syndrome, toxic epidermal necrolysis, and angioedema have been reported. Serious reactions are observed more often in children (8–10 in 1,000) than adults (0.8–3 in 1,000). Rash also appears to be more common in patients receiving concomitant valproic acid or when the recommended dose escalation schedule is exceeded. The increased rate of rash observed in patients taking valproate when lamotrigine is initiated probably reflects reduced metabolism and therefore higher serum levels of lamotrigine (due to enzyme inhibition by valproate). Initiating therapy at the lowest possible dosage and escalating slowly appear to minimize the occurrence of skin rash. Rash should result in prompt discontinuation of lamotrigine therapy and appropriate evaluation. Hypersensitivity reactions, some fatal or life-threatening, have also occurred with lamotrigine. Early manifestations of hypersensitivity (e.g., fever and lymphadenopathy) may be present even though a rash is not evident (Karande et al., 2006; Levy et al., 2002).

A history of another ASM-related rash is a major risk factor for developing rash to lamotrigine (Hirsch et al., 2006), and this drug should not be an early therapeutic choice for patients with a history of hypersensitivity to other ASMs.

Levetiracetam

Cutaneous eruptions rarely occur in patients treated with levetiracetam (Arif et al., 2007).

Oxcarbazepine

Allergic skin reactions such as rash, pruritus, or urticaria may occur with oxcarbazepine use. Approximately 2.5% of patients develop a skin rash (Arif et al., 2007). Other skin conditions reported include erythema multiforme and oral ulceration. Other serious dermatological reactions, including Stevens-Johnson syndrome and toxic epidermal necrolysis, have been reported in both children and adults in association with oxcarbazepine. AHS rarely occurs. Cross-sensitivity between carbamazepine and oxcarbazepine is approximately 25–30% and is likely due to the structural similarity of the two drugs (Misra et al., 2003).

Perampanel

Drug-induced rashes uncommonly occur with perampanel use (Lin et al., 2018).

Phenobarbital

Hypersensitivity reactions to phenobarbital may present as various organ system problems, including blood, liver, renal, and skin disorders. Discontinuation of the drug is necessary but may not be sufficient to reverse progression of any serious hypersensitivity reaction because of the slow metabolism and excretion of phenobarbital.

Cutaneous reactions occur in 1–2% of patients and include scarlatiniform or morbilliform maculopapular rash. Angioedema, bullous rash, exfoliative dermatitis, lupus-like symptoms, photosensitivity, purpura, serum sickness, Stevens-Johnson syndrome, and toxic epidermal necrolysis are rare but serious adverse effects of phenobarbital. Although uncommon, AHS has been reported with phenobarbital.

Avoid the use of phenobarbital in patients with a history of barbiturate hypersensitivity. Injectable solutions may also contain propylene glycol and should be avoided in patients with a hypersensitivity to propylene glycol. A history of hypersensitivity reactions should be obtained for a patient and the immediate family members. If hypersensitivity histories are positive, caution should be used in prescribing phenobarbital. Hypersensitivity reactions have been reported in patients who previously experienced phenytoin or carbamazepine hypersensitivity (Facts and Comparisons, 2007; Levy et al., 2002). Patients who have experienced reactions due to phenobarbital therapy should not be further exposed to the drug.

Phenytoin

Adverse dermatological reactions to phenytoin occur in 5–10% of patients and usually present as a maculopapular rash. More serious responses such as bullous rash, exfoliative dermatitis, purpura, erythema multiforme, Stevens-Johnson syndrome, or toxic epidermal necrolysis can occur but are rare. Minor reactions, such as rash, more often develop in the first few weeks of therapy, in contrast to more serious reactions that more often develop later. Skin hyperpigmentation has been reported and is more common in women than in men. Phenytoin can produce hypertrichosis or hirsutism. Coarsening of the facial features and enlargement of the lips are among the adverse effects.

Hypersensitivity reactions have been reported in patients who previously experienced other hydantoin hypersensitivity (e.g., fosphenytoin), barbiturate hypersensitivity (e.g., hypersensitivity to phenobarbital), or carbamazepine hypersensitivity (Facts and Comparisons, 2007; Levy et al., 2002).

Pregabalin

The incidence of rash is low with this drug. Pregabalin is contraindicated in patients who have a demonstrated or suspected hypersensitivity to the drug or its inactive ingredients. It is not known if cross-hypersensitivity exists between gabapentin and pregabalin, but the drugs are chemically and structurally similar. Use pregabalin with caution in patients with a known hypersensitivity to gabapentin (Facts and Comparisons, 2007; Levy et al., 2002).

Rufinamide

Rash, pruritus, Stevens-Johnson syndrome, and AHS have been reported rarely in association with rufinamide therapy. All patients who develop a rash while taking rufinamide must be closely supervised. If any severe reaction (e.g., AHS) is suspected, rufinamide should be discontinued and an alternative treatment started.

Tiagabine

Approximately 2.5% of patients develop a skin rash (Arif et al., 2007). Maculopapular rash, vesicular rash, and, rarely, Stevens-Johnson syndrome have been reported with tiagabine use (Facts and Comparisons, 2007; Levy et al., 2002).

Topiramate

Approximately 1% of patients develop a rash with topiramate use (Arif et al., 2007). Topiramate is contraindicated in any patient hypersensitive to the drug or any of the product's components. Rarely, serious and potentially fatal exfoliative dermatologic reactions have been reported (Facts and Comparisons, 2007; Levy et al., 2002).

Valproic Acid, Valproate, Divalproex Sodium

Dermatological reactions have been seen in patients receiving valproic acid. These reactions include transient alopecia, skin rash, pruritus, photosensitivity, erythema multiforme, and Stevens-Johnson syndrome (Facts and Comparisons, 2007; Levy et al., 2002). Approximately 1% of patients develop a rash (Arif et al., 2007). Multiorgan hypersensitivity reactions (AHS) have been rarely reported with valproate use. Cross-sensitivity with other drugs that produce this syndrome is unclear but may be possible (Facts and Comparisons, 2007; Levy et al., 2002).

Vigabatrin

Angioedema, maculo-papular rash, pruritus, Stevens-Johnson syndrome, and toxic epidermal necrolysis have been reported by patients taking vigabatrin.

Zonisamide

Approximately 4.5% of patients develop a rash (Arif et al., 2007). Zonisamide is a sulfonamide and can rarely produce severe, possibly fatal reactions such as toxic epidermal necrolysis, Stevens-Johnson syndrome, fulminant hepatic necrosis, and blood dyscrasias. Once sensitization to sulfonamides has occurred, a recurrence can be precipitated by administration of sulfonamides by any route. Zonisamide should be discontinued if there is any sign of a hypersensitivity reaction. Rash usually develops early (2–16 weeks) in the course of treatment with zonisamide.

Recommended Antiseizure Medications in Patients with History of Drug-Induced Skin Rash

- *Generalized epilepsies*: Levetiracetam, lacosamide, topiramate, valproate
- *Focal epilepsies*: Brivaracetam, gabapentin, lacosamide, levetiracetam, perampanel, topiramate

Note: The risk for cutaneous adverse effects (e.g., Stevens-Johnson syndrome and toxic epidermal necrolysis) with phenytoin, phenobarbital, and carbamazepine is increased during radiotherapy. When treatment is indicated, a drug with a lower potential for allergic cutaneous reactions (e.g., brivaracetam, levetiracetam, or topiramate) is preferred (Michelucci, 2006).

References

Alvestad S, Lydersen S, Brodtkorb E. Rash from antiepileptic drugs: Influence by gender, age, and learning disability. *Epilepsia*. 2007;48:1360–1365.

Arif H, Buchsbaum R, Weintraub D, et al. Comparisons and predictors of rash associated with 15 antiepileptic drugs. *Neurology*. 2007;68:1701–1709.

Asconapé JJ. Some common issues in the use of antiepileptic drugs. *Semin Neurol*. 2002;22:27–39.

Dubakiene R, Kupriene M. Scientific problems of photosensitivity. *Medicina*. 2006;42:619–628.

Facts and Comparisons. *Drug Facts and Comparisons*. Wolters Kluwer Health/Facts and Comparisons, St. Louis; 2007.

Fleming P, Marik PE. The DRESS syndrome: The great clinical mimicker. *Pharmacotherapy*. 2011;31(3):45e–49e.

Fowler T, Bansal AS, Lozsádi D. Risks and management of antiepileptic drug induced skin reactions in the adult out-patient setting. *Seizure*. 2019;72:61–70.

Hirsch LJ, Weintraub DB, Buchsbaum R, Spencer HT, Straka T, Hager M, Resor Jr SR. Predictors of lamotrigine-associated rash. *Epilepsia*. 2006;47:318–322.

Ihtisham K, Ramanujam B, Srivastava S, et al. Association of cutaneous adverse drug reactions due to antiepileptic drugs with HLA alleles in a north Indian population. *Seizure*. 2019;66:99–103.

Karande S, Gogtay NJ, Kanchan S, Kshirsagar NA. Anticonvulsant hypersensitivity syndrome to lamotrigine confirmed by lymphocyte stimulation in vitro. *Indian J Med Sci*. 2006;60:59–63.

Knowles SR, Shapiro LE, Shear NH. Anticonvulsant hypersensitivity syndrome: Incidence, prevention and management. *Drug Safety*. 1999;21:489–501.

Kocaoglu C, Cilasun C, Solak ES, Kurtipek GS, Arslan S. Successful treatment of antiepileptic drug-induced DRESS syndrome with pulse methylprednisolone. *Case Rep Pediatr*. 2013;2013:928910.

Kwong KL, Lam SY, Lui YS, Wong SN, So KT. Cross-sensitivity in a child with anticonvulsant hypersensitivity syndrome. *J Paediatr Child Health*. 2006;42:474–476.

Lammintausta K, Kortekangas-Savolainen O. The usefulness of skin tests to prove drug hypersensitivity. *Br J Dermatol*. 2005;152:968–974.

Levy RH, Mattson RH, Meldrum BS, Perucca E. *Antiepileptic Drugs*, 5th ed. Philadelphia: Lippincott Williams and Wilkins; 2002.

Lin KL, Lin JJ, Chou ML, et al. Efficacy and tolerability of perampanel in children and adolescents with pharmacoresistant epilepsy: The first real-world evaluation in Asian pediatric neurology clinics. *Epilepsy Behav*. 2018;85:188–194

Ljunggren B, Bojs G. A case of photosensitivity and contact allergy to systemic tricyclic drugs, with unusual features. *Contact Dermat*. 1991;24:259–265.

Michelucci R. Optimizing therapy of seizures in neurosurgery. *Neurology*. 2006;67;S14–S18.

Misra UK, Kalita J, Rathore C. Phenytoin and carbamazepine cross reactivity: Report of a case and review of literature. *Postgrad Med J*. 2003;79:703–704.

Moore DE. Drug-induced cutaneous photosensitivity. *Drug Safety*. 2002;25:345–372.

Neuman MG, Cohen L, Nanau RM, Hwang PA. Genetic and immune predictors for hypersensitivity syndrome to antiepileptic drugs. *Transl Res*. 2012;159(5):397–406.

Pirmohamed M, Park BK. Genetic susceptibility to adverse drug reactions. *Trends Pharmacol Sci*. 2001;22:298–305.

Reddy RB, Shekar PC, Chandra KL, Aravind R. Oral lesions associated with Nevirapine-induced Stevens-Johnson syndrome and toxic epidermal necrolysis: A report of 10 cases. *J Oral Maxillofac Pathol*. 2013;17(3):431–435.

Sperling MR, Klein P, Aboumatar S, et al. Cenobamate (YKP3089) as adjunctive treatment for uncontrolled focal seizures in a large, phase 3, multicenter, open-label safety study. *Epilepsia*. 2020;61:1099–1108.

Zaccara G, Franciotta D, Perucca E. Idiosyncratic adverse reactions to antiepileptic drugs. *Epilepsia*. 2007;48:1223–1244.

Online Resources

Brivaracetam (Briviact). www.briviact.com/2020

Cannabidiol (Epidiolex). www.epidiolex.com/2020

Cenobamate (Xcopri). https://reference.medscape.com/drug/xcopri-cenobamate-1000328/2020

Eslicarbazine acetate (Aptiom). www.aptiom.com/2014.

Ezogabine (Potiga). www.potiga.com/ 2014.

Lacosamide (Vimpat). www.vimpat.com/2014.

Perampanel (Fycompa). us.eisai.com/wps/wcm/connect/Eisai/Home/Our.../FYCOMPA/ 2014.

Rufinamide (Banzel). www.banzel.com/ 2014.

Vigabatrin (Sabril). www.lundbeck.com/upload/us/files/.../Sabril/2014.

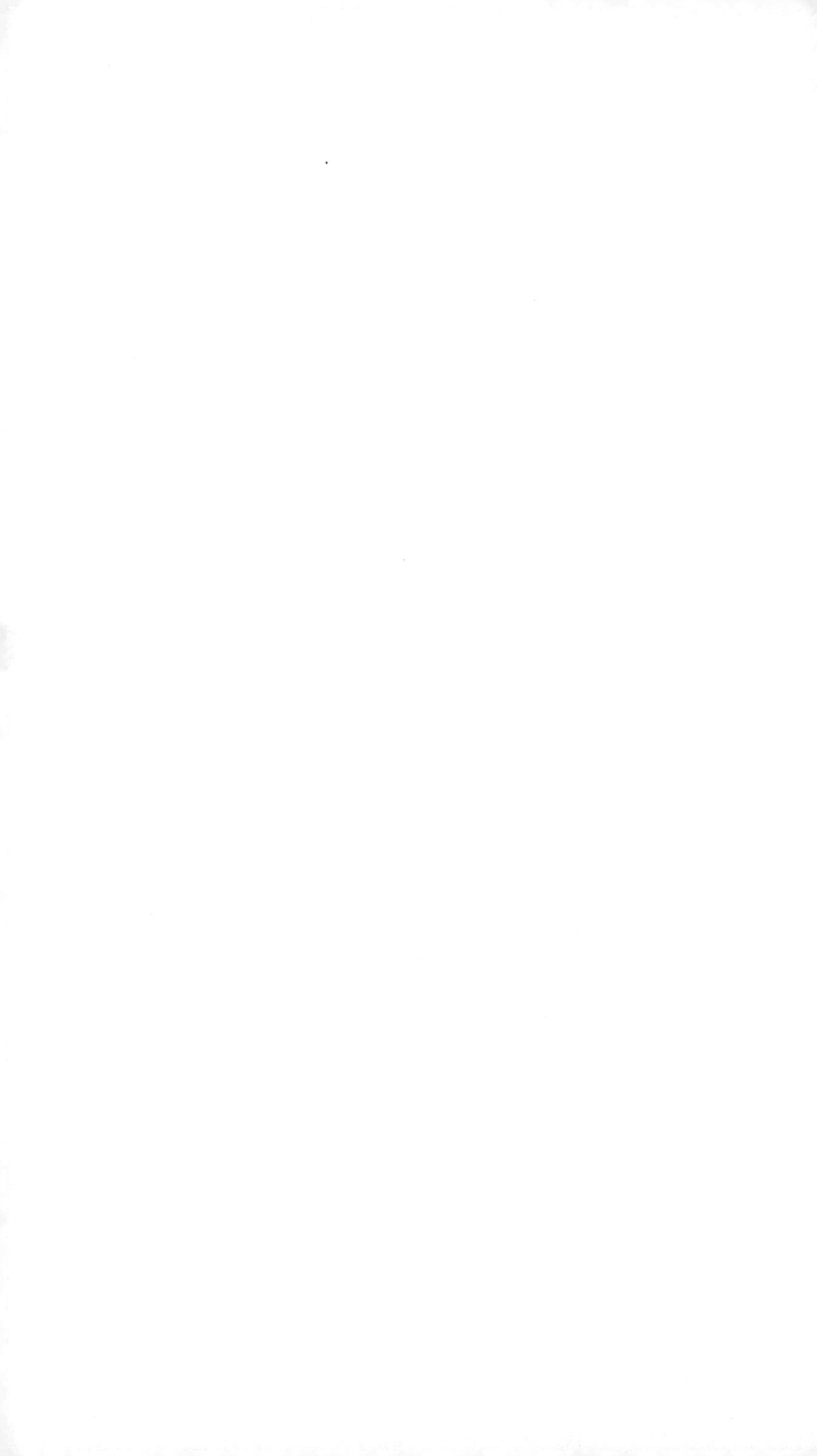

Chapter 28

Antiseizure Medications and Ophthalmologic Problems

Ophthalmologic problems in patients with epilepsy may be due to either the disease process or therapy with antiseizure medications (ASMs). Visual disturbances such as blurred vision, diplopia, and oscillopsia are generally benign, reversible, dose-dependent neurotoxic adverse effects of ASMs. The dose of medication simply needs to be reduced or the dosing frequency increased to abolish this complaint in most instances. However, some patients have visual complaints at relatively low serum levels, and the offending ASM must be stopped and replaced with another.

Other ocular complaints may be related to the unique mechanistic properties of the drug and can occur when they are administered at therapeutic levels. This is true of vigabatrin and ezogabine, which have special retinal toxicity that has greatly limited their use.

Antiseizure Medications and Ophthalmologic Problems

Ezogabine

Production of ezogabine was discontinued in June 2017. Ezogabine can cause abnormalities of the retina. These abnormalities have funduscopic features similar to those seen in retinal pigment dystrophies that are known to result in damage to photoreceptors and vision loss. Approximately one-third of those patients who had ophthalmologic examinations performed after 4 years of treatment were found to have retinal pigmentary abnormalities. Funduscopic abnormalities have most commonly been described as perivascular pigmentation (bone spicule pattern) in the retinal periphery and/or as areas of focal retinal pigment epithelium clumping. The rate of progression of retinal abnormalities and the reversibility after drug discontinuation are unknown.

Vigabatrin

Vigabatrin causes a visual disturbance (Bhattacharyya and Basu, 2005; Hilton et al., 2004). This is due to the concentration of vigabatrin in retinal glial cells that results in toxicity, ultimately affecting foveal and peripheral cone cells. Other ASMs that act on γ-aminobutyric acid (GABA)ergic pathways do not accumulate in the retina to the same extent as vigabatrin and do not have retinal toxicity.

The onset of vision loss from vigabatrin is unpredictable and can occur at any time after starting treatment. Symptoms of vision loss from vigabatrin are unlikely to be recognized by patients or caregivers before vision loss is severe. Vigabatrin-associated visual disturbances can be identified with electroretinograms and visual field perimetry. Perimetry defects characteristically present as bilateral concentric nasal constriction with temporal and central sparing, a pattern rarely seen in other conditions. Approximately, 30% (20–50%) of patients receiving the drug at normal therapeutic doses have visual field abnormalities (You et al., 2006). Men receiving vigabatrin are more susceptible to visual field constriction than are women, and adults are probably more susceptible than are children. The vast majority of patients with vigabatrin-associated visual field constriction are asymptomatic. In clinical practice, patients with visual field defects often remain asymptomatic until the defect impinges on, or is close to, fixation; this is particularly likely in the case of binasal defects where the preserved temporal visual field in each eye enables patients to retain good mobility. Longitudinal investigations of vigabatrin-associated visual field loss have reported the defects to be permanent, persisting even after patients are withdrawn from the drug (Hilton et al., 2004). However, visual field defects were found to be reversible in two children treated with vigabatrin when the drug was withdrawn (Nabbout, 2001).

For this reason, *vigabatrin is reserved for situations when no other drug offers hope* or when a short-term course of therapy is planned. *For children with tuberous sclerosis who have infantile spasms, the benefits of vigabatrin monotherapy appear to outweigh the risks* (Hilton et al., 2004; Nabbout, 2001; You et al., 2006). It is not clear that other conditions warrant the use of this agent. When treatment with vigabatrin is indicated, visual field testing (e.g., perimetry) should be carried out at the start of treatment (within 4 weeks of the start of treatment) and at regular time intervals (every 3 months); electroretinography may help detect abnormalities as well, perhaps before field loss appears (Figure 28.1). Finally, vigabatrin should be withdrawn from patients with drug-resistant focal seizures within 3 months of initiation and within 2–4 weeks of initiation for patients with infantile spasms who fail to show substantial clinical benefit.

Other Antiseizure Medications

Benzodiazepines

Benzodiazepines are reportedly contraindicated in patients with acute closed-angle glaucoma according to recommendations of the official drug information materials. However, a systematic review of the literature reveals that this contraindication is based on only one published case, while 22 other investigations, some of them controlled, found that benzodiazepines reduce intraocular pressure (Fritze et al., 2002). Hence, this recommendation is probably not valid and benzodiazepines may be used in patients with glaucoma.

Ophthalmoplegia has been reported consequent to administration of phenytoin, phenobarbital, primidone, and carbamazepine. Phenytoin can induce external ophthalmoplegia whether administered orally or intravenously.

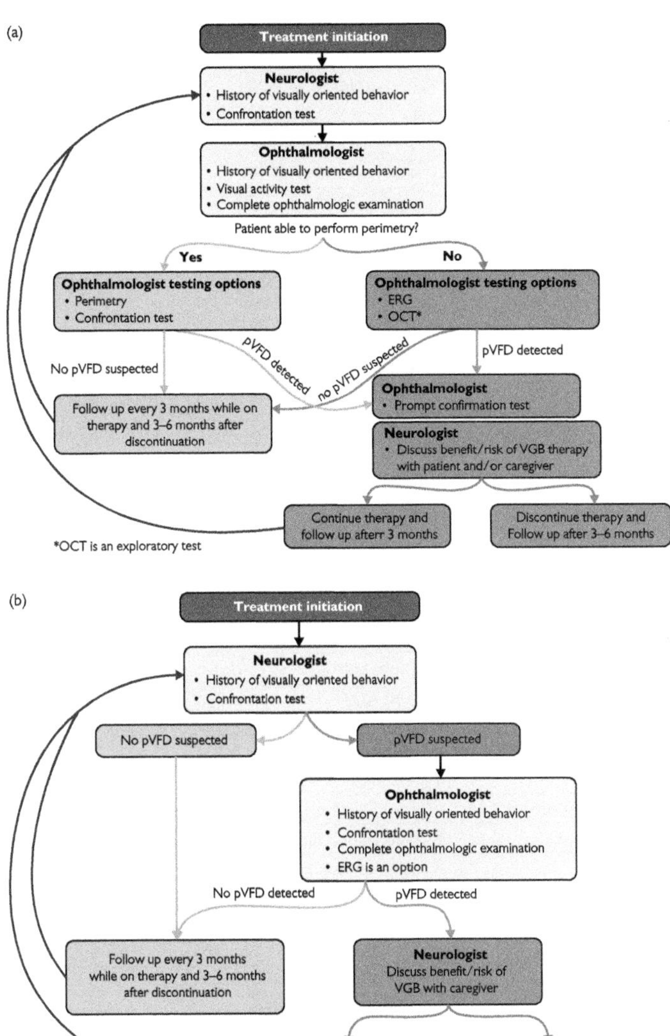

Figure 28.1. Recommended screening algorithm for patients with (a) focal seizures and (b) infantile spasms, taking vigabatrin.

ERG, Electroretinography; OCT, Optical coherence tomography; VGB, Vigabatrin; pVFD, Peripheral visual field defect.

Adapted from: Sergott RC, Wheless JW, Smith MC, Westall CA, Kardon RH, Arnold A, Foroozan R, Sagar SM. Evidence-based review of recommendations for visual function testing in patients treated with vigabatrin. *Neuro-Ophthalmol*. 2010; 34: 20–35.

Table 28.1 Visual adverse effects of antiseizure medications

Antiseizure medication	Visual adverse effects
Acetazolamide	Enhanced ocular blood flow, decreased intra ocular pressure
Benzodiazepine	Blurred vision, visual electrophysiological changes, maculopathy
Brivaracetam	–
Cannabidiol	–
Carbamazepine	Blurred vision, diplopia, abnormal color perception, nystagmus, oscillopsia (illusionary movements of objects), altered visual evoked potentials (VEPs), ophthalmoplegia
Cenobamate	Diplopia, blurred vision, impaired vision, nystagmus
Eslicarbazepine acetate	Diplopia, blurred vision, impaired vision, nystagmus
Ethosuximide	Photophobia, myopia
Ezogabine	Retinal pigmentary abnormalities, blurred vision, diplopia, nystagmus
Felbamate	Blurred vision, diplopia, miosis, hemianopia, conjunctivitis
Gabapentin	Amblyopia, blurred vision, nystagmus, diplopia, visual electrophysiological changes, impaired critical flicker frequency
Lacosamide	Diplopia, blurred vision, nystagmus
Lamotrigine	Blurred vision, diplopia, visual electrophysiological disturbances, nystagmus
Levetiracetam	Blurred vision, diplopia
Oxcarbazepine	Diplopia, blurred vision
Perampanel	Diplopia, blurred vision
Phenobarbital	Blurred vision, miosis, mydriasis, ophthalmoplegia
Phenytoin	Nystagmus, ophthalmoplegia, blurred vision, diplopia, disturbed color perception
Pregabalin	Blurred vision, diplopia, nystagmus, conjunctivitis
Primidone	Blurred vision, diplopia, nystagmus, ophthalmoplegia
Rufinamide	Diplopia, blurred vision, nystagmus
Tiagabine	Abnormal color perception, blurred vision, nystagmus, diplopia
Topiramate	Blurred vision, diplopia, acute myopia, acute angle closure glaucoma, suprachoroidal effusions, nystagmus, conjunctivitis
Valproate	Abnormal color perception, altered VEPs, blurred vision, diplopia, nystagmus
Vigabatrin	Diplopia, nystagmus, peripheral visual field loss, color perception abnormalities, retinal abnormalities, optic nerve pallor, visual electrophysiological changes, reduced contrast sensitivity, reduced ocular blood flow
Zonisamide	Blurred vision, diplopia, nystagmus, acute angle closure glaucoma

See individual drug websites listed in the Online Resources.

Incomplete as well as complete ophthalmoplegia has been reported with phenytoin even within therapeutic range (Fredericks et al., 1976; Puri and Chaudhry, 2004; Spector et al., 1976; see also individual drug websites listed in the Online Resources section of this chapter).

Topiramate

This drug can rarely cause acute myopia and secondary closed-angle glaucoma without pupillary block, likely related to carbonic anhydrase inhibition. This is more common in females, occur when serum levels are within a normal therapeutic range, and usually appear within the first month of therapy. The symptoms include an acute onset of decreased visual acuity and/or ocular pain; topiramate should be discontinued immediately. Ophthalmologic examination may reveal myopia, ocular hyperemia, shallowing of the anterior chamber, and elevated intraocular pressure, with or without pupil dilation; choroidal effusions have also been described. It has been suggested that supraciliary effusion and ciliary body swelling may displace the lens and iris anteriorly, secondarily resulting in angle closure glaucoma (Bhattacharyya and Basu, 2005; Hilton et al., 2004).

Zonisamide

Like topiramate, this drug is a sulfonamide and carbonic anhydrase inhibitor and there are rare case reports of closed-angle glaucoma and myopic shift (Weiler, 2015).

References

Bhattacharyya KB, Basu S. Acute myopia induced by topiramate: Report of a case and review of the literature. *Neurol India*. 2005;53:108–109.

Facts and Comparisons. *Drug Facts and Comparisons*. Wolters Kluwer Health/ Facts and Comparisons, St. Louis; 2007.

Fredericks CA, Giannotta SL, Sadun AA. Dilantin-induced long-term bilateral total external ophthalmoplegia. *Clin Neuro-Ophthalmol*. 1986;6:22–26.

Fritze J, Schneider B, Weber B. Benzodiazepines and benzodiazepine-like anxiolytics and hypnotics: The implausible contraindication of angle-closure glaucoma. *Nervenartz*. 2002;73:50–53.

Hilton EJR, Hosking SL, Betts T. The effect of antiepileptic drugs on visual performance. *Seizure*. 2004;13:113–128.

Nabbout R. A risk-benefit assessment of treatment for infantile spasms. *Drug Safety*. 2001;24:813–828.

Puri V, Chaudhry N. Total external ophthalmoplegia induced by phenytoin: A case report and review of literature. *Neurol India*. 2004;52:386–387.

Sergott RC, Wheless JW, Smith MC, et al. Evidence-based review of recommendations for visual function testing in patients treated with Vigabatrin. *Neuro-Ophthalmol*. 2010;34:20–35.

Spector RH, Davidoff RA, Schwartzman RJ. Phenytoin-induced ophthalmoplegia. *Neurology*.1976;26:1031.

Weiler DL. Zonisamide-induced angle closure and myopic shift. *Optomol Vis Sci*. 2015;92:e46–51.

You SJ, Ahn HS, Ko TS. Vigabatrin and visual field defects in pediatric epilepsy patients. *J Korean Med Sci*. 2006;21:728–732.

Online Resources

Brivaracetam (Briviact). www.briviact.com/2020

Cannabidiol (Epidolex). www.epidiolex.com/2020

Cenobamate (Xcopri). https://reference.medscape.com/drug/xcopri-cenobamate-1000328/2020

Eslicarbazine acetate (Aptiom). www.aptiom.com/2014

Ezogabine (Potiga). www.potiga.com/2014

Lacosamide (Vimpat). www.vimpat.com/2014

Perampanel (Fycompa). us.eisai.com/wps/wcm/connect/Eisai/Home/Our.../FYCOMPA/2014

Rufinamide (Banzel). www.banzel.com/2014

Vigabatrin (Sabril). www.lundbeck.com/upload/us/files/.../Sabril/2014

Chapter 29

Antiseizure Medications and Weight Change

Many patients experience weight change after starting an antiseizure medication (ASM). Some ASMs are associated with weight loss, some with weight gain, and others have no effect on weight. Weight gain is associated with an increased risk of comorbidities (e.g., type 2 diabetes, mellitus, and heart diseases) and impairs quality of life and self-esteem. Weight loss is also associated with comorbidity (e.g., osteoporosis and immune and metabolic problems) (Pickrell et al., 2013). Depending on comorbid conditions (i.e., chiefly obesity, diabetes, and, at times, poor appetite), one might consider choosing an ASM that may influence weight in a positive way. For example, an obese patient, particularly one who is diabetic, might secondarily benefit by taking an ASM that causes weight loss (e.g., topiramate). A patient with poor appetite who is underweight might profit by taking an ASM that causes weight gain. In any case, one must have knowledge of this ASM side effect and consider that it can be used to advantage in select patients.

The treating physician should adequately explain to patients the risks of weight change with ASM use; if not, patients may lose the opportunity to ameliorate the risk via prospectively monitoring their weight and executing early lifestyle changes. In addition, subsequent weight change may contribute to discontinuation of the associated ASM (Pickrell et al., 2013). Table 29.1 summarizes the effects of the various ASMs on weight and can be used as a guide.

Antiseizure Medications and Weight Change

Cannabidiol

In cannabidiol-treated patients, 16% had a decrease in weight of 5% or more from their baseline body weight, compared to 8% of patients on placebo. The decrease in weight appeared to be dose-related.

Carbamazepine

Weight gain has been reported in 2–25% of patients during carbamazepine therapy. This wide range suggests that the true incidence is not known. In the experience of the authors, significant weight gain is rare. Weight gain with carbamazepine could be related to water retention; however, increased appetite and increase in weight without edema have also been described (Jallon and Picard, 2001).

Table 29.1 Antiseizure medications and weight change

Weight gain	Weight loss	No effect on weight	Not defined
Valproate	Topiramate	Phenytoin	Phenobarbital
Pregabalin	Zonisamide	Lamotrigine	Ethosuximide
Gabapentin	Felbamate	Levetiracetam (?)	Brivaracetam
Vigabatrin	Acetazolamide (?)	Oxcarbazepine	—
Carbamazepine	Rufinamide	Tiagabine	—
Ezogabine	Cannabidiol	Eslicarbazepine	—
Perampanel	Cenobamate (?)	Lacosamide	—

From Futagi et al. (1996), Hogan et al. (2000), Jallon and Picard (2001), Asconapé (2002), Biton (2006), and Connor et al. (2006); see also individual drug websites listed in the Online Resources list at the end of this chapter.

Cenobamate

This drug may rarely be associated with weight loss.

Eslicarbazepine Acetate

No significant weight changes have been reported in patients taking this drug.

Ethosuximide

There is no evidence that ethosuximide affects weight.

Ezogabine

Ezogabine was associated with dose-related weight gain.

Felbamate

In clinical trials with felbamate, anorexia and weight loss were among the most common adverse events. Anorexia was reported in approximately 10–20% of patients; weight loss, which can be transient, is reported in up to 3–6% of patients. Weight loss with felbamate varies in severity. Among those older than 15 years, mean weight loss was almost 4% of the baseline weight. The mechanism by which felbamate affects weight is unknown. Patients who lose weight with felbamate nearly always report anorexia; therefore, reduction in caloric intake may be responsible for the reduction in weight (Biton, 2003).

Gabapentin

Weight gain up to more than 10% of the baseline weight during gabapentin therapy has been reported in about 6% of patients. The mechanisms of body weight gain with gabapentin could reflect the enhancement of γ-aminobutyric acid (GABA)-mediated inhibition in the medial hypothalamus (Jallon and Picard, 2001). Weight loss associated with anorexia has rarely been reported in some patients.

Lacosamide

No significant weight changes have been reported in patients taking this drug.

Lamotrigine

No significant weight changes have been reported in patients taking this drug.

Levetiracetam

No significant weight changes have been reported in patients taking this drug in most studies. One study reported significant weight gain associated with levetiracetam (Pickrell et al., 2013).

Oxcarbazepine

Weight gain or weight loss has infrequently been reported.

Perampanel

Perampanel-treated adults gained an average of 1.1 kg (2.5 lbs) compared to an average of 0.3 kg (0.7 lbs) in placebo-treated adults. The percentages of adults who gained at least 7% and 15% of their baseline body weight in perampanel-treated patients were 9.1% and 0.9%, respectively.

Phenobarbital

The effects of phenobarbital on weight change have not been studied well. No systematic changes have been observed.

Phenytoin

Phenytoin does not have significant effects on weight.

Pregabalin

Since the time pregabalin became available for routine clinical use, reports of weight gain associated with its use have been published. Studies suggest significant weight gain (>7%) in 15–20% of patients, depending on the dose (Elger et al., 2005).

Rufinamide

Decreased weight has been reported in patients receiving rufinamide both in the presence and absence of gastrointestinal symptoms.

Tiagabine

Weight gain was observed in 2% of patients taking tiagabine in preclinical trials, which is probably not significant.

Topiramate

Topiramate has been shown to have hypothalamic effects, which could explain the reduction in appetite (Eliasson et al., 2007). The anorectic effect of topiramate may be due to its antagonism of glutamate (Ioannides-Demos et al., 2005). Patients treated with topiramate experienced mean percent reductions in weight that were dose-dependent. Nine percent of patients taking 200–400 mg/day and up to 13% of patients receiving doses of greater than 600 mg/day will experience weight loss. Weight loss is highest in patients with a high body mass index (Biton, 2003). The weight loss may not persist over a period of years, however, and may be transient.

Valproic Acid, Valproate, Divalproex Sodium

As many as 50% of patients taking valproate experience weight gain (Isojarvi et al., 1996). The magnitude of weight gain varied substantially between studies from approximately 5 to 50 kg. Valproate may increase appetite for carbohydrates and reduce energy expenditure by enhancing GABA-mediated neurotransmission. It is not clear that whether this effect is dose-dependent. Rarely, anorexia with weight loss has been reported in patients taking this drug (Biton, 2003; Jallon and Picard, 2001).

Vigabatrin

As many as 47% of patients taking vigabatrin experience weight gain. Weight gain is not related to the occurrence of edema.

Zonisamide

More than one-quarter of patients taking zonisamide lost more than 5 lbs in one study. Zonisamide displays dose-dependent serotonergic and dopaminergic activities that may contribute to its anorectic effect (Gadde et al., 2003; Ioannides-Demos et al., 2005).

Recommended Antiseizure Medications in Obese Patients with Epilepsy

- *Generalized epilepsies*: Lamotrigine, cannabidiol (in patients with Lennox-Gastaut syndrome or Dravet syndrome), rufinamide (in patients with Lennox-Gastaut syndrome), topiramate, zonisamide
- *Focal epilepsies*: Brivaracetam, eslicarbazepine acetate, cenobamate, lacosamide, lamotrigine, phenytoin, topiramate, zonisamide

References

Asconapé JJ. Some common issues in the use of antiepileptic drugs. *Semin Neurol.* 2002;22:27–39.

Biton V. Effect of antiepileptic drugs on bodyweight: Overview and clinical implications for the treatment of epilepsy. *CNS Drugs*. 2003;17:781–791.

Biton V. Weight change and antiepileptic drugs. *Neurologist*. 2006;10:163–167.

Connor KM, Davidson JRT, Weisler RH, Zhang W, Abraham K. Tiagabine for posttraumatic stress disorder: Effect of open-label and double-blind discontinuation treatment. *Psychopharmacology*. 2006;184:21–25.

Elger CE, Brodie MJ, Anhut J, Lee CM, Barrett JA. Pregabalin add-on treatment in patients with partial seizures: A novel evaluation of flexible-dose and fixed-dose treatment in a double-blind, placebo-controlled study. *Epilepsia*. 2005;46:1926–1936.

Eliasson B, Gudbjornsdottir S, Cederholm J, Liang Y, Vercruysse F, Smith U. Weight loss and metabolic effects of topiramate in overweight and obese type 2 diabetic patients: randomized double-blind placebo-controlled trial. *Int J Obesity*. 2007;31:1140–1147.

Futagi Y, Otani K, Abe J. Growth suppression in children receiving acetazolamide with antiepileptic drugs. *Pediatr Neurol.* 1996;15:323–326.

Gadde KM, Franciscy DM, Wagner HR, et al. Zonisamide for weight loss in obese adults. *JAMA*. 2003;289:1820–1825.

Hogan RE, Bertrand ME, Deaton RL, Sommerville KW. Total percentage body weight changes during add-on therapy with tiagabine, carbamazepine and phenytoin. *Epilepsy Res*. 2000;41:23–28.

Ioannides-Demos LL, Proietto J, McNeil JJ. Pharmacotherapy for obesity. *Drugs*. 2005;65:1391–1418.

Isojarvi JI, Laatikainen TJ, Knip M, Pakarinen AJ, Juntunen KT, Myllyla VV. Obesity and endocrine disorders in women taking valproate for epilepsy. *Ann Neurol*. 1996;39:579–584.

Jallon P, Picard F. Bodyweight gain and anticonvulsants: A comparative review. *Drug Safety*. 2001;24:969–978.

Pickrell WO, Lacey AS, Thomas RH, Smith PE, Rees MI. Weight change associated with antiepileptic drugs. *J Neurol Neurosurg Psychiatry*. 2013;84(7):796–799.

Online Resources

Brivaracetam (Briviact). www.briviact.com/2020

Cannabidio (Epidiolex). www.epidiolex.com/2020

Cenobamate (Xcopri). https://reference.medscape.com/drug/xcopri-cenobamate-1000328/2020

Eslicarbazine acetate (Aptiom). www.aptiom.com/2014

Lacosamide (Vimpat). www.vimpat.com/2014

Micromedex Healthcare Series. Internet Database. Greenwood Village, CO: Thompson Healthcare. Updated periodically.

Perampanel (Fycompa). us.eisai.com/wps/wcm/connect/Eisai/Home/Our.../FYCOMPA/2014

Rufinamide (Banzel) www.banzel.com/2014

Tiagabine (Gabitril). Cephalon, Inc. Gabitril. http://www.gabitril.com/download/148–3230 EnlargedPI.pdf

Topiramate (Topamax). Janssen Pharm. Inc. http://www.topamax.com/topamax/assets/topamax.pdf/ 2012

Vigabatrin (Sabril). www.lundbeck.com/upload/us/files/.../Sabril/2014

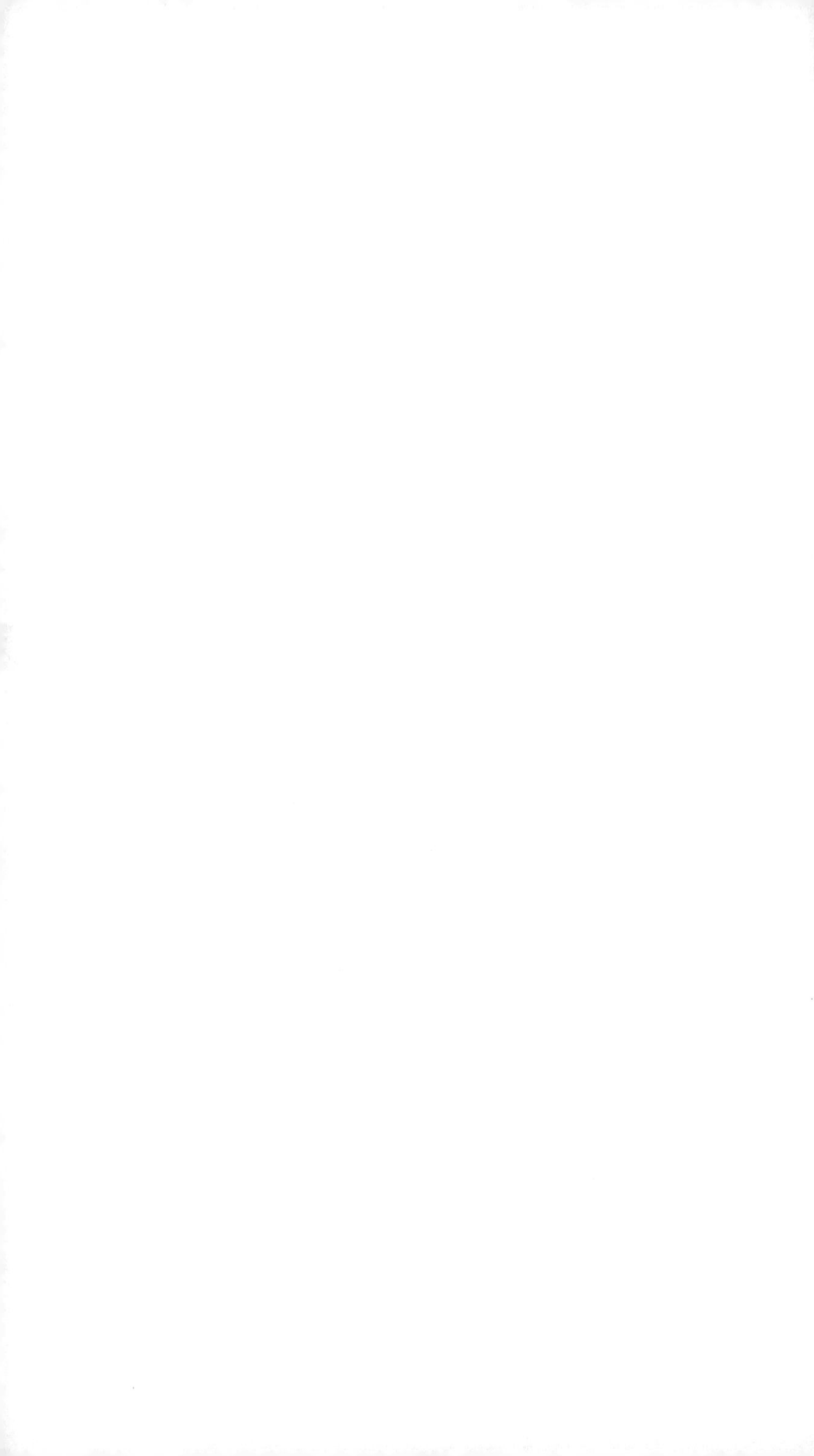

Chapter 30

Antiseizure Medications and Bone Health

Patients taking antiseizure medications (ASMs) have higher rates of osteopenia, osteoporosis, and bone fractures than the general population (Beniczky et al., 2012; Gissel et al., 2007). Bone loss mediated by ASMs affects patients of all ages, irrespective of sex. Studies evaluating bone density in patients recruited from epilepsy clinics suggest that the rate of osteopenia and osteoporosis generally is 40–75% and that the magnitude of the reduction in real bone mineral density may be as high as 16% (Petty et al., 2005); although other studies have found varying percentages, all have found a relatively high prevalence of bone demineralization in people with epilepsy. Decrease in bone mineral density leads to increased bone fragility and, hence, greater risk of fracture. When one considers that people with epilepsy have a greater propensity for falls as well, the reduction in bone density has even greater importance than usual.

There are probably multiple causes of the increased rate of osteopenia and osteoporosis in people with epilepsy. They may be caused in part by effects of the disease on lifestyle and income. People with epilepsy may have reduced activity levels compared with the general population and tend to have lower incomes, which might impact dietary habits. However, ASMs probably cause reduced bone density by virtue of their metabolic effects. Most of the available data describe bone density and metabolism in patients taking older ASMs (phenytoin, phenobarbital, carbamazepine, and valproate), although information is becoming available about some of the newer ASMs (Beniczky et al., 2012; Mintzer et al., 2006). This chapter briefly reviews how ASMs can produce bone demineralization and how this might be prevented.

Evidence suggests that ASMs may have negative effects on bone mineral density through a variety of mechanisms (Ali et al., 2004). Decrease in bone mineral density is thought to be related to decreased intestinal absorption of calcium, accelerated vitamin D hydroxylation to inactive forms, increased bone turnover, impairment of parathyroid hormone (PTH)-induced calcium mobilization, interference with vitamin K metabolism, inhibition of osteocalcin, increased urinary loss of calcium and phosphorus due to renal tubular dysfunction, and probably other mechanisms. There is an extensive body of literature that suggests that ASMs can produce hypocalcemia, hypophosphatemia, increased alkaline phosphatase levels, a slight increase in the parathormone level, and a decrease in biologically active vitamin D levels.

The mechanism of bone loss is uncertain. Many of the above-cited adverse effects can be attributed to induction of the cytochrome P-450 system enzymes by many ASMs. Carbamazepine, phenytoin, phenobarbital, and primidone, all enzyme inducers, increase the metabolism of vitamin D and its active metabolite, lowering their serum levels. Decreased vitamin D levels may result in decreased calcium absorption, secondary hyperparathyroidism, and decrease in bone density (Babayigit et al., 2006). Oxcarbazepine also significantly reduces 25-hydroxy vitamin-D levels and increases bone-specific alkaline phosphatase, which is a marker of bone formation (Mintzer et al., 2006). The effects of ASMs may be additive (when used as polytherapy) (Farhat et al., 2002; Shen et al., 2014). While the theoretical basis for enzyme-inducing ASMs causing decreased bone density seems strong, the association of valproate, a cytochrome P-450 inhibitor (Babayigit et al., 2006; Gissell et al., 2007), and non–enzyme-inducing ASMs (e.g., gabapentin) with osteoporosis raises the possibility that a more complex picture exists (Ensrud et al., 2008; Shen et al., 2014). Valproic acid, as an inhibitor of hepatic microsomal enzymes, exerts its detrimental effects on bone health through several mechanisms, including induction of vitamin D catabolism, reduction of osteoblast proliferation, and decrease in collagen synthesis (Miziak et al., 2019). Some data suggest that lamotrigine may not have a deleterious effect on metabolic indices (Pack et al., 2005; Sheth and Hermann, 2007). Levetiracetam, which has no effect on hepatic microsomal enzymes, also may have harmful effects on bone (El-Haggar et al., 2018). However, data regarding the effects of levetiracetam and oxcarbazepine on bone health in human and animal studies are conflicting (Beniczky et al., 2012; Fekete et al., 2013; Koo et al., 2013, 2014). Data regarding the effects of the newer ASMs (e.g., brivaracetam, lacosamide, perampanel, etc.) on bone health are not available yet.

What advice can a physician offer patients who take ASMs? Table 30.1 summarizes recommendations for patient care.

Table 30.1 Recommendations for patients taking antiseizure medications

General recommendations for all patients	Engage in daily regular weight-bearing physical activity (provided medically safe). Maintain a balanced diet rich in protein, calcium and vitamin D. Stop smoking. Minimize caffeine intake. Minimize alcohol intake. Take 1,000–1,500 mg of calcium (nutrition and supplement) daily Check serum vitamin D levels and, if low, take 1,000 IU vitamin D supplement with non–enzyme-inducing ASMs and 2,000 IU with enzyme-inducing ASMs daily.
Additional recommendations for patients with osteopenia or osteoporosis	Follow all the general recommendations. Take higher doses of vitamin D daily. For osteoporosis, treat with an appropriate pharmaceutical agent to enhance bone formation (e.g., bisphosphonate, alendronate, denosumab, teriparatide, and others). Consult an endocrinologist if needed.

From: Petty et al. (2005), Mintzer et al. (2006), Gissel et al. (2007), and Meier & Kraenzlin (2011).

Given the tendency of many ASMs to produce bone loss, measurement of bone density may be useful during the course of therapy. A baseline dual-energy x-ray absorptiometry (DEXA) scan might be performed at the start of therapy for patients at significant risk for osteopenia or osteoporosis. Risks for decreased bone density include being nonambulatory or relatively inactive, institutionalized, or excessively thin. Postmenopausal women and patients with other medical risk factors such as concomitant steroid therapy are also at high risk. For patients not at risk, controversy exists over the value of a baseline DEXA scan, and one might wait until ASM therapy has been taken for 5 years before performing this test. In children, some have recommended performing a DEXA scan even sooner, after 1 year of ASM therapy in low-risk patients and after 6 months in high-risk patients (Kothare and Kaleyias, 2007). If there is evidence for decreased bone density on the DEXA scan, measure serum calcium, alkaline phosphatase, and 25-hydroxy vitamin D levels and consider increasing doses of calcium and vitamin supplementation. When patients take either agents presently known to cause osteoporosis or safer agents, serial scans during the course of therapy are prudent and should be done every 1.5–3 years, depending on the results of the baseline DEXA scan.

A systematic review and meta-analysis showed that use of ASMs was associated with an 86% increase in the risk of fractures at any site and a 90% increase in the risk of hip fractures. When the authors restricted the analysis to osteoporosis-related fractures, the risk remained higher, confirming the detrimental effect of ASMs on bone health. Among users of enzyme-inducing ASMs and users of non–enzyme-inducing ASMs, they found a significant difference in fracture risk, though the risks in both groups were higher compared with those in non-user controls (Shen et al., 2014).

For the patient who must be started on drug therapy, the higher potential for development of osteoporosis with enzyme-inducing ASMs provides an impetus to prescribe an ASM such as lamotrigine that has not been associated with increased bone turnover. This may cause less bone turnover and pose less risk for bone health. Should a patient presently take an enzyme-inducing drug or valproate, extra attention should be paid to bone health and calcium intake. In the absence of a problem, the commonsense measures already advised should be taken.

If a physician diagnoses osteoporosis or osteopenia in a patient who is presently taking an enzyme-inducing drug or valproate, what should be done? If the seizures are well-controlled, there may be more risk of seizure recurrence if the ASM is changed, and patients may be reluctant to switch drugs. In that case, calcium and vitamin D supplements should be prescribed at a minimum, in combination with a pharmaceutical agent to enhance bone formation (e.g., bisphosphonate or alendronate) (Table 30.1). A follow-up DEXA scan should be performed in 1 year to assess response. If bone density is improved, then therapy does not need to be altered, and bone density can be monitored over the succeeding years. However, should these medical measures prove ineffective without improvement on subsequent bone density scans, then it is advisable to switch the patient to a safer, non–enzyme-inducing ASM.

References

Ali II, Schuh L, Barkley GL, Gates JR. Antiepileptic drugs and reduced bone mineral density. *Epilepsy Behav*. 2004;5:296–300.

Babayigit A, Dirik E, Bober E, Cakmakci H. Adverse effects of antiepileptic drugs on bone mineral density. *Pediatr Neurol*. 2006;35:177–181.

Beniczky SA, Viken J, Jensen LT, Andersen NB. Bone mineral density in adult patients treated with various antiepileptic drugs. *Seizure*. 2012;21(6):471–472.

El-Haggar SM, Mostafa TM, Allah HMS, Akef GH. Levetiracetam and lamotrigine effects as mono- and polytherapy on bone mineral density in epileptic patients. *Arq Neuropsiquiatr*. 2018;76:452–458.

Farhat G, Yamout B, Mikati MA, Demirjian S, Sawaya R, El-Hajj Fuleihan G. Effect of antiepileptic drugs on bone density in ambulatory patients. *Neurology*. 2002;58:1348–1353.

Fekete S, Simko J, Gradosova I, Malakova J, Zivna H, Palicka V, Zivny P. The effect of levetiracetam on rat bone mass, structure and metabolism. *Epilepsy Res*. 2013;107(1–2):56–60.

Gissel T, Poulsen CS, Vestergaard P. Adverse effects of antiepileptic drugs on bone mineral density in children. *Exp Opin Drug Safety*. 2007;6:267–278.

Koo DL, Hwang KJ, Han SW, et al. Effect of oxcarbazepine on bone mineral density and biochemical markers of bone metabolism in patients with epilepsy. *Epilepsy Res*. 2014;108(3):442–447.

Koo DL, Joo EY, Kim D, Hong SB. Effects of levetiracetam as a monotherapy on bone mineral density and biochemical markers of bone metabolism in patients with epilepsy. *Epilepsy Res*. 2013;104(1–2):134–139.

Kothare SV, Kaleyias J. The adverse effects of antiepileptic drugs in children. *Exp Opin Drug Safety*. 2007;6:251–265.

Meier C, Kraenzlin ME. Antiepileptics and bone health. *Ther Adv Musculoskelet Dis*. 2011;3(5):235–243.

Mintzer S, Boppana P, Toguri J, DeSantis A. Vitamin D levels and bone turnover in epilepsy patients taking carbamazepine or oxcarbazepine. *Epilepsia*. 2006;47:510–515.

Miziak B, Chroscinska-Krawczyk M, Czuczwar S J. An update on the problem of osteoporosis in people with epilepsy taking antiepileptic drugs. *Expert Opin Drug Safety*. 2019;18:679–689.

Pack AM, Morrell MJ, Marcus R, et al. Bone mass and turnover in women with epilepsy on antiepileptic drug monotherapy. *Ann Neurol*. 2005;57:252–257.

Petty SJ, Paton LM, O'Brien TJ, et al. Effect of antiepileptic medication on bone mineral measures. *Neurology*. 2005;65:1358–1365.

Shen C, Chen F, Zhang Y, Guo Y, Ding M. Association between use of antiepileptic drugs and fracture risk: A systematic review and meta-analysis. *Bone*. 2014;64:246–253.

Sheth RD, Hermann BP. Bone mineral density with lamotrigine monotherapy for epilepsy. *Pediatr Neurol*. 2007;37:250–254.

Chapter 31

Antiseizure Medications in Patients with HIV Infection/AIDS

Central nervous system (CNS) complications occur in 39–70% of patients with HIV/AIDS (Siddiqi and Birbeck 2013). The incidence of seizures may be as high as 11% in HIV-infected patients (Kellinghaus et al., 2007; Liedtke et al., 2004). The etiology of seizures among patients with HIV/AIDS has a long list, including acute symptomatic (provoked) causes, CNS opportunistic infections, malignancy, stroke, dementia, and immune reconstitution inflammatory syndrome, among others. Though generalized seizures certainly exist in patients with HIV/AIDS, these are almost certainly due to preexisting genetic risks. Focal seizures more often occur in these individuals and may or may not be related to HIV. Since provoked seizures are especially common among patients with HIV/AIDS, it is important to thoroughly evaluate the underlying cause of the seizure. A clinical assessment looking for sources of infection is needed, and investigations should include serum glucose, sodium, calcium, magnesium, and creatinine levels; liver function tests; complete blood count; CD4 count; blood cultures; urine cultures; a toxicology screen; a chest X-ray; neuroimaging; and cerebrospinal fluid (CSF) examination. Electroencephalography (EEG) may be helpful in evaluating seizure recurrence risk and can distinguish encephalopathy from nonconvulsive status epilepticus in patients with a decreased level of consciousness (Leitinger et al., 2015; Siddiqi and Birbeck 2013).

Although it is more common for patients with HIV/AIDS to subsequently develop epilepsy, people with epilepsy can certainly contract HIV. It is recommended that antiretroviral drugs be initiated in all HIV-infected individuals, thus antiretroviral and antiseizure medication (ASM) coadministration is nearly unavoidable in this population. A discussion with the HIV physician is warranted. Ideally, an effective antiretroviral drug regimen with no clinically important drug interaction with the patient's established effective ASM therapy should be selected. When this is not possible, a transition to another ASM (discussed later) is needed. Recurrent seizures or increased seizure frequency should be evaluated more carefully in patients with epilepsy and HIV. One should maintain a low threshold for repeat neuroimaging and lumbar puncture in a person with HIV and epilepsy to ensure that no underlying HIV-related pathology is contributing to seizure recurrence or exacerbation (Siddiqi and Birbeck 2013).

When a patient with HIV/AIDS presents with an acute seizure, controlling the seizure is more important than concerns of compromising HIV therapy. Status epilepticus should be managed with a standard, routinely applied protocol. After controlling the acute seizure, an evaluation must commence to assess the underlying etiology, risk of seizure recurrence, and the need to start an ASM. If seizure recurrence, abnormal imaging, or abnormal EEG findings support chronic ASM therapy, then careful consideration must be given to drug selection. The patient may need transition from the medication used acutely to something suitable for long-term use (Figure 31.1) (Siddiqi and Birbeck, 2013).

The combination regimens used to treat HIV infection often include substrates, inducers, and inhibitors of several cytochrome P-450 isoenzymes. Complex interactions may occur when some ASMs are administered to patients receiving treatment for HIV infection (see Chapter 6). The choice of an appropriate ASM can therefore be challenging. For example, phenobarbital, phenytoin, and carbamazepine have complex drug-drug interactions and are suboptimal in these patients (Asconapé, 2018; Liedtke et al., 2004). In contrast, levetiracetam, lacosamide, gabapentin, and brivaracetam are ideal ASMs for patients with HIV/AIDS (Asconapé, 2018; Siddiqi and Birbeck, 2013). Although the choice of ASM must consider efficacy against a seizure type or syndrome, it is equally important to address comorbid illnesses and comedications (Liedtke et al., 2004; Mullin et al., 2004; Romanelli et al., 2000). When ASMs that have pharmacokinetic interactions must be used, dose adjustments of antiretroviral agents may be needed and closer monitoring of this therapy is advised.

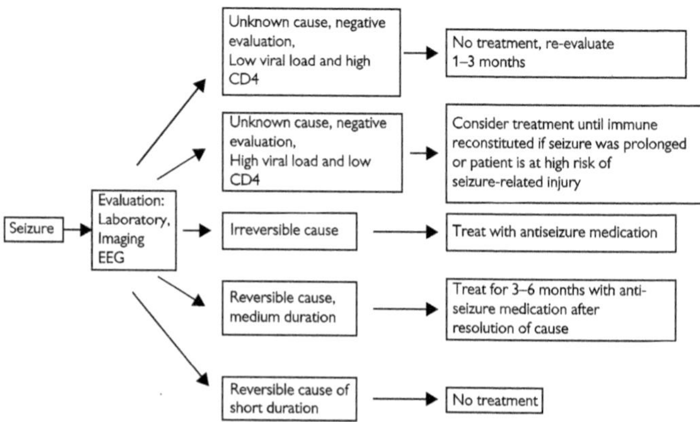

Figure 31.1 Algorithm for treatment of seizure in patients with HIV/AIDS.

ASM: Antiseizure medication; ARV: Antiretroviral; CSF: Cerebrospinal fluid; EEG: Electroencephalography.

Adapted from: Siddiqi O, Birbeck GL. Safe treatment of seizures in the setting of HIV/AIDS. *Curr Treat Options Neurol.* 2013;15: 529–543.

Recommended Antiseizure Medications in Patients with HIV Infection/AIDS

- *Generalized epilepsies*: Levetiracetam, lacosamide
- *Focal epilepsies*: Brivaracetam, gabapentin, lacosamide, levetiracetam

References

Asconapé JJ. Pharmacokinetic considerations with the use of antiepileptic drugs in patients with HIV and organ transplants. *Curr Neurol Neurosci Rep*. 2018;18:89.

Kellinghaus C, Engbring C, Kovac S, et al. Frequency of seizures and epilepsy in neurological HIV-infected patients. *Seizure*. 2008;17(1):27–33.

Leitinger M, Beniczky S, Rohracher A, Gardella E, Kalss G, Qerama E, et al. Salzburg Consensus Criteria for non-convulsive status epilepticus: Approach to clinical application. *Epilepsy Behav*. 2015;49:158–163.

Liedtke MD, Lockhart SM, Rathbun RC. Anticonvulsants and antiretroviral interactions. *Ann Pharmacother*. 2004;38:482–489.

Mullin P, Green G, Bakshi R. Special populations: The management of seizures in HIV-positive patients. *Curr Neurol Neurosci Rep*. 2004;4:308–314.

Romanelli F, Jennings HR, Nath A, Ryan M, Berger J. Therapeutic dilemma: The use of anticonvulsants in HIV-positive individuals. *Neurology*. 2000;54:1404–1407.

Siddiqi O, Birbeck GL. Safe treatment of seizures in the setting of HIV/AIDS. *Curr Treat Options Neurol*. 2013;15(4):529–543.

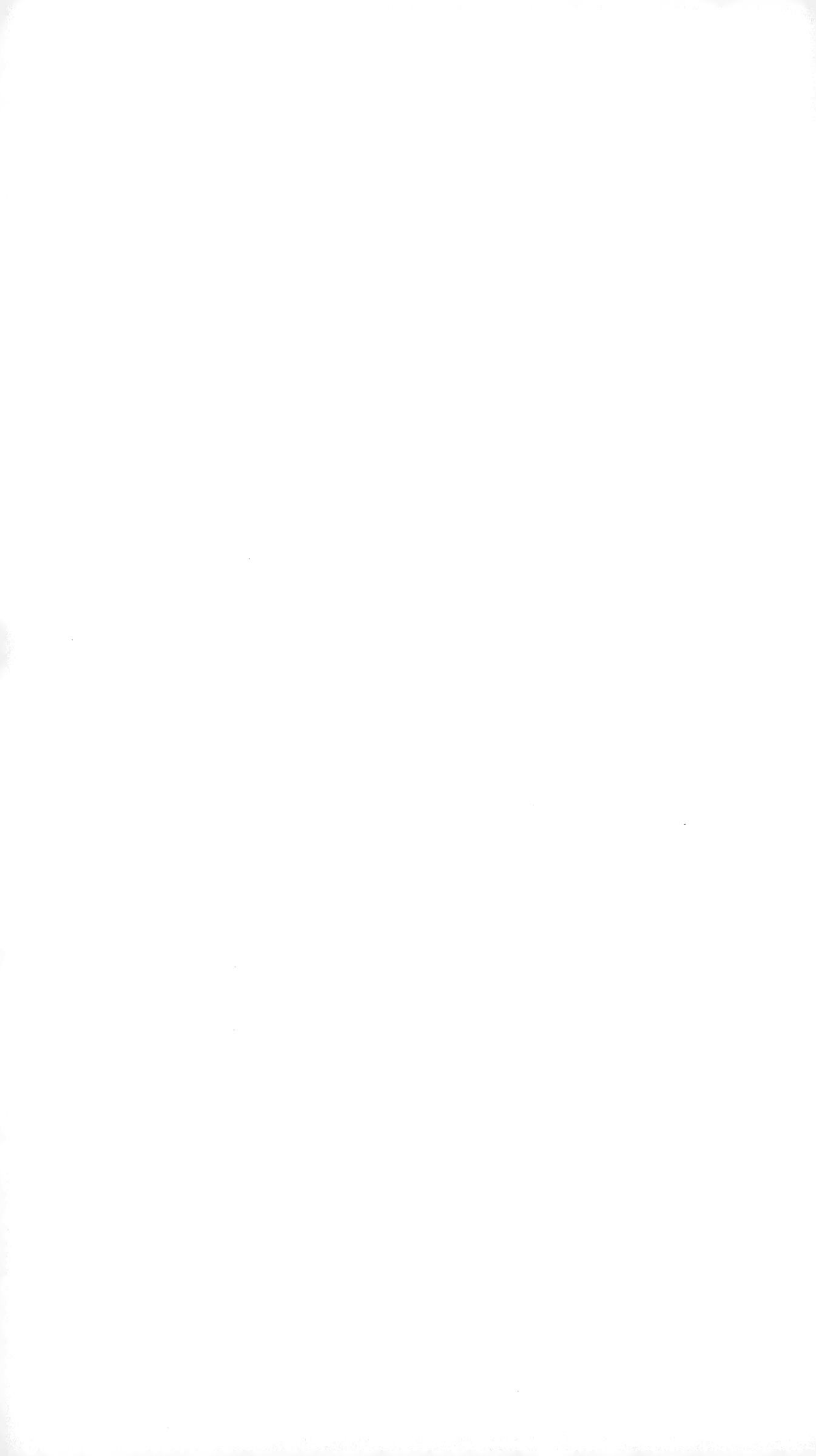

Chapter 32

Antiseizure Medications in Patients with Coronavirus Infections

Coronavirus is one of the major viruses that primarily targets the human respiratory system, but it may invade the central nervous system (CNS), spreading from nasal mucosa or respiratory tract to the CNS itself. Previous epidemics or pandemics of coronaviruses include the severe acute respiratory syndrome (SARS) in 2002 and the Middle East respiratory syndrome (MERS) in 2012. The most recent pandemic of coronavirus infection is coronavirus disease (COVID-19) that is caused by SARS-CoV2 (Wiersinga et al., 2020). Common symptoms of COVID-19 illness include fever, cough, and fatigue. In the most severe cases, patients may develop pneumonia, acute respiratory distress syndrome, acute cardiac problems, and multiorgan failure.

In general, it appears that people with COVID-19 are unlikely to develop seizures (Lu et al., 2020). However, patients critically ill with COVID-19 may develop seizures as a consequence of hypoxia, metabolic derangements, organ failure, or cerebral damage (Asadi-Pooya and Simani 2020). In critically ill patients, isolated seizures can quickly escalate to generalized convulsive status epilepticus or, more frequently, nonconvulsive status epilepticus (NCSE), which is associated with a high morbidity and mortality (Ch'ang and Claassen, 2017). When examining a patient who is critically ill and has a change in mental status, one should ensure that NCSE is not present (Sutter et al., 2016). Salzburg Consensus Criteria for Non-Convulsive Status Epilepticus is a helpful guide to make a diagnosis of NCSE in critically ill patients (Leitinger et al., 2015).

In a critically ill patient, seizures add to the burden of morbidity and increase mortality rates; seizures should be aborted immediately and prevented from recurring. In such circumstances, the treating physician should try to determine the cause of the seizure and promptly manage that cause (e.g., hypoxia, metabolic derangements). However, it is often necessary to start antiseizure medication (ASM) therapy as well to abort prolonged seizures and also to prevent further seizures from happening. In the case of serial seizures or status epilepticus, general management principles should be applied. Rescue treatment (with benzodiazepines) and an ASM should be started to abort the seizure and also prevent further seizures. In case of a single seizure lasting less than 5 minutes, there is no need for a rescue treatment (with benzodiazepines; these drugs should be used with caution in patients with compromised respiratory function), and an ASM should be started to prevent further. Ideally, these drugs are loaded so that a therapeutic level is reached quickly and then a suitable maintenance dose can be given. Since these patients are critically ill, a drug with IV formulation is preferable. However, because these patients suffer from severe respiratory and/or cardiac problems, drugs with significant respiratory or cardiac adverse effects (e.g., phenytoin, phenobarbital) should be avoided. Lacosamide, brivaracetam, and levetiracetam are safe treatment options in these patients. Dosage adjustment of brivaracetam is recommended for all stages of hepatic impairment. Dosage adjustment of levetiracetam and lacosamide is necessary in patients with renal impairment (Brigo et al., 2019; Trinka et al., 2017).

Recommended Antiseizure Medications in Patients with Coronavirus Infections

Brivaracetam, lacosamide, levetiracetam

Coronavirus Infection in People with Epilepsy

Management of COVID-19 in patients with epilepsy is complicated. Remdesivir and steroids appear to provide benefit for people with COVID-19. But remdesivir is metabolized by liver, and therefore drug exposure could be reduced in patients taking ASMs that induce hepatic microsomal enzymes (Yang, 2020) (review Table 6.1 for ASM effects on liver metabolism).

Antibodies used as treatment for COVID-19 are unlikely to be affected by ASMs. In addition, cardiac (see Chapter 17), hepatic (see Chapter 13) or renal (see Chapter 12) derangements, which may happen in patients with severe COVID-19, may require adjustment to ASMs in people with epilepsy. Finally, some therapies currently under investigation for the treatment of COVID-19 have significant cardiovascular adverse effects (e.g., QT prolongation). Similarly, many ASMs have significant cardiovascular adverse effects (see Chapter 17). In any patient with epilepsy who is being treated for COVID-19, therapeutic drug monitoring could provide valuable information to adjust the drug dosages (see Chapter 4). Close clinical monitoring of the patient is warranted to ensure adequate efficacy and limit toxicity.

References

Asadi-Pooya AA, Simani L. Central nervous system manifestations of COVID-19: A systematic review. *J Neurol Sci*. 2020 Apr 11;413:116832. doi:10.1016/j.jns.2020.116832.

Brigo F, Lattanzi S, Nardone R, Trinka E. Intravenous brivaracetam in the treatment of status epilepticus: A systematic review. *CNS Drugs*. 2019;33:771–781.

Ch'ang J, Claassen J. Seizures in the critically ill. *Handb Clin Neurol*. 2017;141:507–529.

Leitinger M, Beniczky S, Rohracher A, Gardella E, Kalss G, Qerama E, et al. Salzburg Consensus Criteria for Non-Convulsive Status Epilepticus: Approach to clinical application. *Epilepsy Behav*. 2015;49:158–163.

Lu L, Xiong W, Liu D, et al. New onset acute symptomatic seizure and risk factors in coronavirus disease 2019: A retrospective multicenter study. *Epilepsia*. 2020;61:e49–e53.

Sutter R, Semmlack S, Kaplan PW. Nonconvulsive status epilepticus in adults: Insights into the invisible. *Nat Rev Neurol*. 2016;12:281–293.

Trinka E, Kälviäinen R. 25 years of advances in the definition, classification and treatment of status epilepticus. *Seizure*. 2017;44:65–73.

Wiersinga WJ, Rhodes A, Cheng AC, Peacock SH, Prescott HC. Pathophysiology, transmission, diagnosis, and treatment of coronavirus disease 2019 (COVID-19). *JAMA*. 2020;324:782–793.

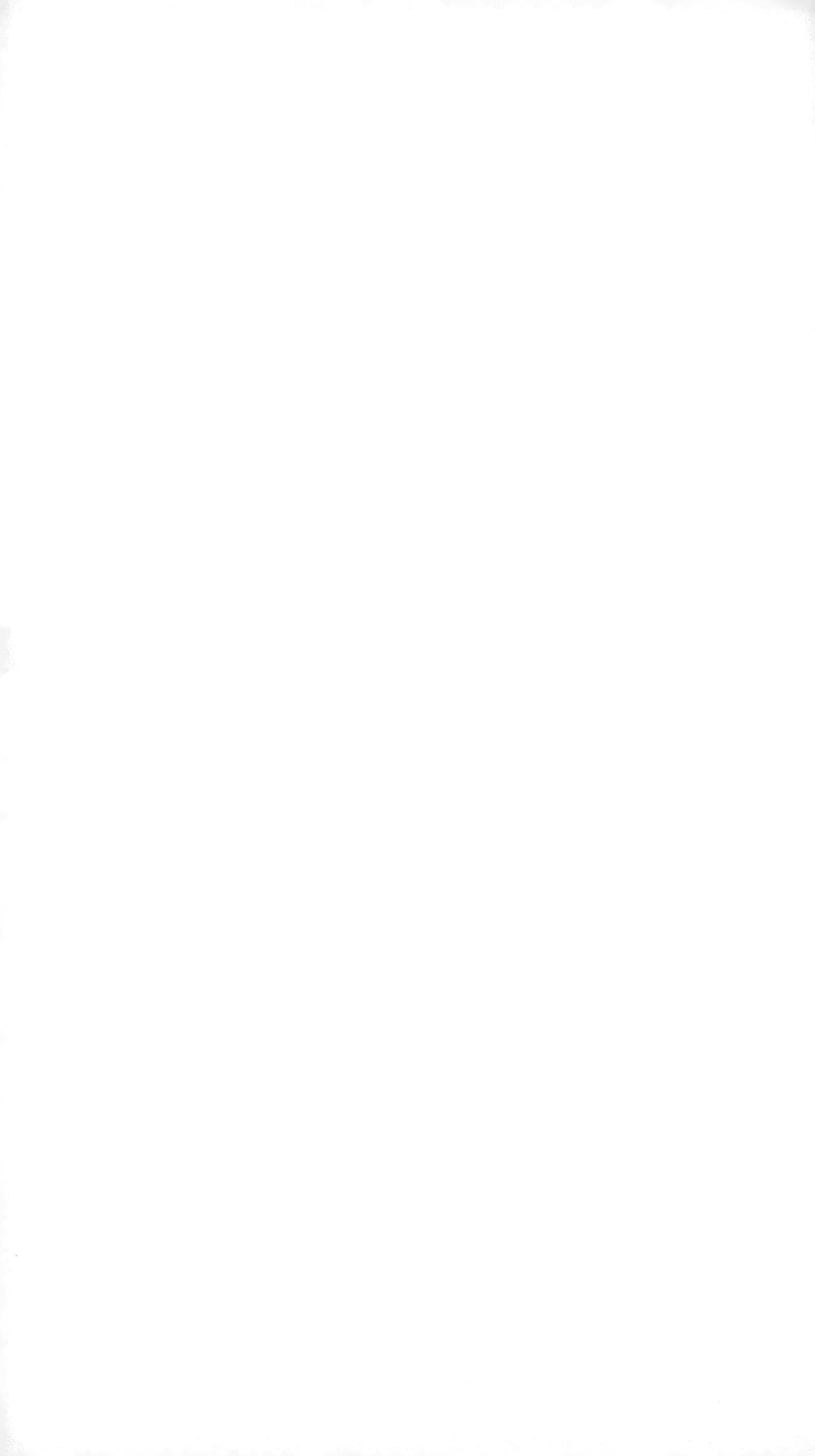

Chapter 33

Antiseizure Medications in the Pipeline

More than 30% of people with epilepsy have persistent seizures despite the use of appropriate therapies: these patients have drug-resistant epilepsy (Chen et al., 2018). Therefore investigating and discovering new medications to treat epilepsy is of paramount significance. There are multiple dugs in the pipeline to treat epilepsy. In this chapter, we briefly review some of these new antiseizure medications (ASMs).

Alprazolam

Alprazolam has long been used for treatment of anxiety. An inhaled formulation is in investigational trials as a rescue medication for seizure clusters or prolonged seizures. This drug is delivered via a novel approach, the *Staccato inhalation system*, that aerosolizes the drug and delivers it to the lungs without requiring patient cooperation for inhalation. The large surface area of the lungs allows for rapid absorption, with nearly immediate delivery to the brain without first-pass hepatic metabolism. This drug holds promise for rapid termination of those seizures that occur in clusters and prolonged seizures.

CVL-865

This agent is a γ-aminobutyric acid (GABA)-A receptor-positive allosteric modulator under investigation for the treatment of focal seizures. It may reduce the propensity for seizures by enhancing inhibitory mechanisms.

Fenfluramine Hydrochloride (ZX008)

ZX008 (low-dose fenfluramine HCl) is under investigation as an adjunctive treatment of Dravet syndrome. It may also have antiseizure effects in patients with Lennox-Gastaut syndrome (Bialer et al., 2018; Pierce and Mithal, 2020). The most common treatment-related adverse effects of fenfluramine are mild to moderate somnolence, fatigue, and anorexia. The metabolism of fenfluramine is via multiple CYP hepatic enzymes; it may have significant drug interactions (Bialer et al., 2018).

Ganaxolone

Ganaxolone, a synthetic analog of the progesterone metabolite allopregnanolone, is a positive allosteric modulator of the GABA-A receptor (Bialer et al., 2018). Ganaxolone has orphan epilepsy indications for refractory status epilepticus and CDKL5 deficiency disorder. The most frequently reported adverse effects are central nervous system (CNS)-related and included somnolence, dizziness, fatigue, and headache. Drug interactions are not significant (Bialer et al., 2018).

Anakinra

Anakinra, a protein consisting of 153 amino acids, is a recombinant human interleukin (IL)-1 receptor antagonist. Due to its ability to block IL-1β, anakinra may represent a novel therapy to attenuate maladaptive neurogenic inflammation and epileptogenesis (Bialer et al., 2018). The most common adverse effects of anakinra are injection site reaction, headache, nausea, vomiting, pyrexia, and hypersensitivity reactions. Drug interactions are possible (Bialer et al., 2018).

Soticlestat

Soticlestat is an inhibitor of the enzyme cholesterol 24-hydroxylase (CH24H) and may lead to lower glutamate levels in the brain. It is currently under investigation for patients with epileptic encephalopathy, such as Dravet's syndrome and Lennox-Gastaut syndrome.

XEN1101

XEN1101 is a Kv7 potassium channel modulator under investigation for treatment of focal epilepsy. As no approved agents modulate this channel (ezogabine having been withdrawn in 2017), it represent a novel approach to therapy.

Second-Generation Drugs to Valproic Acid

Valnoctamide and sec-butylpropylacetamide have broad-spectrum antiseizure profiles in animal models. These drugs may cause liver toxicity (Bialer et al., 2018).

Everolimus

Everolimus represents an example of precision medicine in epilepsy and the first generation of disease-modifying agents, but data on long-term safety are needed (Mula, 2018). Hyperactivation of the mechanistic target of rapamycin (mTOR) pathway due to loss of function of the tuberous sclerosis complex (TSC) proteins is thought to be the cause of both focal cortical dysplasia and drug-resistant seizures in TSC. Everolimus and sirolimus, both mTOR-inhibiting drugs, were shown to be effective in the treatment of TSC-related renal angiomyolipoma and subependymal giant cell astrocytoma (Overwater et al., 2019). Several studies in TSC patients also showed a reduction in seizure frequency due to mTOR inhibition. The most important adverse effects of mTOR inhibitors are aphthous stomatitis and respiratory infections (Overwater et al., 2019). Table 33.1 shows the current recommendations on epilepsy treatment in patients with TSC (Overwater et al., 2019).

Table 33.1 Current recommendations on epilepsy treatment in patients with tuberous sclerosis complex (TSC)

Epilepsy syndrome	First line	Second line	Third line	Fourth line
West syndrome (infants)	Vigabatrin	Steroids (ACTH/ prednisolone)	Ketogenic diet	ASM combination
Focal seizures in infants	Vigabatrin	Topiramate Carbamazepine Oxcarbazepine Other ASMs	Consider epilepsy surgery	Ketogenic diet ASM combination
Focal seizures in patients >2 years	Carbamazepine Oxcarbazepine Other ASMs	Consider epilepsy surgery, if not an option try second ASM	Everolimus	Consider ASM combination ketogenic diet VNS

ASM, antiseizure medication; VNS, vagal nerve stimulation; ACTH, adrenocorticotropic hormone.

Adapted from: Overwater IE, Rietman AB, van Eeghen AM, de Wit MCY. Everolimus for the treatment of refractory seizures associated with tuberous sclerosis complex (TSC): Current perspectives. *Ther Clin Risk Manag.* 2019; 15: 951–955.

References

Chen Z, Brodie MJ, Liew D, Kwan P. Treatment outcomes in patients with newly diagnosed epilepsy treated with established and new antiepileptic drugs: A 30-year longitudinal cohort study. *JAMA Neurol*. 2018;75:279–286.

Bialer M, Johannessen SI, Koepp MJ, et al. Progress report on new antiepileptic drugs: A summary of the Fourteenth Eilat Conference on New Antiepileptic

Drugs and Devices (EILAT XIV). II. Drugs in more advanced clinical development. *Epilepsia*. 2018;59:1842–1866.

Mula M. Emerging drugs for focal epilepsy. *Expert Opin Emerg Drugs*. 2018;23:243–249.

Overwater IE, Rietman AB, van Eeghen AM, de Wit MCY. Everolimus for the treatment of refractory seizures associated with tuberous sclerosis complex (TSC): Current perspectives. *Ther Clin Risk Manag*. 2019;15:951–955.

Pierce JG, Mithal DS. Fenfluramine: New treatment for seizures in Dravet syndrome. *Pediatr Neurol Briefs*. 2020;34:8.

Index

Tables, figures, and boxes are indicated by *t*, *f*, and *b* following the page number

B

D

E

F

G

H

I

Q

R

U

V